Snoring and Obstructive Sleep Apnea

Second Edition

Snoring and Obstructive Sleep Apnea

Second Edition

Editors

David N.F. Fairbanks, M.D.

Clinical Professor of Otolaryngology-Head and Neck Surgery
George Washington University School of Medicine
Ear, Nose, and Throat Medical Group of Washington, D.C.
Co-Director, Sleep Disorders Center
Sibley Memorial Hospital
Washington, D.C.

Shiro Fujita, M.D. (1929–1993)

Former Director of Neuro-otology
Department of Otolaryngology-Head and Neck Surgery
ENT Consultant
Sleep Disorder and Research Center
Henry Ford Hospital
Detroit, Michigan
Clinical Associate Professor of Otolaryngology
University of Michigan Medical School
Ann Arbor, Michigan

Raven Press   *New York*

Raven Press, Ltd., 1185 Avenue of the Americas, New York, New York 10036

Made in the United States of America

Library of Congress Cataloging-in-Publication Data

Snoring and obstructive sleep apnea / [edited by] David N. F. Fairbanks,
    Shiro Fujita. — 2nd ed.
       p. cm.
    Includes bibliographical references and index.
    ISBN 0-7817-0196-1
    1. Sleep apnea syndromes—Surgery. 2. Snoring. I. Fairbanks,
David N. F. II. Fujita, Shiro (1929–1993).
    [DNLM: 1. Sleep Apnea Syndromes—therapy. 2. Snoring—therapy.
WF 143 S673 1994]
RF484.S66 1994
616.2—dc20
DNLM/DLC
for Library of Congress   94-2841
                                            CIP

9 8 7 6 5 4 3 2 1

Contents

Contributing Authors

Mary K. Craddock, M.D. *Department of Anesthesia, Sibley Memorial Hospital, 5255 Loughboro Road, N.W., Washington, D.C. 20016*

Jack A. Coleman, M.D. *Department of Otolaryngology, Vanderbilt University Medical Center, Nashville, Tennessee 37232-2559*

Robert I. Dickson, M.D., F.R.C.S. *Clinical Associate Professor, Division of Otolaryngology, University of British Columbia, 888 West 8th Avenue, Vancouver, British Columbia V6J 4G7, Canada*

David N. F. Fairbanks, M.D. *Clinical Professor of Otolaryngology-Head and Neck Surgery, George Washington University School of Medicine, 3 Washington Circle, Washington, D.C. 20037*

Shiro Fujita, M.D. (deceased) *Director of Neuro-otology, Department of Otolaryngology-Head and Neck Surgery, ENT Consultant, Sleep Disorder and Research Center, Henry Ford Hospital, Detroit, Michigan 48202; and Clinical Associate Professor of Otolaryngology, University of Michigan Medical School, Ann Arbor, Michigan*

Christian Guilleminault, M.D. *Stanford Sleep Disorders Clinic, 211 Quarry Road, N2A, Stanford, California 94305*

Takenosuke Ikematsu, M.D. (deceased) *Ikematsu Clinic of Otorhinolaryngology, 226, Nakanodai, Noda City, Chiba Pref., Japan*

George P. Katsantonis, M.D. *Clinical Professor of Otolaryngology, Saint Louis University Hospital, 6125 Clayton Avenue, Suite 430, St. Louis, Missouri 63139*

David E. Lees, M.D. *Professor and Chairman, Department of Anesthesia, Georgetown University Medical Center, 3800 Reservoir Road, N.W., Washington, D.C. 20007*

Roger R. Marsh, Ph.D. *Director, ORL Research, Department of Otolaryngology and Human Communication, The Children's Hospital of Philadelphia, 3400 Civic Center Boulevard, Philadelphia, Pennsylvania 19104*

Michael J. Papsidero, M.D., F.A.C.S. *Associate Director, Mount Sinai Nasal/Sinus Center, One Mount Sinai Drive, Cleveland, Ohio 44106; and Cleveland Ear, Nose, Throat & Facial Surgery Group, Inc., 12000 McCracken Road, Garfield Heights, Ohio 44125*

Samuel J. Potolicchio, Jr., M.D. *Associate Professor of Neurology, Department of Neurology, Georgetown University Hospital, 3800 Reservoir Road, NW, Washington, D.C. 20007*

William P. Potsic, M.D.   *Professor of Otolaryngology/Head and Neck Surgery, Department of Otolaryngology and Human Communication, The Children's Hospital of Philadelphia, University of Pennsylvania, 3400 Civic Center Boulevard, Philadelphia, Pennsylvania 19104*

Nelson B. Powell, M.D.   *Clinical Assistant Professor of Sleep Disorders Medicine and Research, Department of Psychiatry and Behavioral Sciences, Stanford University Medical Center, Stanford, California 94305*

Susan Redline, M.D., M.P.H.   *Assistant Professor of Medicine, Cleveland Veterans Administration Medical Center, 10701 East Boulevard, Cleveland, Ohio 44106*

Robert W. Riley, M.D.   *Clinical Assistant Professor of Sleep Disorders Medicine and Research, Department of Psychiatry and Behavioral Sciences, Stanford University Medical Center, Stanford, California 94305*

Thomas Roth, Ph.D.   *Chief, Sleep Disorders Medicine, Sleep Research and Disorders Center, Henry Ford Hospital, 2921 West Grand Boulevard, Detroit, Michigan 48202; and Department of Medicine, Case Western Reserve University School of Medicine, 2109 Adelbert Road, Cleveland, Ohio 44106*

Mark H. Sanders, M.D.   *Associate Professor of Medicine and Anesthesiology, Department of Medicine, University of Pittsburgh Medical Center, 440 Scaife Hall, Pittsburgh, Pennsylvania 15261*

Aaron E. Sher, M.D.   *Clinical Associate Professor of Surgery and Pediatrics, Division of Otolaryngology—Head and Neck Surgery, Albany Medical College, 980 Western Avenue, Albany, New York 12203; and Director of Apnea Program and Associate Medical Director, Capital Region Sleep Wake Disorders Center of Albany Medical Center and St. Peter's Hospital, Albany, New York 12203*

F. Blair Simmons, M.D.   *Division of Otolaryngology, Head and Neck Surgery, Stanford University Medical Center, Stanford, California 94305*

Arthur M. Strauss, D.D.S.   *Sleep Disorders Center, Crozer-Chester Medical Center, One Medical Center Boulevard, Upland, Pennsylvania 19013-3995*

Kingman P. Strohl, M.D.   *Professor of Medicine and Physiology and Biophysics, Department of Medicine, Case Western Reserve University School of Medicine, 2109 Adelbert Road, Cleveland, Ohio 44106; and Department of Medicine, Division of Pulmonary and Critical Care Medicine, University Hospitals of Cleveland, 2074 Abington Road, Cleveland, Ohio 44106*

B. Tucker Woodson, M.D.   *Assistant Professor of Surgery, Department of Otolaryngology and Human Communication, Medical College of Wisconsin, 9200 West Wisconsin Avenue, Milwaukee, Wisconsin 53226*

Preface

A certain excitement in the medical and scientific community comes with the recognition and naming of a new syndrome, especially one such as obstructive sleep apnea, with such common elements as snoring and sleepiness. Yet, with that excitement comes the humbling realization that physicians have observed the co-existing symptoms of snoring and sleepiness for over a century but did not understand their interrelationship.

Research into sleep-breathing disorders began in earnest in the last third of this century, and is documented in the monumental work of Guilleminault and Dement (1). In 1974, Simmons and Hill (2) introduced into the otolaryngology literature a new syndrome "hypersomnia caused by upper airway obstructions", which would become known as obstructive sleep apnea syndrome.

Some twenty years earlier, Ikematsu (3) was developing a highly successful surgical operation for snoring. It would not be heard of in the English-speaking medical world until Fujita (4) introduced it in 1979 as an alternative to tracheostomy in the treatment of obstructive sleep apnea. Simmons et al. (5) promptly validated the effectiveness of the operation (uvulopalatopharyngoplasty) that revolutionized the management of that disease.

The First Edition of this book brought together Fujita, Ikematsu, and Simmons—the pioneers in the field of surgery for sleep-related breathing disorders. Dr. Ikematsu died in 1990, after publication of the First Edition, and Dr. Fujita died on May 24, 1993. Their chapters in the Second Edition are reprinted from the First Edition in recognition of their historical and educational significance.

Other contributors to both editions have been early workers and thoughtful observers in the field; and many other investigators and clinicians in the specialties of otolaryngology—head and neck surgery, neurology, pulmonology, and sleep medicine—have also contributed substantially to the body of knowledge regarding snoring and sleep apnea. They are cited in the reference lists at the end of each chapter.

This book provides the otolaryngologist–head and neck surgeon with a condensed, practical guide for the management of patients with snoring and obstructive sleep apnea.

David N. F. Fairbanks

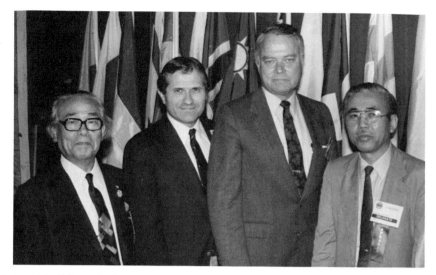

Left to right: Takenasuke Ikematsu, David N. F. Fairbanks, F. Blair Simmons, and Shiro Fujita at the Symposium on Sleep Apnea and Snoring, XIII World Congress of Otorhinolaryngology, May 1985.

REFERENCES

1. Lugaresi E, Cirignotta F, Coccagna G, Baruzzi A. Snoring and the obstructive apnea syndrome. *Electroencephalogr Clin Neurophysiol (Suppl)* 1982; 35:421–430.
2. Boulware MH. *Snoring, new answers to an old problem.* Rockaway, New Jersey: American Faculty Press, 1974: 18.
3. Lugaresi E, Coccagna G, Baruzzi A. Snoring and its clinical implications. In: Guilleminault C, Dement WC, eds. *Sleep apnea syndromes.* New York: Alan R. Liss, 1978: 13–21.
4. Immelmann K. *Schlafverhalten bei Mensch und Tier.* Konstanz, Byk-Gulden-Lomberg, 1964.
5. Singleton WB. Partial velum palatiectomy for relief of dyspnea in brachycephalic breeds. *J Sm Anim Pract* 1962; 3:215–216.
6. Dugan, H. Bedlam in the boudoir. *Collier's* 1947 Feb 22.
7. McWhirter N, ed. *Guinness book of world records.* New York: Bantam Books, 1986: 38.
8. Seifert P. Snoring. *South Med J* 1980; 73:1035–1037.
9. Afzelius L, Elmqvist D, Hougaard K, Laurin S, Nilsson B, Risberg AM. Sleep apnea syndrome—an alternative treatment to tracheostomy. *Laryngoscope* 1981; 91:285–291.
10. Soll BA. Treatment of obstructive sleep apnea with a nocturnal airway-patency appliance. *N Engl J Med* 1985; 313:386–387.
11. Cartwright RD. Predicting response to the tongue retaining device for sleep apnea snydrome. *Arch Otolaryngol* 1985; 111:385–388.
12. Trachtman P. In: Constable G, ed. Chapter 5. *The gunfighters.* New York: Time-Life Books, 1974: 188.
13. Dallas police holding woman in death of man who snored. *Washington Post* 1983 Dec 4: A9.

Snoring and
Obstructive Sleep Apnea

Second Edition

Snoring and Obstructive Sleep Apnea, Second Edition,
edited by D.N.F. Fairbanks and S. Fujita.
Raven Press, Ltd., New York © 1994.

1

Snoring

An Overview with Historical Perspectives

David N. F. Fairbanks

*Department of Otolaryngology, George Washington University School of Medicine,
Washington, D.C. 20037; and Sleep Disorders Center, Sibley Memorial Hospital,
Washington, D.C. 20016*

Snoring, the lay term for obstructive breathing during sleep, is one of the most prevalent of obnoxious human habits. In a 30- to 35-year-old population, 20% of men and 5% of women will snore; by age 60, 60% of men and 40% of women will snore habitually (1). No reason is known for the preponderance of male snoring, but an old legend held that primitive men defended their women even at night, by making terrifying noises to frighten away beasts of prey (2).

Snoring is three times more common in obese persons than in thin ones (3). Yet many thin, athletic persons snore.

Snoring is almost exclusively found in humans, as opposed to the rest of the animal kingdom. "Wild animals do not snore," write Immelmann (4), the German naturalist. "They sleep either in the ventral position or on the side so that the lower jaw is always somehow sustained, thus preventing its falling back." But when humankind's primate ancestors developed the alternative of sleeping on their backs, they became snorers.

Most animals do not sleep on their backs, so they do not snore. However, bulldog owners would challenge that statement. Bulldogs (and other brachycephalic dogs) snore terribly, and they often require surgical resection of the soft palate and uvula to keep them from strangling while asleep (5).

"The annals of medical history afford solace to the snorer," wrote H. Dugan (6) in his article "Bedlam in the Boudoir." "Twenty of thirty-two Presidents of the United States are proved or believed on a thick web of circumstances to have been nocturnal nuisances in the White House. The list is bipartisan and consoling. Washington, both Adamses, Van Buren, Fillmore, Pierce, Buchanan, Lincoln, Johnson, Grant, Hayes, Arthur, Cleveland, Hoover, and FDR all snored."

President Theodore Roosevelt once snored so loudly in a hospital that complaints were filed by almost every patient in the wing where he was recuperating (2).

1

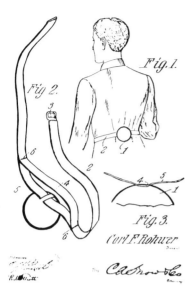

FIG. 1. "Snore ball," remedy designed to keep snorer from sleeping on his or her back.

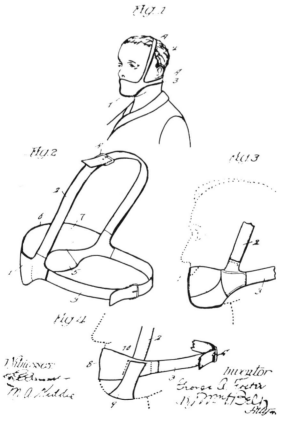

G. A. FOSTER.
DEVICE FOR PREVENTING SNORING.
APPLICATION FILED AUG 13 1915.

1,216,679.

Patented Feb. 20 1917.

FIG. 2. Chin and mouth strap designed to keep mouth shut, on assumption that snoring is result of mouth breathing.

Foreign Prime Ministers and Potentates in the distinguished snorers club would fill the dictionary of biography. The historian Plutarch said that the Emperor Otho snored; Lord Chesterfield snored, and so did Beau Brummel, the ladies' man. According to the memoirs of ladies who knew him, Mussolini was an astounding snoring artist; and Winston Churchill was a 35-decibel snorer by the report of the naval officer who auditioned him onboard a ship in August 1944 (2).

The Guinness Book of World Records (7) states, "The highest measured sound level recorded by any chronic snorer is a peak of 87.5 decibels at Hever Castle, Kent, England, in the early hours of June 28, 1984. Melvyn Switzer of Hampshire was 1 ft from the meter." Similar sound levels have been recorded in the medical setting—up to 80 decibels (8), which is about as loud as the diesel engine one hears when riding toward the rear of a Greyhound bus.

There is no lack of would-be snoring remedies. The U.S. Patent and Trademark Office has over 300 of them listed. Some are variations on the old idea of taping a marble on the snorer's back to force him or her to sleep on his side (Fig. 1), because snoring is often worse when the person sleeps supine. Chin straps to keep the mouth closed (Fig. 2), whiplash neck-sprain collars, and neck extender pillows (Fig. 3) to keep the chin up are usually disappointing as snore cures. Nasopharyngeal tubes (9) and mouth inserts to pull the tongue forward (10,11) have been reported as successful, but patient compliance in wearing such uncomfortable devices is a limiting

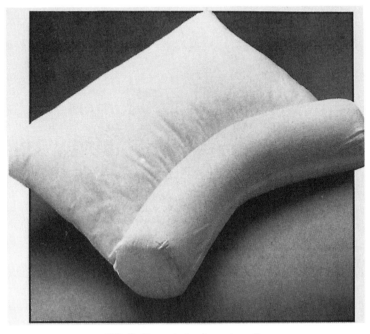

FIG. 3. Purported anti-snoring pillow.

PATENTED OCT 3 1972   3,696,377

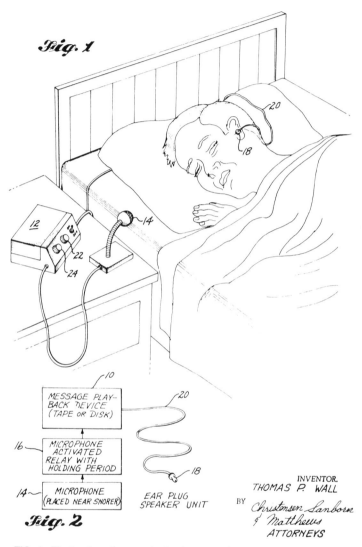

FIG. 4. Electronic anti-snore device instructs sleeper to "stop snoring."

factor. A number of ingenious electronic gadgets have been devised (Figs. 4 and 5) which deliver painful or unpleasant stimuli to patients when they snore—as if they could be trained or conditioned (Pavlovian style) to desist. Unfortunately, snoring is purely an involuntary phenomenon, and if these devices work, it is most likely because they keep the patient from going to sleep altogether.

FIG I

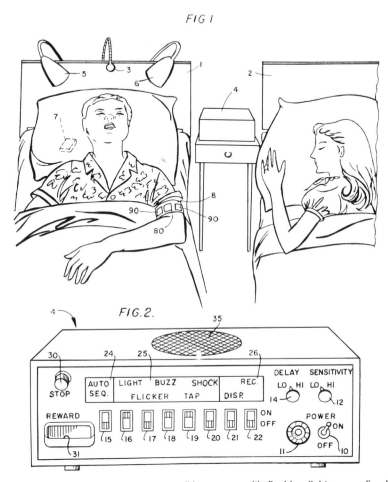

FIG. 5. Anti-snore trainer purports to condition snorer with flashing lights, sounding buzzer, muscular stimulator, and—finally—electric shock.

SOCIAL EFFECTS OF SNORING

Snoring may be a minor annoyance in some households, but in others it is disruptive to family life, makes the snorer an object of ridicule, and commits other household members to sleepless nights filled with resentment. Hapless bedpartners become consumed with the plotting of strategies to get to sleep (i.e., sleeping pills, ear plugs, ear muffs, pushing the snorer out of bed, etc.).

History books tell us that John Wesley Hardin, the legendary Texas gunfighter of the American frontier, is said to have become so upset with the loud snoring of a guest in the hotel room next to his that he shot through the wall and killed the poor fellow (12). It is quite possible that many spouses have contemplated similar drastic actions. At least one did: On December 3, 1983, United Press International reported that Dallas police had taken into custody Ms. Joanne Robinson, who "grabbed a pistol from under her bedcovers and fired five shots," killing a man "who snored too loudly" (13).

A list of complaints expressed by snorers seeking help in our office (Table 1) gives poignant testimony to the hardships that snoring imposes on the lives of snorers and their companions. While some spouses can easily fall asleep in a noisy environment (including close proximity to a snorer), others cannot. The noises of snoring are difficult to ignore because of their inherent irregularity. Listeners have been known to lie awake for hours simply marveling at the kaleidoscopic variety of sounds that can be produced by the snorer, and some snorers make truly frightening sounds suggesting that each breath may be their last.

TABLE 1. *Snoring-related complaints*

Drives wife from bedroom (18 responses)
Drives roommate (3) or husband (2) from bedroom
Girlfriend won't marry me (3)
Boyfriend has "had it" with me
Keeps wife awake (5)
Disturbs wife (2)
Frightens wife
Drives wife crazy
Troubles everyone in house
Wife and son harrass me unmercifully
I'm the big joke to my grandchildren
I feel ostracized
Children are intolerant (4)
Terribly embarrassing at campouts, at slumber parties, or in dormitory
Intolerable to associates on business trips (4)
Had to leave the boat for friends to sleep
Shakes entire house
Can be heard through two walls (6), upstairs and downstairs (2)
Because I snore so loud at movies and church, they ask me to leave
I kick and flail (2), struggle, shout, and sleepwalk
Cannot sleep restfully, shake the bed
Snorting is intolerable
Morning headaches (3)
Drowsy all day (4)
Fall asleep on the job (4)
Fall asleep driving the car (9)
Fell asleep driving and struck a telephone pole
Fall asleep waiting for red light to change (3)
Cannot drive at night
Fall asleep watching TV
Fall asleep eating dinner
Fall asleep talking to wife

Most spouses, at least in their more rational daytime hours, recognize the involuntary nature of the snoring problem, but at night, in their yearning for sleep, they cannot help but feel resentment. The listener conjures up anguished recollections of past sleepless nights and ruined days that followed. Such thoughts are not conducive to drifting off to sleep.

Despite the obviously disruptive effect of snoring on the lives of married partners, most professionals have assumed that one spouse's intolerance to the other's snoring is not the *cause* of a disturbed relationship, but rather an outward *manifestation* of some other cause. This may be an incorrect assumption. Legal courts have traditionally trivialized the significance of snoring (2), not considering it as grounds for divorce—until recently (14).

Couples who have learned to cope with a snoring problem have usually established separate sleeping quarters—but not without some anguish, because some spouses consider this an abandonment of their marital expectations. At least 10 patients have come to me already divorced from their first marriages and faced with fiancés who would not consummate the marriage until the snoring problem had been solved.

PATHOPHYSIOLOGY OF SNORING

Snoring is one sign of a number of different disorders. The sounds of snoring originate in the collapsible part of the airway where there is no rigid support—that is, from the epiglottis to the choanae (Fig. 6). It involves the soft palate, uvula, tonsils, tonsillar pillars, base of the tongue, and pharyngeal muscles and mucosa. Four factors, singly or in combination, contribute to snoring (Fig. 7, Table 2):

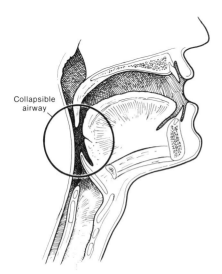

Collapsible
airway

FIG. 6. Cutaway anatomical view to show collapsible portion of airway where no rigid support exists and where snoring originates.

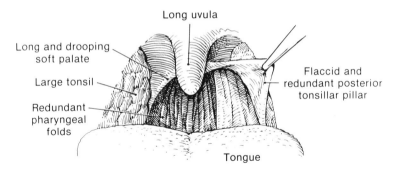

FIG. 7. Intra-oral view demonstrates some common anatomical features of snorers.

1. Incompetent tone of palatal, lingual, and pharyngeal muscles is the cause of most adult-onset snoring. In deep-sleep stages, such musculature fails to participate in the respiratory cycle to keep the airway open during inspiration. Specifically, the dilator effect of the pharyngeal muscles and the protrusive effect of the genioglossus muscle are inadequate (15,16). Thus the tongue falls backward into the airway and vibrates against the flaccid soft palate, uvula, and pharyngeal folds. This is exaggerated when the person has consumed alcoholic beverages, sedative-hypnotics, tranquilizers, or antihistamines before retiring. Hypothyroidism also contributes to poor muscle tone, snoring, and apnea, as do neurological disorders such as cerebral palsy, muscular dystrophy, and myasthenia.

Unfortunately, inadequate muscle tone is often not very apparent on physical examination of the awake patient. However, a characteristic finding in some patients is redundant vertical folds in the tissues of the posterior pharynx, making it look more like the interior of an intestine than an airway (Fig. 7).

2. Space-occupying masses impinging on the airway can contribute to snoring. In children, snoring is almost always from enlarged tonsils and adenoids. One-third of adult snorers also have tonsils large enough to contribute to the airway problem (17) (Fig. 8). Bulky pharyngeal tissues are notable in obese persons. A receding chin may be unable to keep the tongue sufficiently forward. Retro- or micrognathia produces a tongue that is large relative to the space available for it to occupy, but Down's syndrome and acromegaly produce an absolute tongue enlargement. Cysts and tumors are uncommon causes, but they need to be ruled out with mirror exam or endoscopy.

TABLE 2. *Anatomical factors contributing to snoring*

1. *Incompetent tone of palatal, pharyngeal, and glossal muscles* which fail to maintain airway patency during the inspiratory phase of the respiratory cycle.
2. *Space-occupying masses* (i.e., tonsils, adenoids, cysts, tumors, tongue, etc.) which compromise the size of the pharyngeal airway.
3. *Excessive length of the soft palate and uvula* such that they decrease the anterior–posterior dimension of the nasopharyngeal airway and also vibrate during respiration.
4. *Obstructive nasal breathing* which creates excessive negative pressure in the collapsible pharyngeal airway to achieve inspiratory airflow.

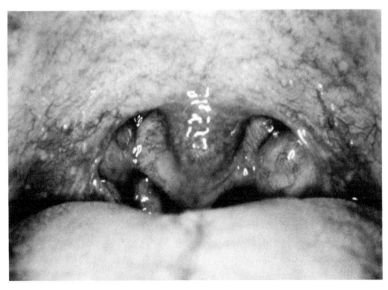

FIG. 8. Large tonsils, drooping soft palate, and bulky uvula in an obstructive sleep apnea patient. (From ref. 40, with permission.)

3. Excessive length of the soft palate and uvula narrows the nasopharyngeal aperture, because the palate descends not only inferiorly in direction, but posteriorly as well (Fig. 6). Often the snorer exhibits no more than a slit-like opening from the nose into the pharynx. Thus, he or she must breathe through a one-way valve. This is most apparent to the examiner when the patient is placed in the supine position.

4. Restriction of airflow in the nose creates increased negative pressure during inspiration which draws together the flaccid tissues in the collapsible part of the airway, where they vibrate and cause snoring. This explains the common observation that many persons who ordinarily do not snore may do so when they have a cold or an allergy attack. Nasal, septal, or turbinate deformity, nasal tumor, and sinusitis with nasal polyps are also possible causes of snoring (18).

APNEA AND THE MEDICAL EFFECTS OF SNORING

Snoring is both a social and a medical problem. Heavy snorers are more likely to be hypertensive, and to suffer strokes and angina pectoris, than nonsnorers of a similar age and weight (19,20). The most advanced stage of snoring is obstructive sleep apnea which causes profound cardiac, pulmonary, and behavioral problems. ("Apnea" comes from the Greek term meaning "want of breath.") This condition may affect as many as 2% of adult women and 4% of adult men.

Spouses and roommates describe this as not just snoring but snorting and choking as well, a frightening struggle to breathe while asleep. Whereas snoring means partial obstruction of the airway, apnea means total obstruction. It interrupts the loud snoring with episodes of silence during which time the snorer struggles with unsuccessful respiratory effort (obstructive apnea). After a number of seconds a loud snort (the so-called "resuscitative snort") occurs as the patient awakens (at least partially), forces open his airways, and resumes breathing. This is often accompanied by kicking or flailing of the arms or a body spasm. Various contorted body positions are assumed to reopen the airways, and the half-awake victim may rise up in bed or fall out of it entirely. These snorts and body motions almost invariably drive any companion to different sleeping quarters.

Occasional brief obstructive events are harmless and are quite common in the normal adult population. However, it is considered pathological when apnea episodes last over 10 seconds each and occur over 7–10 times per hour (or 30 times per night) (21). Significant apnea occurs in 35% of habitual snorers. In many apnea patients, episodes last over 30 seconds each and occur hundreds of times during a night. Patients may spend over half of their sleep time in total airway obstruction.

Another common phenomenon in apneic patients is not-quite-complete obstructive events—that is, ones in which some air squeaks through. When such airflow is reduced to 30% of normal, the event is termed a *hypopnea* or a *hypopneic episode*. An alternative definition is reduction of respiratory flow that is associated with oxygen desaturation and/or some degree of sleep arousal.

In sleeping apneic patients who are already bordering on hypoxemia, a hypopneic episode can trigger significant oxygen desaturation rather like a full apneic episode can. And because the consequences of hypopneas are comparable to those of apneas, the frequency of each should be added together when severity of disease is being assessed. The sum of apneas (A) and hypopneas (H) that occur in 1 hour of typical sleep is termed the *apnea–hypopnea index* (AHI) or the *respiratory disturbance index* (RDI).

Apneic patients generally are not aware of these obstructive events; their bedpartners are more likely to be, but not always. Thus diagnostic confirmation requires an overnight sleep study (polysomnography) that will enumerate the type, duration, and frequency of respiratory disturbances. It will also assess their impact on sleep and oxygenation (see Figs. 9 and 10).

Augmented ventilatory effort in response to increased internal airway resistance (from snoring with or without apnea/hypopnea) results in repetitive arousals from sleep (22,23). These are usually partial arousals, from deeper stages into lighter stages of sleep. Afflicted patients do not enjoy sufficient deep-stage (restorative) sleep to feel refreshed when morning comes. This sleep deprivation makes them sleepy during waking hours. Such patients may fall asleep while driving an automobile or while working on the job. They suffer serious employment problems and are hazardous drivers. They fall asleep while trying to read, watch television, or carry on conversation. Irritability and personality changes (e.g., emotional depression) are common consequences of sleep deprivation. Excessive daytime sleepiness is named as the most consistent sign and symptom of obstructive sleep apnea—that is, after loud snoring (20,24) (Table 3).

Additionally, chronic nocturnal hypoxemia has some predictable cardiovascular

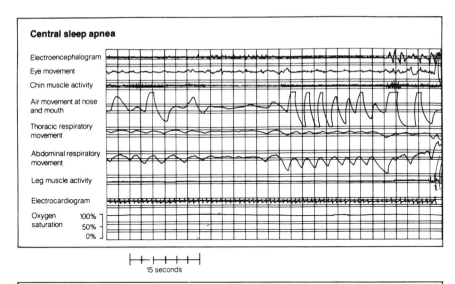

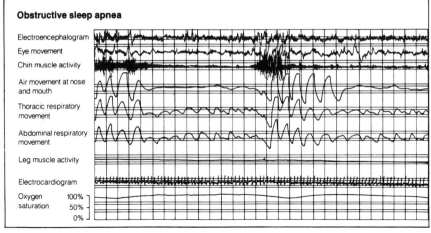

FIG. 9. Polysomnographic tracings contrast central versus obstructive sleep apnea. Note more pronounced thoracic and abdominal respiratory movements in obstructive sleep apnea patient (**bottom**) as well as decreases in oxygen saturation. (From ref. 41.)

consequences. Hypoventilation leads to pulmonary hypertension, then to increased cardiac workload and to systemic hypertension in at least 50% of apneic patients (25). Indeed, the prevalence of sleep apnea among patients with essential hypertension is over 25% (26).

Significant aberrations in blood oxygen and carbon dioxide levels lead to cardiac arrhythmias in half of apneic patients during sleep. The risk of myocardial infarction is 23 times higher for men with obstructive sleep apnea (over 5.3 episodes per hour) than for comparable nonapneic men (27). Furthermore, repetitious hypoxemia

SibleyMemorial Hospital
POLYSOMNOGRAM REPORT

NAME: _____   STUDY DATE: Jan 14, 1993

REF. PHYSICIAN: Fairbanks _____   LOG NO.: 93-005   SEX: Male

HISTORY: Suspected sleep apnea ___   D.O.B. 2-2-42   AGE: 50

_____   HEIGHT: 5' 12"   WEIGHT: 201

SLEEP STAGING:

Stage 1:	66	min.	20	% TST
Stage 2:	171	min.	50	% TST
Stage 3:	9	min.	3	% TST
Stage 4:	0	min.	0	% TST
Stage 5:	93	min.	27	% TST

A

Total Recording Time: _____375_____ min.
Total Sleep Time: _____339_____ min.

SLEEP VARIABLES:

Sleep onset time: 2 min   Number of awakenings 1 min: 3
Rem latency: 40 min   Number of awakenings by tech: ____
Time to first stage 4 not obtnd   Wake after sleep onset (WASO) 27 min
Number of REM periods: 4   Number of body movements: ____
Penile tumescence: ____   (per/hr.) ____

SLEEP DISORDERED BREATHING:

	Non REM	REM	Total	
Total number of apneas:	309	64	373	**B**
Central:				
Obstructive:	309	64	373	
Mixed:				
Number of hypopneas:	32	0	32	
Apnea plus hypopnea index:	60/hr	11/hr	71/hr	**C**
Mean duration of apnea:	27 sec	33 sec		
Longest duration of apnea:	33 sec	50 sec	**D**	
Mean SaO$_2$ decrease:	98-75%	below 60%		
Peak SaO$_2$ decrease:	below 60%	below 60%	**E**	
Cardiac arrhythmias:	NONE	**F**		

MSLT DATA:

	Nap I	Nap II	Nap III	Nap IV	Nap V	
Sleep onset:						mean onset: ____
Rem onset:						mean onset: ____

INTERPRETATION: This study shows severe obstructive sleep apnea _____

FIG. 10. What to look for in a polysomnogram report. **A:** Compare sleep time spent in light stages (1 and 2) versus deep stages (3, 4, and REM). Normal would be close to equivalent. **B:** Note types and numbers of apneas. Over 30 is abnormal. **C:** Note apnea + hypopnea index (number of events per hour). Over 10 is abnormal. **D:** Note duration of apneas. Over 10 seconds is abnormal. **E:** Note peak oxygen desaturation (Sao$_2$). Below 90% is significant. Below 60% is life-threatening. **F:** Note cardiac arrhythmias (from hypoxemia).

TABLE 3. *Signs and symptoms of obstructive sleep apnea*

Loud snoring (notable in all patients)
Hypersomnolence (notable in most patients)
Abnormal motor activity during sleep
Obesity (frequent but not necessarily)
Hyperactivity and antisocial behavior (children)
Personality changes, depression
Impaired intellectual performance
Hypertension (frequent)
Nocturnal cardiac arrythmias (frequent)
Cor pulmonale (in advanced cases)
Morning headaches
Sexual impotence

in severe apneics contributes to general intellectual deterioration (impairment of verbal fluency, attention, memory, and executive functions) which may not be fully reversible (28).

Morning headaches in apneics are probably caused by serum hypercarbia, a trigger of vascular cephalgia.

Obstructive sleep apnea is related (in some cases) to the Pickwick syndrome (29) described as obesity, hypersomnolence, periodic breathing with alveolar hypoventilation, and cor pulmonale. As early as 1906, Sir William Osler (30) alluded to it when he observed, "An extraordinary phenomenon in excessively fat young persons is an uncontrollable tendency to sleep—like the fat boy in Pickwick." He was referring to Joe, a character in one of Charles Dickens' famous novels, *The Posthumous Papers of the Pickwick Club* (31). Pickwick syndrome is generally thought of as an adult disorder, but the Dickens character was actually a child, who probably suffered airway obstruction from large tonsils and adenoids.

As early as 1889, William Hill (32) made similar observations as follows: "The stupid-looking lazy child who frequently suffers from headaches at school, breathes through his mouth instead of his nose, snores and is restless at night, and wakes up with a dry mouth in the morning is well worthy of the solicitous attention of the school medical officer." He advocated relief of nasal obstructions (such as large adenoids) in order to lessen the number of "stupid children."

Snoring children with massively enlarged tonsils and adenoids are at risk for significant cardiovascular, developmental, educational, and behavioral consequences of snoring and the sleep apnea syndrome (33,34). Sleepiness in a child is often manifested as hyperactivity or antisocial behavior.

MANAGEMENT

For adults who are mild or occasional snorers, the self-help remedies listed in Table 4 are worth trying. Some stimulating products (i.e., those containing caf-

TABLE 4. *Self-help suggestions for snorers*[a]

---

1. Adopt an athletic life-style and exercise daily to develop good muscle tone and to lose weight.
2. Avoid alcoholic beverages within 4 hours of retiring.
3. Avoid tranquilizers, sleeping pills, and antihistamines before bedtime.
4. Sleep sideways rather than on your back. (Pin a "snore-sock" to your pajama back: a stocking with a tennis ball in it.)
5. Tilt the entire bed with the head upwards four inches: Place bricks under the bedposts at the bedhead.
6. Try wearing a whiplash collar at night to keep your chin extended, and avoid use of a thick pillow that would kink your neck.
7. Drink a cola or cup of coffee before you retire so your companion can get to sleep first.

---

[a]Adapted from ref. 42, with permission.

feine) taken at bedtime might be helpful to allow the nonsnorer to fall asleep first. However, the snoring is often made worse when the stimulant wears off.

Similarly, a tricyclic antidepressant such as protriptylene (Vivactyl) is helpful to some patients (35). It acts by decreasing the amount of time the sleeper spends in rapid eye movement (REM) sleep, which is when snoring and apnea are the worst.

However, the side effects of stimulating and mood-elevating drugs are often quite intolerable to patients; these include insomnia, prolonged dreaming with unpleasant nightmares, constipation, hesitancy with micturation, urinary retention, altered libido, painful ejaculations, and elevation of blood pressure and pulse rate. Furthermore, even when these medications are effective, it means a lifetime of medications, which the patient may not view favorably.

Heavy snorers, those who snore in any position, so-called "obnoxious snorers," and any snorer whose life is disrupted by snoring should have a thorough examination of the nose, mouth, palate, nasopharynx, hypopharynx, and larynx. Additionally, studies in a sleep laboratory (polysomnograms) are essential in adult patients who are hypersomnolent or who produce interrupted snoring sounds that are suggestive of apnea episodes. In fact, apnea of significant degrees can be present in patients who claim not to suffer sleepiness, and their apnea might be detected only by polysomnography (36).

Patients whose snoring (or mild apnea) comes from nasal congestion may benefit from treatment of allergy or infection, or they may need surgical correction of structural deformities (18). Patients with receding chins may require surgical advancement of the mandible and maxilla, but mild cases are sometimes helped with nightly use of oral inserts that thrust the tongue or mandible forward.

Nightly use of continuous positive airway pressure (CPAP), delivered through a nasal mask, helps keep the airway from collapsing. It is a remarkably effective treatment for apnea (especially severe cases) if the nasal airways are clear and if the patient will use it every night, presumably for the rest of his or her life.

Surgery can remove and tighten up redundant pharyngeal tissue and shorten a long floppy uvula and soft palate. This operation, known as *uvulopalatopharyngoplasty* (UPPP), is successful in treatment of "obnoxious snorers" and many obstructive sleep apnea patients when the orovelopharynx is the obstructive site (24,25,37,38).

From time to time, anecdotes are heard about snorers cured with simple uvulectomy, but it has never emerged as a consistently successful treatment (38). New interest (and lay publicity) about uvulectomy ("uvuloplasty") is being generated by advocates of laser surgery.

Tracheostomy was the original treatment for patients with far-advanced and life-threatening sleep apnea, but many patients and spouses find the appearance, the sounds, and the care of a tracheotomy to be objectionable. CPAP has almost eliminated the need for tracheostomy.

Neurostimulation of the upper airway dilating muscles (creating an "airway pacemaker") makes for interesting research, the objective being a more physiologic restoration of airway patency (39).

Every chronically snoring child should be examined thoroughly. Snoring and obstructive breathing are never normal in childhood. If no other specific cause for the snoring is discovered, tonsillectomy and adenoidectomy will usually bring prompt and dramatic relief of snoring and will probably make an important difference in the health and well-being of the child.

SUMMARY

Snoring is an extremely prevalent disorder which often leads to medical problems and also imposes significant impediments to good interpersonal relationships. It is a complaint that should not be ignored or belittled. Snoring means obstructive breathing, and its most exaggerated form is obstructive sleep apnea.

An anonymous wit once said, "Laugh and the world laughs with you—snore and you sleep alone." Snoring is not funny to those whose lives are severely disturbed by this breathing disorder, and with today's expanded medical understanding about it, snoring is not hopeless either.

REFERENCES

1. Lugaresi E, Cirignotta F, Coccagna G, Baruzzi A. Snoring and the obstructive apnea syndrome. *Electroencephalogr Clin Neurophysiol [Suppl]* 1982;35:421–430.
2. Boulware MH. *Snoring, new answers to an old problem.* Rockaway, NJ: American Faculty Press, 1974.
3. Lugaresi E, Coccagna G, Baruzzi A. Snoring and its clinical implications. In: Guilleminault C, Dement WC, eds. *Sleep apnea syndromes.* New York: Alan R Liss, 1978;13–21.
4. Immelmann K. *Schlafverhalten bei Mensch und Tier.* Konstanz: Byk–Gulden–Lomberg, 1964.
5. Singleton WB. Partial velum palatiectomy for relief of dyspnea in brachycephalic breeds. *J Small Anim Pract* 1962;3:215–216.
6. Dugan H. Bedlam in the boudoir. *Colliers* 1947;Feb 22.
7. McWhirter N, ed. *Guinness book of world records.* New York: Bantam Books, 1986;38.
8. Seifert P. Snoring. *South Med J* 1980;73:1035–1037.
9. Afzelius L, Elmqvist D, Hougaard K, Laurin S, Nilsson B, Risberg AM. Sleep apnea syndrome— an alternative treatment to tracheostomy. *Laryngoscope* 1981;91:285–291.
10. Soll BA. Treatment of obstructive sleep apnea with a nocturnal airway-patency appliance. *N Engl J Med* 1985;313:386–387.
11. Cartwright RD. Predicting response to the tongue retaining device for sleep apnea syndrome. *Arch Otolaryngol* 1985;111:385–388.

12. Trachtman P. *The gunfighters.* Constable G, ed. New York: Time–Life Books, 1974;176.
13. Dallas police holding woman in death of man who snored. *Washington Post* 1983;Dec 4:A9.
14. Shapiro SL. On the causes and treatment of snoring. *Eye Ear Nose Throat Monthly* 1971;50:75–79.
15. Suratt PM, Dee P, Atkinson RL, Armstrong P, Wilhoit SC. Fluoroscopic and computed tomographic features of the pharyngeal airway in obstructive sleep apnea. *Am Rev Respir Dis* 1983;127: 487–492.
16. Haponik EF, Smith PL, Bohiman ME, Allen RP, Goldman SM, Bleecker ER. Computerized tomography in obstructive sleep apnea. *Am Rev Respir Dis* 1983;127:221–226.
17. Fairbanks DNF. Snoring: surgical *vs.* nonsurgical management. *Laryngoscope* 1984;94:1188–1192.
18. Ellis PDM, Harries MLL, Ffowcs Williams JE, Shneerson JM. The relief of snoring by nasal surgery. *Clin Otolaryngol* 1992;17:525–527.
19. Koskenvuo M, Partinen M, Sarna S, et al. Snoring as a risk factor for hypertension and angina pectoris. *Lancet* 1985;April 23;893–896.
20. Palomaki H, Partinen M, Juvela S, Kaste M. Snoring as a risk factor for sleep-related brain infarction. *Stroke* 1989;20:1311–1315.
21. Chaudhary BA, Speir WA. Sleep apnea syndromes. *South Med J* 1982;75:39–45.
22. Strollo PJ, Sanders JH. Significance and treatment of nonapneic snoring. *Sleep* 1993;16:403–408.
23. Guilleminault C, Stoohs R, Clerk A, Simmons J, Labanowski M. From obstructive sleep apnea syndrome to upper airway resistance syndrome: consistency of daytime sleepiness. *Sleep* 1992;15: S13–S16.
24. Fujita S, Conway W, Zorick F, Roth T. Surgical correction of anatomic abnormalities in obstructive sleep apnea syndrome: uvulopalatopharyngoplasty. *Otolaryngol Head Neck Surg* 1981;89:923–934.
25. Simmons FB, Guilleminault C, Silvestri R. Snoring, and some obstructive sleep apnea, can be cured by oropharyngeal surgery. *Arch Otolaryngol* 1983;109:503–507.
26. Partinen M, Telakivi T. Epidemiology of obstructive sleep apnea syndrome. *Sleep* 1992;15:S1–S4.
27. Hung J, Whitford EG, Parsons RW, Hillman DR. Association of sleep apnoea with myocardial infarction in men. *Lancet* 1990;336:261–264.
28. Montplaisir J, Bedard MA, Richer F, Rouleau I. Neurobehavioral manifestations in obstructive sleep apnea syndrome before and after treatment with continuous positive airway pressure. *Sleep* 1992;15:S17–S19.
29. Burwell DS, Robin ED, Whaley RD, Bickelmann AG. Extreme obesity associated with alveolar hypoventilation—a Pickwickian syndrome. *Am J Med* 1956;21:811–818.
30. Osler W. *The prinicples and practice of medicine.* New York: Appleton, 1906;431–433.
31. Dickens C. *The posthumous papers of the Pickwick club.* London: Chapman & Hall, 1837.
32. Hill W. On some causes of backwardness and stupidity in children. *Br Med J* 1889;2:711–712.
33. Luke MJ, Mehrizi A, Folger GM, Rowe RD. Chronic nasopharyngeal obstruction as a cause of cardiomegaly, cor pulmonale, and pulmonary edema. *Pediatrics* 1966;37:762–768.
34. Talaat AM, Nahhas MM. Cardiopulmonary changes secondary to chronic adenotonsillitis. *Arch Otolaryngol* 1983;109:30–33.
35. Series F, Marc I. Effects of protriptyline on snoring characteristics. *Chest* 1993;104:14–18. (Also see page 2.)
36. Moran WB, Orr WC, Fixley MS, Wittels EE. Nonhypersomnolent patients with obstructive sleep apnea. *Otolaryngol Head Neck Surg* 1984;92:608–610.
37. Gislason T, Lindholm C, Almqvist M, Birring E, Boman G, Eriksson G, Larsson SG, Lidell C, Svanholm H. Uvulopalatopharyngoplasty in the sleep apnea syndrome, predictors of results. *Arch Otolaryngol Head Neck Surg* 1988;114:45–51.
38. Zohar Y, Finkelstein Y, Strauss M, Shvili Y. Surgical treatment of obstructive sleep apnea: technical variations. *Arch Otolaryngol Head Neck Surg* 1993;119:1023–1029.
39. Fairbanks DW, Fairbanks DNF. Neurostimulation for obstructive sleep apnea: investigations. *Ear Nose Throat J* 1993;72:52–57.
40. Fairbanks DNF. Snoring: not funny—not hopeless. *Am Fam Physician* 1986;33:205–211.
41. Becker K, Cummiskey J. Managing sleep apnea: what are today's options? *J Respir Dis* 1985;6:50–71.
42. Fairbanks DNF. *Snoring: not funny, not hopeless* [leaflet]. American Academy of Otolaryngology—Head and Neck Surgery.

Snoring and Obstructive Sleep Apnea, Second Edition,
edited by D.N.F. Fairbanks and S. Fujita.
Raven Press, Ltd., New York © 1994.

2

Obstructive Sleep Apnea

Diagnosis by History, Physical Examination, and Special Studies

Aaron E. Sher

Division of Otolaryngology—Head and Neck Surgery, Albany Medical College, Albany, New York 12203; and Capital Region Sleep Wake Disorders Center of Albany Medical Center and St. Peter's Hospital, Albany, New York 12203

HISTORY

In evaluating a patient with obstructive sleep apnea (OSA), it is important to obtain a history from the patient, but also from his bed partner or family. The pathognomonic event—the obstructive apnea—is hidden from the patient's consciousness because it occurs while he is asleep. The patient is usually not aware of the loud snoring, irregular breathing patterns, and other physical concomitant events such as thrashing about in bed, all of which characterize this disorder. Therefore, the patient's own history must be supplemented whenever possible, by the observations of those who observe his nocturnal behavior. Most of the electroencephalographic (EEG) "arousals" which terminate the apneic event do not bring the patient to full wakefulness, but rather to a superficial level of sleep adequate to recruit muscle tone and open the airway. Only on rare occasions, perhaps numbering three or four out of hundreds of apneas through the night, will the patient actually reach a level of alertness that will allow recognition of the event. It is on those occasions that the patient will report awakening in the middle of a snore or gasp, or with the sensation of choking. Frequently the patient believes that he aroused several times during the night to void, but there is no demonstrable urological or metabolic explanation for the nocturia, and the arousal was actually apnea-induced. While some adult patients will present with enuresis with no documentable urological etiology, this presentation is far more common in the pediatric population.

Interestingly, patients with predominantly central apnea (i.e., apnea on a neurological or cardiopulmonary basis rather than on the basis of airway compromise) more frequently are aware of their disturbed sleep and their arousals. These patients will complain of insomnia—unlike OSA patients, who generally perceive their sleep as being sound.

OSA patients often complain of having a dry throat or dry mouth in the morning, because many of them mouth breathe when they sleep. They awaken unrefreshed, feeling as though they had been awake all night.

The patient or his bed partner may have noted that all of these complaints are exacerbated by consumption of even small quantities of alcohol the previous evening or by the use of hypnotic agents to induce sleep. Alcohol and many hypnotic and sedative drugs exacerbate the airway obstructive phenomenon characteristic of OSA.

Frequently the patient has little or no insight into the cause of his morning complaints, because he has no perception of what occurred during the night when he slept.

Excessive daytime sleepiness (EDS) represents a principal sequela of the sleep disruption characteristic of OSA. Even EDS often remains partially or totally hidden from the patient's perception, and the patient may deny EDS despite reports to the contrary from his family or employer. In such denial, men typically dismiss as insignificant their sleepiness, even if they have had to significantly modify their lives or work to stay awake. They may have to stay in physically active jobs rather than advance to cognitive or management positions.

It is not uncommon for patients who may have had multiple automobile accidents caused by their EDS, or who may have lost employment because of their EDS, to deny EDS. Their misfortunes may be attributed instead to external forces. In such cases, the physician must rely heavily on the history given by the patient's family.

On the other hand, there are patients with OSA whose subjective perception of their degree of EDS exceeds that which would be predicted from objective testing. While this may suggest the presence of other sleep/wake pathology, it may be that the patient is unusually sensitive to the effects of sleep disruption. This group of patients, highly aware of their disability of EDS, may represent a minority of OSA patients.

There is no universally applicable explanation for the frequent discrepancy between the patient's perception of his EDS, that reported by his family or associates, and that documented objectively. The lack of accurate subjective assessment may result from the fact that OSA tends to progress in small increments of severity over relatively long periods of time. The concomitantly slow progression of severity of EDS may go unrecognized by the patient. In some cases, the level of EDS ultimately reached may be perceived by the patient as his "normal" state, as the consequences of his EDS (i.e., road accidents or job difficulties) may be wrongly blamed on extraneous environmental or personal factors.

In children, while EDS may result from OSA, the daytime complaint may take the form of inattentiveness, attention deficit disorder, hyperirritability, or hyperactivity.

Other sequelae of OSA, such as nocturnal arrhythmia, myocardial infarction, cerebrovascular accident, hypertension, morning headache, seizure, or onset of cor pulmonale, may *not* be appropriately attributed to the patient's underlying and causative OSA if the physician relies solely on the *patient's* history, and if the patient himself is unaware of his OSA. Similarly, sexual impotence, a complication of OSA, may remain without an appropriate explanation, if the patient does not realize the nature of his disorder.

Skillful questioning by the physician can sometimes uncover a clinical picture suggestive of OSA that would have been passed over by a physician with less knowledge of the symptoms of OSA or a lower level of clinical suspicion. Nonetheless, the importance of the patient's bed partner or family in the history ascertainment process is to be emphasized. In reality, it is often these people who insist that the patient seek medical attention in the first place, often over protestation by the patient.

Aspects of the history that may serve as a red flag to alert the physician to the diagnosis of OSA are the presence of other upper airway symptoms and the presence of known upper airway pathology. Known pathology may be structural (craniofacial anomaly, hypertrophic tonsils, and adenoids) or neoplastic (benign or malignant). It may be on a metabolic basis (pharyngeal soft tissue abnormalities of acromegaly, hypothryoidism, mucopolysaccharidoses) or on a traumatic basis (mandibular deformity, temporomandibular displacement, or pharyngeal or neck scarring—either accidental or postsurgical).

Progressive weight gain during the period of symptom progression is important to note, because it may be the former that results in the latter. While weight gain can be the cause of OSA in adults and children, children will sometimes present with failure to thrive rather than obesity. This eventuality results from growth hormone deficiency secondary to OSA, because growth hormone secretion is sleep-entrained and suppressed by severe OSA.

Onset or progression of neurological dysfunction which results in pharyngeal muscular hypotonia or incoordination of respiratory effort should also alert the physician to the possibility of secondary OSA—that is, OSA resulting from neurological dysfunction.

The history of past ventilatory difficulties during the perioperative period of previous surgical procedures—that is, prior to endotracheal intubation for general anesthesia, or immediately following extubation—should suggest, or lend support for, the diagnosis of underlying OSA. Loss of upper airway patency in such situations results from the use of sedating or paralyzing agents which interact unfavorably with an already compromised upper airway. In essence, loss of pharyngeal muscle support induced by these drugs represents an exaggerated form of the muscular hypotonia induced normally by the sleeping state.

PHYSICAL EXAMINATION

There are no physical findings that are pathognomonic for OSA. In his chapter on pharyngeal surgery (chapter 6), Dr. Fujita provides descriptions and photographs of anatomical features he observed in OSA patients. In years gone by, such findings may have been dismissed by examiners as not so abnormal, because they were rather prevalent. But then, snoring and apnea are also prevalent; and the relationship between the disorder and the anatomical findings (especially in the awake patient) might be apparent only to a seasoned examiner.

Furthermore, some common anatomical variations in the nose or oropharynx might be insignificant were they to appear singly; but combined in one patient, they might create a composite picture of airway incompetence.

Also, a patient visiting a physician for other reasons may not mention symptoms suggestive of OSA, yet exhibit anatomical features that raise the examiner's suspicions. The following leading questions are then worth asking:

1. Do you snore?
2. Is it every night and in every position?
3. Do you gasp, choke, snort, or quit breathing at night?
4. Is it hard to get up in the morning?
5. Do you get drowsy on the job or when driving?

Among the physical findings and properties which characterize the pharynx in OSA are increased collapsibility, increased compliance, increased resistance, and decreased cross-sectional area (1–8).

The effectiveness of the action of the airway supportive muscles depends on their tonicity, the proper coordination of their contraction with that of the diaphragm, the vector angles through which they operate, and the linear distance through which they contract. These latter two parameters relate to the basic anatomical attributes of the individual patient. The amount of force needed to maintain airway patency relates to the degree of negative pressure acting on the pharynx, the dimensions and configuration of the pharynx, and the degree to which the supportive muscle action is coordinated with the onset of inspiration. Muscles which have been demonstrated to support the patency of the pharyngeal airway include the genioglossus, geniohyoid, palatoglossus, palatopharyngeus, stylopharyngeus, and tensor palatini.

Anatomic narrowing of the upper airway creates a situation whereby negative pharyngeal pressure generated in inspiration requires augmented activity from the dilating muscles of the upper airway to maintain patency of the airway.

In wakefulness, the contraction of these dilating muscles is adequate to overcome anatomic narrowing in sleep apnea patients. However, there is a normal sleep-related decrease in the tonicity of these muscles, and this results in OSA. The activity of these muscles is further modulated by the peripheral and central mechanisms of respiratory function; therefore, not only will neural control abnormalities of these muscles lead to apnea, but so too may alterations in neural regulation of breathing and reflex responses to airway occlusion (9–15).

Therefore, physical examination must focus on the physical properties and spatial relationships of the pharyngeal airway, head, and neck, as well as on the neuromuscular integrity of the airway and mechanisms of breathing control.

A relative narrowing of the upper airway anywhere from the nose to the hypopharynx would exacerbate a neurophysiologic tendency toward OSA. Many specific pathologic lesions have been identified in the nose, nasopharynx, oropharynx,

TABLE 1. *Pathologic conditions associated with obstructive sleep apnea syndrome*[a]

Nose	*Larynx*
Deviated septum	Edema of supraglottic structures
Polyposis	Vocal cord paralysis
Septal hematoma	
Septal dislocation	*Neuromuscular*
	Cerebral palsy
Nasopharynx	Myotonic dystrophy
Carcinoma	Muscular dystrophy
Adenoidal hypertrophy	Myasthenia gravis
Lymphoma	Multiple sclerosis
Stenosis	Hypothyroidism
Pharyngeal flap	Chiari malformation
Papillomatosis	syringomyelobulbia
	Cerebral palsy
Mouth and Oropharynx	Myotonic dystrophy
Hypertrophic tonsils	Shy-Drager syndrome
Lymphoma of tonsils	Acquired nonprogressive
Lingual cyst	dysautonomia
Lingual tonsillar hypertrophy	Olivopontocerebellar
Macroglossia	degeneration
Acromegaly	Spinal cord injury
Micrognathia	Bulbar stroke
Congenital	
Acquired	
Lipoma of neck	
Hunter syndrome	
Hurler syndrome	
Head and neck burns	
Papillomatosis	

[a]From ref. 58, with permission.

hypopharynx, and larynx of individual patients with OSA (Table 1). Such lesions can be benign or malignant neoplasms or can be post-traumatic or inflammatory lesions, or they may develop from metabolic abnormalities.

In children with no facial dysmorphia, craniofacial anomaly, or neurological abnormality, hypertrophic tonsils and adenoid are frequently implicated as the underlying etiology for OSA (1,16,17).

In the vast majority of adults with OSA, no specific focus of pathology can be identified. In one series of approximately 200 patients with OSA, only three patients had a single anatomic problem that could be surgically corrected. The remainder had a combination of "disproportionate anatomic relationships" of the upper airway (18). While the cause of these disproportionate anatomic relationships in otherwise "normal" individuals may be multifactorial, it is clear that the angles and distances within the upper airway and the vectors of action of the airway supporting muscles are determined by the dimensions and spatial relationships of the underlying craniofacial skeleton.

Many well-defined craniofacial anomalies result in OSA. Frequently the anatomic basis for the upper airway obstruction is multifactorial, involving complex skeletal abnormalities translated into pharyngeal soft tissue abnormalities (19).

Factors that may contribute to upper airway obstruction include, but are not limited to, micrognathia, maxillary hypoplasia, decreased size of the nasal capsule, choanal atresia or stenosis, decreased pharyngeal circumference, and distorted pharyngeal orientation caused by abnormal angulation of the cranial base.

Individual skeletal changes may have profound effects on the upper airway. Patients with an abnormally acute angle at the skull base have the following associated changes: decreased anterior–posterior dimensions of the cranial base, decreased anterior–posterior length of the bony pharynx, decreased width of the bony pharynx (reduced inter-pterygoid distance), and decreased anterior–posterior length of the nasal and oral airway.

The associated soft tissue changes include diminished cross-sectional area of the pharynx and "verticalization" of the pharynx, such that the palate is suspended straight down into the airway with the tip of the palate often extending to the inferior base of the tongue. This creates a long vertical portion of the posterior tongue, in apposition over an excessively long distance with the soft palate and posterior pharyngeal wall (19).

All of these changes would predispose to pharyngeal collapse. The tendency to pharyngeal collapse would result from the overall diminished cross-sectional area of the pharynx and the altered relationship of the tongue and soft palate and posterior pharyngeal wall.

If a patient who has acute angulation of the skull base also is micrognathic, the long tubular lower pharynx would be even smaller in the anterior–posterior dimension, with an increased likelihood of pharyngeal collapse. Were maxillary hypoplasia or choanal atresia added to the abnormalities, the patient would then be forced into the unstable, unfavorable dynamics of chronic mouth breathing. This would further jeopardize the already highly vulnerable airway. Add generalized muscular hypotonia and the patient loses the sole mechanism of protection against airway collapse in sleep (19).

Until recently, the only craniofacial anomaly recognized with some frequency in the adult OSA population was mandibular malformation. This has been described in adults on a congenital basis, secondary to postoperative changes, and secondary to the destruction of the temporomandibular joints in rheumatoid arthritis (20–24).

Several abnormal patterns of craniofacial development have been recognized in adults who were previously considered morphologically normal but who manifested OSA (25–34). In a study of bony landmarks in lateral cephalograms of patients with OSA, 153 of 155 patients had at least two abnormal landmarks (35). Among the abnormalities identified are acute cranial base angle, hypoplasia of the maxilla, micrognathia, retrognathia, and macroglossia.

The association of obesity with OSA is well-recognized. The majority of adult OSA patients are somewhat obese, although this is not necessarily the case. It has been demonstrated that patients with OSA who are not obese have the most significant craniofacial abnormalities documented by cephalometry. Those with morbid obesity tend to have few abnormal cephalometric measurements. The largest group of patients fall in between, and has an intermediate level of obesity and an intermediate degree of cephalometric abnormality. There is evidence that the effect of obesity on OSA relates to local parapharyngeal fat deposits (31,36,37), but the interrelationship may be more complex.

It can be hypothesized that OSA often results from craniofacial dysmorphia of varying degrees of severity. The most severely dysmorphic patients, recognized early as having anomalous craniofacial development, would present with airway obstruction at birth or in infancy. Those of this group who are most severely affected would have airway problems awake and asleep. Those somewhat less affected would have only OSA. Mildly dysmorphic patients would develop OSA later in life, either as children whose hypertrophic tonsils and adenoids tip the balance in favor of frank OSA, or as adults whose weight and cervical fat deposition reach a critical threshold that converts incipient OSA (i.e., snoring) into frank OSA.

On the other hand, it must be emphasized that abnormalities of respiratory control and muscular hypotonia can have a major etiologic role in OSA. Primary neuromuscular etiology for OSA has been reported in such entities as Chiari malformation, syringomyelobulbia, cerebral palsy, myotonic dystrophy, Shy–Drager syndrome, acquired nonprogressive dysautonomia, olivopontocerebellar degeneration, spinal cord injury, and bulbar stroke.

Thus, any diagnostic approach must take into account the specific craniofacial morphology, the contribution of superimposed pathologic space-occupying lesions, the neuromuscular status, and the degree of obesity.

SPECIAL STUDIES TO DOCUMENT OBSTRUCTIVE SLEEP APNEA

Polysomnography

Polysomnography (PSG) is a continuous recording, generally through a complete night, of the following physiological parameters:

Electroencephalogram (EEG)
Electromyogram (EMG)
Electro-oculogram (EOG)
Nasal airflow
Oral airflow
Thoracic movement
Abdominal movement
Blood oxygen saturation (Sao_2)
Electrocardiogram (EKG)

EEG, EMG, and EOG jointly define the state of sleep versus wakefulness, and they divide sleep into its characteristic pattern of cyclical repetition of stages 1 and 2 (light sleep), 3 and 4 (slow wave or deep sleep), and REM (rapid eye movement sleep).

Nasal and oral airflow and respiratory effort (thoracic and abdominal movement) define normal breathing, central apnea (no airflow at nose or mouth *and* no respiratory effort), and obstructive apnea (no airflow at nose or mouth despite respiratory effort).

Blood oxygen saturation monitors the degree of oxygen desaturation which occurs during apnea.

Electrocardiogram defines the cardiac arrhythmias which result from apnea.

Severity of the OSA in any given patient is partly defined in terms of some or all of the following parameters: frequency of apneas (total lack of breathing) or hypopneas (some air enters the nose and mouth, but in significantly diminished quantity); duration of apneas or hypopneas; degree of oxygen desaturation and duration of such periods of desaturation; abnormalities of cardiac rate and rhythm corresponding to the apneas.

Note that all of these variables are measured with sensors which do not enter the body or violate skin or mucosal surfaces.

Patients with OSA will demonstrate the following: repeated periods of apnea or hypopnea; concomitant oxygen desaturation of variable severity and duration; and concomitant abnormalities in heart rate and rhythm (varying from benign to life-threatening).

Severity of OSA is further defined by the degree of sleep architecture disruption which results from the apnea-induced arousals. It is the disruption of sleep architecture which appears to be the predominant cause of excessive daytime sleepiness. Patients with OSA will demonstrate the following: disruption of the normal cyclical pattern of sleep stage repetition through the night, with increased light sleep, decreased deep (slow wave) sleep, decreased REM sleep, and multiple arousals (terminating the apneas).

Note that formal PSG is generally performed under continuous monitoring and observation by a PSG technologist who not only confirms proper equipment functioning and makes appropriate adjustments and calibrations throughout the night, but who also records his/her observations of patient behavior through the night. The latter observations are correlated with the PSG recordings to provide the comprehensive analysis of a sleep study.

The cost of formal PSG and the desire to maximize patient convenience have resulted in the development of many forms of "ambulatory" or "portable" or "home" sleep monitoring. In most cases, selected variables from among the full PSG montage are monitored in the home setting. The technician's role is to set up the equipment in the patient's home, but the technician does not monitor the overnight study.

While such studies afford the patient the added convenience of sleeping in his own familiar surroundings, these studies have not, to date, been recognized for routine diagnostic purposes by either the American Thoracic Society or the American Sleep Disorders Association. Some systems measure respiratory parameters but do not measure the parameters by which sleep is documented and staged. While such systems may successfully identify apnea, the severity of apnea may not be adequately defined and other sleep aberrations may be overlooked.

While other portable systems afford more comprehensive monitoring, it is not yet clear that this degree of complex monitoring can be routinely achieved in the home without supervision and potential for intervention if needed.

Much attention is currently focused on issues relating to ambulatory or home monitoring because great emphasis is placed on cost containment. At present, the relative cost and effectiveness of ambulatory monitoring as compared to in-laboratory comprehensive PSG has not been adequately defined, and PSG remains the diagnostic tool of choice.

Multiple Sleep Latency Test (MSLT)

After completing a night of well-defined PSG-monitored sleep, the patient is monitored during an 8- to 10-hr period starting the following morning; that is, he is given 20-min opportunities to nap every 2 hr and is monitored for sleep onset and REM onset in each. The results of this test objectively document the patient's level of daytime sleepiness, or drive to sleep, as compared with normals and various abnormals (apneics, narcoleptics, sleep deprived individuals) against whose sleepiness the test is standardized (38).

While MSLT is not necessary to *diagnose* OSA, it does permit an objective assessment of the patient's degree of daytime sleepiness. As pointed out above, the subjective assessment by the patient of his degree of daytime sleepiness is frequently significantly flawed. Furthermore, the degree of severity of the OSA as defined strictly by respiratory parameters does not necessarily correlate in the individual case with the degree of sleepiness; that is, different patients will respond to the same degree of respiratory sleep disturbance with *different* degrees of EDS.

Because EDS represents one of the major parameters of morbidity of OSA, MSLT can help to comprehensively define the severity of OSA in a given patient.

SPECIAL STUDIES WHICH HELP TO IDENTIFY THE LOCATION AND MECHANISM OF AIRWAY COLLAPSE

Recognizing that traditional otolaryngological procedures to augment upper airway dimensions (i.e., tonsillectomy and nasal surgery) were generally not adequate treatment for the adult OSA patient, Fujita adapted an operation formerly applied to diminish snoring (39), and in 1981 he reported on uvulopalatopharyngoplasty (UPPP). UPPP represents the first operative procedure specifically designed to treat OSA (40).

Using as the criterion for "success" decrease in the apnea index (apneas/hour) of at least 50%, UPPP was reported to achieve only a 50% success rate; that is, only half of all patients operated achieved this level of success. However, the apnea index in the successful group was diminished by 88% (41). This encouraged widespread application of UPPP. The English language literature on UPPP consists of over 90 papers, most of these being case series.

A number of investigators have attempted to identify those patient characteristics which predict success at UPPP.

Routine otolaryngological examination, degree of obesity, and severity of apnea were not consistently predictive of success or failure in UPPP.

Attention was turned to selection of patients for UPPP based on aspects of their pharyngeal anatomy.

It had been demonstrated that infants and children with obstructive apnea secondary to anomalous craniofacial development could be classified by mechanism and location of pharyngeal collapse. Using fiberoptic endoscopy with or without Müller maneuver, the pattern and location of pharyngeal collapse was found to be patient-specific rather than syndrome-specific. Furthermore, each patient consistently demonstrated the same pattern of collapse on repeated examinations. The interventional approach was effectively guided by the endoscopic assessment of the pattern of airway collapse (42).

Strikingly similar patterns of pharyngeal collapse have been described in adult patients not identified as being anomalous in craniofacial structure (43).

Cephalometric analysis of OSA patients who were not identified as having anomalies nonetheless revealed distinct craniofacial abnormalities.

As the soft tissue configuration of the pharynx reflects the underlying craniofacial skeletal structures, the functional narrowing of the pharyngeal airway reflects both soft tissue structure and craniofacial skeletal structure.

The diversity of patterns of pharyngeal collapse has been corroborated in OSA patients with endoscopy awake—with and without Müller maneuver, endoscopy asleep, manometry, and rapid-sequence computerized tomography (41,44–53).

Cephalometric parameters have been related to differing patterns of pharyngeal collapse (32,54).

The characterization of airway anatomy and dynamics has resulted in a greater understanding of the limitations of UPPP as a surgical correction for OSA. It has also led to the evolution of surgical techniques to supplement UPPP when more extensive modification of the pharynx is mandated by diffuse and/or severe anatomical compromise (55,56).

Initial efforts to apply these principles focused on preselecting OSA patients who would be more likely to succeed at UPPP and, thereby, boost the success rate above 50%. However, there was, simultaneously, the growing perception that the original criterion for "success" defined by Fujita was not adequately stringent.

For example, by Fujita's "success" criterion of at least a 50% decrease in apnea index, a severely affected patient who just attained this level of improvement postoperatively would be considered a "success" despite a significant level of residual apnea.

As more stringent criteria were applied in defining success, the overall "success rate" declined. Thus, even if one could boost success by preselection of patients, application of stricter definitions of success tended to reverse the gain. For instance, in a series of 50 patients selected for UPPP by fiberoptic endoscopy with Müller maneuver, the "success" rate varied from 85% to 45% depending on how "success" was defined. Using 50% decrease in apnea index, the success rate was 85%. This represented a significantly improved outcome than that reported by Fujita, using the same definition of "success." It was postulated that the increment was achieved by eliminating as surgical candidates those patients whose focus of pharyngeal collapse was documented by Müller maneuver to be unlikely to respond to UPPP. However, in the same series, if "success" was redefined in terms of achieving a "normal" state (i.e., apnea index less than 5), then the success rate dropped from 85% to 45%. Presumably, had patients not been preselected by Müller maneuver, the success rate by this criterion might have been far lower than 45%; that is, large numbers of patients were refused surgery on the basis of a presumably "unfavorable" Müller maneuver (57).

Analysis of the data reported on UPPP suggests that it may be possible to preselect a group of patients who, on the basis of their pharyngeal anatomy and function, have a higher likelihood of success with UPPP. However, if "success" is defined strictly, the fraction of all OSA patients who can achieve such a level of benefit from UPPP remains small.

It was the recognition that OSA patients are a heterogeneous group (having differing locations and patterns of pharyngeal collapse) that resulted in the evolution of new surgical procedures to augment the potential benefit of UPPP. These procedures accomplish this by modifying portions of the pharynx not effectively altered by UPPP, primarily the retrolingual pharynx.

The two leading approaches to correction of retrolingual narrowing differ from each other in that one achieves its goal by skeletal alteration whereas the other relies on primary soft tissue resection (55,56). The two approaches appear to be complementary to one another.

Neither of these approaches replaces UPPP, but along with UPPP and nasal surgery they comprise a complex armamentarium from which procedures can be applied singly, together, or sequentially to reconstruct the upper airway in such a way as to overcome its inherent inadequacy. The overall therapeutic approach is guided by the airway characteristics of the individual patient (55,56).

Fiberoptic endoscopy (awake, with/without Müller maneuver) and lateral cephalometry are probably the most widely applied techniques used to define upper airway characteristics in patients being selected for surgery. Other approaches (outlined above) to assessing the mechanism of airway collapse offer promise and may, in time, supplement or supplant endoscopy and cephalometry.

REFERENCES

1. Anch AM, Remmers JE, Bunce H. Supraglottic airway resistance in normal subjects and patients with occlusive sleep apnea. *J Appl Physiol Respir Environ Exercise Physiol* 1982;53:1158–1163.
2. Brown IG, Bradley TD, Phillipson EA, et al. Pharyngeal compliance in snoring subjects with and without sleep apnea. *Am Rev Respir Dis* 1985;132:211–215.
3. Haponik EF, Smith PL, Bohlman ME, et al. Computerized tomography in obstructive sleep apnea. *Am Rev Respir Dis* 1983;130:221–226.

4. Kuna S, Remmers JE. Neural and anatomic factors in upper airway obstruction. *Med Clin North Am* 1985;69:1221–1242.
5. Rivlin J, Hoffstein V, Kalbfleisch J, et al. Upper airway morphology in patients with idiopathic obstructive sleep apnea. *Am Rev Respir Dis* 1984;129:355–360.
6. Stauffer JL, Zwillich CW, Cadieux RJ, et al. Pharyngeal size and resistance in obstructive sleep apnea. *Am Rev Respir Dis* 1987;136:623–627.
7. Suratt PM, Dee P, Atkinson RL, et al. Fluoroscopic and computed tomographic features of the pharyngeal airway in obstructive sleep apnea. *Am Rev Respir Dis* 1983;127:487–492.
8. Suratt PM, Mctier RF, Wilhoit SC. Collapsibility of the nasopharyngeal airway in obstructive sleep apnea. *Am Rev Respir Dis* 1985;132:967–971.
9. Brouillette RT, Thach BT. Control of genioglossus muscle inspiratory activity. *J Appl Physiol Respir Environ Exercise Physiol* 1980;49:801–808.
10. Brouillette RT, Thach BT. A neuromuscular mechanism maintaining extrathoracic airway patency. *J Appl Physiol Respir Environ Exercise Physiol* 1979;46:772–779.
11. Orr WC, Stahl M. Responses to airway occlusion in symptomatic and asymptomatic patients with sleep apnea [Abstract]. *Chest* 1982;86:236.
12. Jeffries B, Brouillette RT, Hunt CE. Electromyographic study of some accessory muscles of respiration in children with obstructive sleep apnea. *Am Rev Respir Dis* 1984;129:696–702.
13. Onal E, Lopata M, O'Connor T. Pathogenesis of apneas in hypersomnia–sleep apnea syndrome. *Am Rev Respir Dis* 1982;125:167–174.
14. Orr WC. Sleep-related breathing disorders: an update. *Chest* 1983;84:475–480.
15. Orr WC, Stahl M. Responses to airway occlusion in symptomatic and asymptomatic patients with sleep apnea [Abstract]. *Chest* 1982;85:236.
16. Guilleminault C, Korobkin R, Winkle R. A review of 50 children with obstructive sleep apnea syndrome. *Lung* 1981;159:275–287.
17. Brouillette RT, Fernbach SK, Hunt CT. Obstructive sleep apnea in infants and children. *J Pediatr* 1982;100:31–40.
18. Rojewski TE, Schuller DE, Clark RW, et al. Videoendoscopic determination of the mechanism of obstruction in obstructive sleep apnea. *Otolaryngol Head Neck Surg* 1984;92:127–131.
19. Sher AE. Obstructive sleep apnea syndrome: a complex disorder of the upper airway. *Otolaryngol Clin North Am* 1990;23:593–608.
20. Davies SF, Iber C. Obstructive sleep apnea associated with adult acquired micrognathia from rheumatoid arthritis. *Am Rev Respir Dis* 1983;127:245–247.
21. Guilleminault C, Riley R, Powell N. Sleep apnea in normal subjects following mandibular osteotomy with retrusion. *Chest* 1985;88:776–778.
22. Panje WR, Holmes DK. Mandibulectomy without reconstruction can cause sleep apnea. *Laryngoscope* 1984;94:1591–1594.
23. Puckett CL, Pickens J, Reinisch JF. Sleep apnea in mandibular hypoplasia. *Plast Reconstr Surg* 1982;70:213–216.
24. Spier S, Rivlin J, Rowe DR, et al. Sleep in Pierre Robin syndrome. *Chest* 1986;90:711–715.
25. Bacon WH, Krieger J, Turlot JC, et al. Craniofacial characteristics in patients with obstructive sleep apnea syndrome. *Cleft Palate J* 1988;25:374–378.
26. de Berry-Borowiecki B, Kukwa AA, Blanks RHI. Cephalometric analysis for diagnosis and treatment of obstructive sleep apnea. *Laryngoscope* 1988;98:226–234.
27. Djupesland G, Lybert T, Krogstad O. Cephalometric analysis and surgical treatment of patients with obstructive sleep apnea syndrome. *Acta Otolaryngol (Stockh)* 1987;103:551–557.
28. Lowe AA, Santamaria JD, Fleetham JA, et al. Facial morphology and obstructive sleep apnea. *Am J Orthod Dentofacial Orthop* 1986;90:484–491.
29. Lyberg T, Krogstad O, Djupesland G. Cephalometric analysis in patients with obstructive sleep apnea syndrome: soft tissue morphology. *J Laryngol Otol* 1989;103:293–297.
30. Lyberg T, Krogstad O, Djupesland G. Cephalometric analysis in patients with obstructive sleep apnea syndrome: skeletal morphology. *J Laryngol Otol* 1989;103:287–292.
31. Partinen M, Guilleminault C, Quera-Salva MA, et al. Obstructive sleep apnea and cephalometric roentgenograms. The role of anatomic upper airway abnormalities in the definition of abnormal breathing during sleep. *Chest* 1988;93:1199–1205.
32. Riley R, Guilleminault C, Herron J, et al. Cephalometric analysis and flow-volume loops in obstructive sleep apnea patients. *Sleep* 1983;6:303–311.

33. Strelzow VV, Blanks RHI, Basile A, et al. Cephalometric airway analysis in obstructive sleep apnea syndrome. *Laryngoscope* 1988;98:1149–1158.
34. Triplett WW, Lund BA, Westbrook PR, et al. Obstructive sleep apnea syndrome in patients with class II malocclusion. *Mayo Clin Proc* 1989;64:644–652.
35. Jamieson A, Guilleminault C, Partinen M, et al. Obstructive sleep apnea patients have craniomandibular abnormalities. *Sleep* 1986;9:469–477.
36. Horner RL, Mohiaddin RH, Lowell DG, et al. Sites and sizes of fat deposits around the pharynx in obese patients with obstructive sleep apnea and weight matched controls. *Eur J Respir Dis* 1989; 2:613–622.
37. Koenig JR, Thach BT. Effects of mass loading on the upper airway. *J Appl Physiol* 1988;64:2294–2299.
38. Thorpy MJ, et al. The clinical use of the multiple sleep latency test. *Sleep* 1992;15:268–276.
39. Ikematsu T. Study of snoring. 4th report. Therapy [in Japanese]. *J Jpn Otol Rhinol Laryngol Soc* 1964;64:434–435.
40. Fujita S, Conway W, Zorick F, et al. Surgical correction of anatomic abnormalities of obstructive sleep apnea syndrome: uvulopalatopharyngoplasty. *Otolaryngol Head Neck Surg* 1981;89:923–934.
41. Fujita S, Conway WA, Zorick FJ, et al. Evaluation of the effectiveness of uvulopalatopharyngoplasty. *Laryngoscope* 1985;95:70–74.
42. Sher AE, Shprintzen RJ, Thorpy MJ. Endoscopic observations of obstructive sleep apnea in children with anomalous upper airways: predictive and therapeutic value. *Int J Pediatr Otorhinolaryngol* 1986;11:135–146.
43. Finkelstein Y, Talmi Y, Yuval Z. Readaptation of the velopharyngeal valve following the uvulopalatopharyngoplasty operation. *Plast Reconstr Surg* 1988;82:20–30.
44. Borowiecki B, Pollack CP, Weitzman Ed, et al. Fiberoptic study of pharyngeal airway during sleep in patients with hypersomnia obstructive sleep apnea syndrome. *Laryngoscope* 1978;88:1310–1313.
45. de Berry-Borowiecki B, Kukwa AA, Blanks RHI. Indications for palatopharyngoplasty. *Arch Otolaryngol* 1985;111:659–663.
46. Sher AE, Thorpy MJ, Shprintzen RJ, et al. Predictive value of Muller maneuver in selection of patients for uvulopalatopharyngoplasty. *Laryngoscope* 1985;95:1483–1487.
47. Katasantonis GP, Maas CS, Walsh JK. The predictive value of the Mueller maneuver in uvulopalatopharyngoplasty. *Laryngoscope* 1989;99:677–680.
48. Katsantonis GP, Walsh JK. Somnofluoroscopy: Its role in the selection of candidates for uvulopalatopharyngoplasty. *Otolaryngol Head Neck Surg* 1986;94:56–60.
49. Launois SH, Feroah TR, Campbell, et al: Site of obstruction in obstructive sleep apnea: influence on the outcome of uvulopalatopharyngoplasty. *Am Rev Respir Dis* 1993;147:182–189.
50. Hudgel, DW, Hendricks C. Palate and hypopharynx—sites of inspiratory narrowing of the upper airway during sleep. *Am Rev Respir Dis* 1988;138:1542–1547.
51. Hudgel DW. Variable site of airway narrowing among obstructive sleep apnea patients. *J Appl Physiol* 1986;61:1403–1409.
52. Chaban R, Cole P, Hofftein V. Site of upper airway obstruction in patients with idiopathic obstructive sleep apnea. *Laryngoscope* 1988;98:641–647.
53. Stein MG, Gamsu G, De Geer G, et al. Cine CT in obstructive sleep apnea. *AJR* 1987;148:1069–1074.
54. Riley R, Guilleminault C, Powell N, et al. Palatopharyngoplasty failure, cephalometric roentgenograms, and obstructive sleep apnea. *Otolaryngol Head Neck Surg* 1985;93:240–243.
55. Riley RW, Powell NB, Guilleminault C. Obstructive sleep apnea syndrome: a review of 306 consecutively treated surgical patients. *Otolaryngol Head Neck Surg* 1993;108:117–125.
56. Woodson BT, Fujita S. Clinical experience with linguoplasty as part of the treatment of severe obstructive sleep apnea. *Otolaryngol Head Neck Surg* 1992;107:40–48.
57. Gereau S, Sher AE, Glovinsky PB, et al. Results of uvulopalatopharyngoplasty (UPPP) in patients selected by Müller maneuver [Abstract]. *Sleep Res* 1986;15:124.
58. Sher AE. The upper airway in obstructive sleep apnea syndrome: pathology and surgical management. In: Thorpy MJ, ed. *Handbook of sleep disorders*. New York: Marcel Dekker, 1990;311–335.

Snoring and Obstructive Sleep Apnea, Second Edition,
edited by D.N.F. Fairbanks and S. Fujita.
Raven Press, Ltd., New York © 1994.

3

Cardiopulmonary and Neurological Consequences of Obstructive Sleep Apnea

*,[†]Kingman P. Strohl, [†,‡]Thomas Roth, and [§]Susan Redline

*Department of Medicine, Division of Pulmonary and Critical Care Medicine,
University Hospitals of Cleveland, Cleveland, Ohio 44106;
‡Sleep Research and Disorders Center, Henry Ford Hospital, Detroit, Michigan 48202;
§Pulmonary Section, Veterans Administration Medical Center, Cleveland, Ohio 44106; and
†Department of Medicine, Case Western Reserve University, Cleveland, Ohio 44106*

Obstructive sleep apnea is a common event, occurring to a significant degree (≥ 5/ hour of sleep) in 4–9% of the population (1). Severe disease (>20 apneas/hour) is associated with excess mortality (2,3) and presents with complaints related to excessive daytime sleepiness, disturbed sleep, and heavy snoring. Cardiopulmonary consequences of severe obstructive apneas include pulmonary hypertension, cor pulmonale, and cardiorespiratory failure (hypoxemia and hypercapnia) (4). Other reviews have described in detail the mechanical effects of apneic activity on blood pressure and cardiac performance, the influence of abnormal respiratory events on sleep continuity and arousals, and the abnormalities in gas exchange seen during apneas and with severe disease. The purpose of this chapter is to critically review the literature supporting the perspective that sleep apnea syndrome is an illness with basic metabolic and neuropsychological precipitants and consequences.

There is evidence that sleep apnea is associated with the development of a chronic illness with cardiopulmonary and neuropsychological symptoms and signs. There is a spectrum of disease (Fig. 1). Epidemiologically, sleep apnea and snoring are both associated with hypertension, stroke, and myocardial infarction (5). Physiological studies and case reports have implicated excessive sleepiness in impaired job performance, operation of motor vehicles, and social interactions. In this chapter the following questions will be addressed: (a) Are there metabolic risk factors in sleep apnea as commonly found in other cardiovascular illnesses? (b) What factors modulate sleepiness in the apneic patient? (c) How robust is the association between cognitive deficits, in general, and the degree of apneic activity?

Consideration of these issues may result in a greater understanding of the need for therapy or may point to new strategies for management of this common illness.

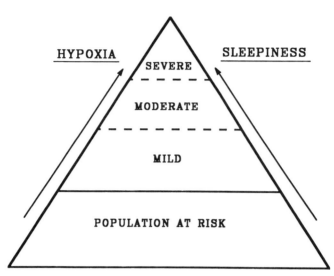

FIG. 1. Spectrum of disease. There is evidence for a spectrum of disease involving hypoxic exposure and sleepiness. At the present time, indications for treatment are clear for those with severe disease, with multiple apneas, and accompanied by disturbing excessive sleepiness or signs of hypoxic stress. There is a larger population with lesser degrees of symptoms and apneic activity who may be at risk for disease progression or who may benefit from treatment in regard to automobile accidents, cognitive deficits, hypertension, and stroke. Our view is that cellular and organ system events result in what is termed *mild, moderate,* or *severe* disease and its potential complications. Understanding these events is necessary for estimating prevalence, identifying risk factors, and creating new and primary therapies.

SLEEP APNEA AS A METABOLIC DISEASE

Alterations in body composition, sleep–wake transitions, and gas exchange can all be linked conceptually and/or experimentally with alterations in metabolism and in regulatory peptides which control metabolism, tissue growth and maturation, and organ function. The associations of sleep apnea with hypothyroidism and with acromegaly (6–8) illustrate how pathological alterations in endocrine function may lead to the development of sleep apnea, and how specific therapy directed at such specific pathology results in resolution of the sleep apnea disorder. A more common risk factor for sleep apnea is obesity. The mechanisms by which obesity causes apneas are thought to be related to mechanical loading of the respiratory system by abdominal girth or pharyngeal mass. One hypothesis to be considered is that alterations in body fat distribution not only may predispose to sleep apnea but may occur as a consequence of apnea-associated alterations in metabolic regulatory peptides. These metabolic factors contribute to the pathogenesis of the disease by altering body composition, increase risk in obstructive sleep apnea syndrome (OSAS) for hypertension, stroke, or myocardial infarction, and possibly lead to central nervous system dysfunction or muscle dysfunction.

Given a perspective that sleep apnea is a chronic disease associated with changes in body composition in adult life, we postulate that sleep apnea may impact on the regulation of growth regulatory peptides. We have preliminary evidence to suggest that in euthryoid patients with moderately severe sleep apnea, cortisol and insulin levels may be elevated (9,10). These hormones interact to regulate not only glucose metabolism but also body mass distribution (11,12). Further support for this concept is suggested by the recent epidemiologic evidence of an association among sleep apnea, hypertension, and cardiovascular disease (2,3,13–15). A common factor for this association could be the "insulin-resistant state" (13,16,17), a syndrome of desensitization of peripheral tissues to the biological actions of insulin. Insulin resistance may be due to genetically programmed disorders of insulin action or might be a result of acquired defects or environmental factors or of increased food or carbohydrate intake (18). With insulin resistance, as in sleep apnea, there are correlations with obesity and hypertension. Epidemiologic studies show associations among (a) insulin resistance and common diseases such as non-insulin-dependent diabetes mellitus (NIDDM), (b) cardiovascular risk factors such as hypertension and lipid abnormalities, and (c) obesity (19).

Waller and Bhopal (20) reviewed eight investigations describing relationships between snoring and vascular disease including hypertension, stroke, and/or myocardial infarction, and they concluded that the apparent excess risk of vascular disease in patients who admit to snoring is probably due to consequences of sleep apnea rather than obesity or simple snoring. Examining 372 snorers with overnight sleep studies, Hoffstein et al. (19) found that the major influence on blood pressure in snorers was via an association with obstructive sleep apnea and nocturnal hypoxemia rather than obesity per se. These and other studies (21–23) indicate potential links between sleep apnea and cardiovascular morbidity that will be important in any evaluation of the impact of sleep apnea on public health.

There is the concept of sleep disorders as leading to a neuroexcitatory state, as defined by sympathetic and humoral stress responses, and resulting in metabolic and cardiovascular adaptations (24). Evidence exists to suggest that the sympathetic nervous system is involved in the pathology of hypertension in sleep apnea (15,25). These observations suggest that sleep apnea is a particularly important and common neuroexcitatory stressor. On the other hand, other studies (26,27) suggest that patients with sleep apnea do not have increased cardiac output and/or fluid retention that would be expected to result from excess catecholamines. Consequently, other events or factors are required to sustain hypertension.

Cushing's disease and acromegaly are two diseases associated with both sleep apnea and insulin resistance. Acromegalics have a high incidence of obstructive sleep apnea (6), and this disease is associated with an insulin-resistant state, presumably due to metabolic factors such as increased growth hormone and insulin-like growth factor 1 (IGF-1). In Cushing's disease, elevated cortisol levels will lead to glucose intolerance, insulin resistance, hyperinsulinemia, and truncal obesity (17, 28,29). The latter is assumed to cause the apnea in Cushing's disease. Obesity, which is a factor associated with the insulin-resistant state, is also present in OSAS not associated with endocrinologic disease (21,23). It is known that high circulating insulin concentrations usually present in the serum of insulin-resistant patients can initiate certain tissue-specific growth effects through intact IGF-1 or IGF-2 receptor–effector systems (18,30). Escouron et al. (31) compared body habitus characteristics and other factors in hypertensive and normotensive patients with sleep apnea presenting to a clinic and found no differences with respect to age and other factors, including weight. Taken together, all these examples suggest the presence of potential association between sleep apnea and the insulin-resistant state based upon factors such as cortisol levels, growth hormone, and possibly catecholamines, acting synergistically to produce changes in vascular tone and resistance.

Our preliminary observations on a clinic-based patient population support a hypothesis that significant degrees of obstructive sleep apnea (apnea–hypopnea index>15) are associated with an increase in insulin levels, whereas severe disease (apnea–hypopnea index>40) is accompanied by fasting hyperglycemia and hyperinsulinemia (10). The data are insufficient to define causal relationships but can support the concept that hyperglycemia and hyperinsulinemia, known cardiovascular risk factors (11,13,16,32), are commonly found in patients with sleep apnea. Further careful studies are needed to determine the degree to which hyperinsulinemia is secondary to events in apnea.

Our working hypothesis is presented in Fig. 2. Three factors interact to produce apneic activity. Traits of genetic (jaw structure, respiratory control, atopy, etc.) and environmental (food availability, allergen, physical activity, sleep deprivation, etc.) origin initiate apneas. Apneas, accompanied by sleep interruption and hypoxia,

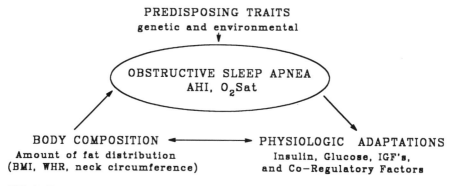

FIG. 2. Factors which interact to propagate apneic activity. Three variables interact to produce apneas. Predisposing traits of genetic and environmental origin lead to the initiation of an obstructive sleep apnea in a given individual. Apneas are then quantifiable by measures such as apnea/hypopnea index (AHI) and oxygen saturation (O_2Sat). Physiologic adaptations to apnea then occur. Cellular adaptations with regard to insulin, glucose, IGF, and their co-regulatory hormones and receptors result in alterations in body composition and also lead to changes in the amount of fat or its distribution. Increases in measures of body-mass index, waist-to-hip ratio, and neck circumference result in more apneas. Hence, a cyclic phenomenon can be produced, propagating apneas over time and leading to the clinical syndromes that are now treatable, and, if this scenario is present, modifiable by recongnition of risk factors and physiologic adaptations.

initiate physiologic adaptations. Adaptations involving regulatory peptides, such as cortisol and insulin, could precipitate changes in body composition, in either the amount of fat or its distribution. Increases in such measures as body mass index (BMI), neck size, or waist circumference are associated with increasing apnea number. Thus, a cycle is initiated that will propagate apneas over time. We believe that from this perspective one might use physiological adaptations or changes in body composition to identify significant apneic effects. Alternatively, preventive measures for apnea might include behavior that reduces obesity or alters body composition and insulin resistance.

MODULATION OF SLEEPINESS IN SEVERE APNEA

Among sleep-disorder patients, nearly half of those with excessive sleepiness regardless of cause report automobile accidents; more than half have had occupational accidents, of which some are life-threatening; many have lost jobs; and many report severely disrupted family life (33). In other words, the patient who complains of excessive sleepiness is, in general, at risk of life-threatening events and appreciable socioeconomic loss and dysfunction.

Objective evaluation associated with multiple apneas has documented the excessive nature of the sleepiness (34–36). The sleepiness as measured by the multiple sleep latency test (MSLT) is very consistent day to day, and it persists throughout the day (37). The average sleep latency on the MSLT of patients with OSAS is less than 5 minutes (which is considered to be pathological) and is similar in severity to that of patients with narcolepsy (36). Successful surgical [e.g., uvulopalato-pharyngoplasty (UPPP)] or medical [e.g., nasal continuous positive airway pressure (CPAP)] treatment of OSAS, as judged by a reduction in respiratory events indices, reverses symptoms of excessive sleepiness and is accompanied by improved MSLT scores (38,39).

The cause of the excessive sleepiness in OSAS is thought to be related to sleep fragmentation and/or nocturnal hypoxemia. Both are sequelae of an apneic event: A progressive oxygen desaturation occurring during the apnea (as recorded by ear oximetry) and the brief arousal from sleep (as seen on the electroencephalogram) that terminates the apnea result in a disruption of the normal progression of sleep staging (i.e., sleep fragmentation). Three lines of evidence now suggest that sleep fragmentation is the cause of the sleepiness in OSAS. Fragmentation of sleep with brief arousals in healthy normal persons can produce excessive sleepiness (40–42). Furthermore, administration of nocturnal oxygen in OSAS patients (which improves their hypoxemia but does not eliminate the apnea and resultant sleep fragmentation) does not alter objective measurements of sleepiness (43). Similarly, UPPP failures with continued apnea and fragmented sleep do show improved nocturnal hypoxemia, but do not have improved sleepiness (38). Conversely, apnea-associated sleep fragmentation has been improved without improving nocturnal hypoxemia, and yet alertness was improved (44). While it seems clear that sleep fragmentation is the cause of diurnal sleepiness in OSAS, how the recovery process for sleep and alertness proceeds following successful treatment of the apnea and reversal of the fragmentation is not known. It is clinically important because OSAS patients often do not fully comply with medical treatment (i.e., CPAP) or partially respond to surgical treatment (i.e., UPPP) (38,45).

Correlational studies in patients with OSAS suggest that hypoxemia does not contribute to sleepiness seen in OSAS (37,46). This also seems true if one compares the nature and extent of neuropsychological deficits among patient groups with differing amounts of sleepiness and hypoxemia. In patients with narcolepsy (with sleepiness similar to OSAS, but no hypoxemia), memory deficits can be acutely reversed as alertness improves with medical therapy (47). On the other hand, recovery of neurocognitive impairment in COPD patients (with no sleepiness, but hypoxemia) may continue up to 6 months (K.A. Adams, *personal communication*, 1992). Thus one expects sleepiness-related areas of deficit in OSAS to reverse rapidly with effective therapy.

Another issue in understanding and managing the sleepiness of OSAS is recognizing other common factors which exacerbate sleepiness. Insufficient sleep, secondary to multiple jobs, shift work, or work demands, is the most common reason for daytime sleepiness in the general population. Hence, sufficient time should be programmed by the patient for sleep. To date, no studies have documented the impact of insufficient sleep superimposed upon the presence of mild apneic activity.

Ethanol is another important factor that exacerbates sleepiness. In a questionnaire study of a large sample of OSAS patients, approximately 50% of the patients noted that alcohol worsens their sleepiness (37). To date, all of the studies of OSAS and ethanol have focused on the interaction of nocturnal alcohol with apnea frequency (48–51). The extent to which daytime ethanol worsens daytime sleepiness in OSAS has not been evaluated. Studies support an interaction between basal levels of sleepiness and functionally disruptive effects of ethanol. Using the MSLT, laboratory performance tests, and, most recently, simulated automobile driving measures, our studies have found that moderate sleep restriction increases the impairing effects of ethanol (52–54). Hence, alcohol use by patients with OSAS will not only increase apneic activity, but will also be expected to affect daytime performance by its interactions with basal sleepiness and inattention.

NEUROPSYCHOLOGICAL DEFICITS IN SLEEP APNEA

The overall impact of sleep apnea relates to the degree to which it causes significant behavioral and medical morbidity, the degree to which any such morbidity may be attenuated, and the relative cost to society (55). Clearly, multiple sleep apneas associated with daytime sleepiness are potentially lethal, associated with significant relative risks for automotive accidents (56,57). The clinical significance of milder degrees of apnea is much less clear. Early studies have demonstrated that apnea indices greater than 5 were rare in healthy young and middle-aged volunteers (often hospital employees) (58). These initial observations led to the use of this value (5 events/hour) as a "cutoff" point to discriminate those with and without "disease." However, more recent studies have demonstrated that this degree of apneic activity is common in the elderly and, in our experience, in noncomplaining family members of subjects with sleep apnea syndrome (59). Designating the majority of these populations as "diseased" on the basis of apneic activity alone is not appropriate. However, there are no studies that have specifically addressed correlations between various levels of apneic activity and consequences with measures of sleepiness, cognitive complaints, or health status. The potential interactions between apneas and neuropsychological sequallae are shown in Fig. 3. There are some studies, reviewed below, which address one or another aspect of this puzzle. We believe that this state of affairs has resulted in overspeculation and wide differences in "clinical opinion" of the impact of apneas on neuropsychological consequences.

There is an extensive literature in normal subjects that relates neuropsychological deficits to experimental sleep restriction and disruption (60). Profound sleep deprivation causes substantial deficits in psychomotor and cognitive performance (61). However, milder degrees of sleep deprivation also significantly impair vigilance, memory and learning, and executive functions (62–66), and selective deprivation of slow-wave and rapid eye movement (REM) sleep (sleep structural changes found in sleep apnea) also has been associated with sleepiness, attention deficits, and impaired executive functioning (67). Affective changes have been noted after total

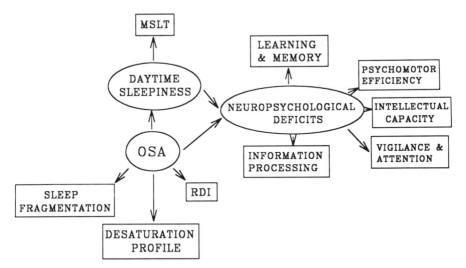

FIG. 3. Model of interactions. A general form of the model is outlined below, with circles representing hypothetical variables and the squares representing measured variables. In this diagram, we see that daytime sleepiness is measured with MSLTs, and neuropsychological function is measured by tests that can be grouped into several dimensions. *Arrows* indicate hypothesized causal paths. MSLT, multiple sleep latency test; OSA, obstructive sleep apnea; RDI, respiratory disturbance index (number of events/hour of sleep).

sleep deprivation (62) as well as after selective sleep deprivation (68). Learning and memory impairments also have been noted after selective deprivation of REM sleep (69) and/or stage II sleep (70). The degree to which these neuropsychological deficits are attributable to sleepiness, a fairly ubiquitous consequence of sleep restriction (71,72) and sleep fragmentation (73), however, is unclear. The relative contributions of total sleep deprivation, selective sleep restriction, and sleep fragmentation to neuropsychological deficits (and the degree to which any such effects are confounded by sleepiness) also are not well defined in these physiological studies of sleep.

The extent to which the findings of experimental sleep disruption can be extrapolated to sleep apnea can be debated. Habituation, which may occur after experimental sleep disruption, is unlikely to occur in patients with sleep apnea who continually breathe against an obstructed airway (68). Also, although a linear association between the number of arousals experimentally produced and physiological sleepiness has been demonstrated (74), a threshold (i.e., arousal rate) at which this occurs is not clearly evident. Most neurophysiological studies have imposed sleep disruptions at rates of one/minute (which may correspond to arousal rates in subjects with approximately 60 events/hour); few address neuropsychological deficits that occur consequent to disruptions at rates less than this, because often both symptomatic and asymptomatic deficits occur in apneics.

There are several pathophysiological processes that may occur as a consequence of sleep disruption and could lead to neuropsychologic deficits. Alterations in brain protein synthesis during sleep have been postulated to be a consequence of arousals and sleep fragmentation (75). Alterations in cerebral metabolism, including reductions in cerebral metabolic rates in central gray areas, have been reported in subjects who are sleep-deprived (76). A correlation of these latter findings with decrements in vigilance (assessed with a continuous performance task) have been interpreted as supporting an effect of sleep deprivation on brain arousal mechanisms.

Hypoxemia itself can produce alterations in cerebral blood flow and neurotransmitter metabolism (77). The relationship between chronic hypoxemia and neuropsychological deficits is best considered in the literature on patients with chronic obstructive pulmonary disease (COPD). Executive functions, psychomotor performance, and attention may be significantly impaired in severely hypoxic COPD patients (78). In comparison to nonhypoxemic controls, participants in the IPPB trial with COPD and relatively mild hypoxemia (pO_2 66 torr) also have demonstrated impairments in abstract reasoning, memory, and psychomotor performance (79). In this study, a dose–response relationship was suggested between degree of neuropsychological impairment and level of resting pO_2. The effects of chronic hypoxia on neuropsychological deficits may be partially reversible; that is, hypoxic patients with COPD have shown significant improvement in a broad range of neuropsychological tests (including tests in intellectual aptitude, memory, psychomotor performance, and executive functions), as well as improvement in mood, following treatment with oxygen therapy for 1 month (78).

In contrast to patients with COPD, subjects with sleep apnea often are hypoxic only intermittently during sleep. Understanding the role of intermittent hypoxemia in the pathogenesis of neuropsychological deficits has been limited by difficulties in separating the influences of daytime hypoxemia from those of nocturnal hypoxemia, as well as in separating the influences of sleep fragmentation from those of hypoxemia. For example, impairments in memory, vigilance, and psychomotor performance have been demonstrated to be more profound in patients with severe sleep apnea associated with both resting and sleep-related hypoxemia than in apneic patients who were less hypoxemic over time (80). However, one recent study of neuropsychological function and sleepiness in heavy snorers suggests that even mild desaturations are associated with fatigue as well as with impaired daytime performance, memory, and perceptual organization (81). It should be noted that these studies utilized limited numbers of subjects and were not controlled for the potential population-based deficits related to blood pressure, age, socioeconomic status, and education.

Neuropsychological deficits have been demonstrated most convincingly in patients with severe disease (>25 events/hour). Among 50 patients with sleep apnea severe enough to warrant tracheostomy, a majority demonstrated deficits in a number of cognitive processes, including intellectual abilities, executive functions, memory, and learning (82). Depression, hypochrondriasis, and conversion-hysteria were present in 56%, 35%, and 29% of these patients, respectively. The majority of patients reported poor social functioning, marital problems, and school or work performance problems (including falling asleep on the job), suggesting that the consequences of severe sleep apnea include substantial impairments in daytime functioning and quality of life. Depression also has been demonstrated in 40–45% of patients with sleep apnea who were the subjects of two other studies (83,84). Depression appears to be greater in those subjects with greatest apneic activity, and it may improve following CPAP treatment (83). A broad range of neuropsychological deficits also has been demonstrated by Greenberg et al. (85) in 14 patients with severe sleep apnea (mean apnea index = 48), as compared to control subjects. In this study, the degree of hypoxemia in the apneic subjects (lowest mean desaturation 68%) correlated with the magnitude of impairments in motor and perceptual–organizational skills. One study to assess specifically neuropsychological functions in sleep apnea subjects with less-than-severe disease was recently reported (86). In this study, moderate-to-severe neuropsychological deficits were observed in 10 subjects with moderate sleep apnea (10–30 events/hour of sleep).

A few studies have examined the effects of therapy on neuropsychologic functions in treated patients (87–89). These studies generally have had little statistical power because of small sample sizes or inappropriate control groups. Even fewer studies have evaluated the efficacy of treatment of subjects with mild and moderate sleep apnea. A recent study by Guilleminault et al. (90) demonstrating improvement in sleep latency after administration of CPAP therapy to heavy snorers suggests that daytime alertness may be impaired in subjects with low levels of apneic activity, presumably a mild disorder, and that treatment may result in beneficial effects. Clearly, further data are needed to evaluate better the benefit of treating the large

(40–60%) proportion of the middle-aged population that reports heavy snoring. It will be important to determine the degree to which neuropsychological deficits observed in snoring and sleep apnea are simple functions of sleepiness and impaired vigilance rather than attributable to more complex or irreversible pathophysiological processes (e.g., due to chronic hypoxemia or sleep fragmentation).

CONCLUSIONS

Viewed from the perspective of sleep apnea as a prevalent, chronic illness, the cardiopulmonary and neurological manifestations of the disease deserve (a) careful consideration of the impact of apneas over time on metabolic and psychological function and (b) critical review of potential confounding events (weight, alcohol, age, sleep deprivation, or medical co-morbidity) that could lead to overestimation of apneic consequences. Current therapy, if directed only at sleep-disordered breathing, may be inadequate unless the metabolic, psychological, or co-morbid substrate for the illness is also addressed. Current treatment "failures" could result from inadequate attention to these other features; alternatively, current treatment "success" could be increased. Finally, attention to primary and preventive therapy and prevention of overtreatment will be needed given apnea's frequent occurrence in the population.

REFERENCES

1. Young TB, Palta M, Dempsey J, et al. Occurrence of sleep disordered breathing among middle-aged adults. *N Engl J Med* 1993;328:1230–1235.
2. He J, Kryger MH, Zorick FJ, Conway W, Roth T. Mortality and apnea index in obstructive sleep apnea: experience in 385 male patients. *Chest* 1988;94(1):9–14.
3. Partinen M, Guilleminault C. Daytime sleepiness and vascular morbidity at seven-year follow-up in obstructive sleep apnea patients. *Chest* 1990;97:27–32.
4. Strohl KP, Saunders NA, Sullivan CA. Clinical aspects of sleep apnea syndromes. In: Sullivan C, Saunders NA, eds. *Sleep and breathing. Lung biology in health and disease*, vol 14, (Lenfant C, series ed.). New York: Marcel Dekker, 1984;365–402.
5. McNamara SG, Cistulli PA, Strohl KP, Sullivan CE. Clinical aspects of sleep apnea. In: Sullivan C, Saunders NA, eds. *Sleep and breathing, 2nd ed.* edited by C Lenfant, *Lung biology in health and disease*, vol 14 (Lenfant C, series ed.). New York: Marcel Dekker, 1993;493–528.
6. Grunstein RR, Ho KY, Sullivan CE. Sleep apnea in acromegaly. *Ann Intern Med* 1991;115:527–532.
7. Perks WH, Horrocks PM, Cooper RA, Bradbury S, Allen A, Baldock N, Prowse K, van't Hoff W. Sleep apnea in acromegaly. *Br Med J* 1980;280:894–897.
8. Strohl KP, Cherniack NS, Gothe B. Physiological basis of therapy for sleep apnea. *Am Rev Respir Dis* 1986;134:791–802.
9. Cahan C, Arafah B, Decker MJ, Arnold JL, Strohl KP. Adrenal steroids in sleep apnea before and after NCPAP treatment. *Am Rev Respir Dis* 1991;143:A382.
10. Cahan C, Denko C, Arnold J, Decker M, Haacke L, Strohl KP. Insulin levels in sleep apnea syndromes. *Chest* 1990;98:122s.
11. Modan M, Halkin H, Almog S, Lusky A, Eshkol A, Shefi M, Shitrit A, Fuchs Z. Hyperinsulinemia: a link between hypertension, obesity, and glucose intolerance. *J Clin Invest* 1985;75:809–817.
12. Roberts CT, LeRoith D. Interactions in the insulin-like growth factor system. *News Physiol Sci* 1992;7:69–75.

13. Ferrannini E, Haffner SM, Mitchell BD, Stern MP. Hyperinsulinemia: the key feature of a cardio-vascular and metabolic syndrome. *Diabetologia* 1991;34:416–422.
14. Ferrannini E, De Frango RA. The association of hypertension, diabetes, and obesity: a review. *J Nephrol* 1989;1:3–15.
15. Fletcher EC, De Behnke RD, Lovoi MS, Gorin AB. Undiagnosed sleep apnea in patients with essential hypertension. *Ann Intern Med* 1985;103:190–195.
16. Landsberg L. Obesity, metabolism, and hypertension. *Yale J Biol Med* 1989;62(5):511–519.
17. Landsberg L, Krieger DR. Obesity, metabolism, and the sympathetic nervous system. *Am J Hypertens* 1989;2:125S–132S.
18. Gerrner ME, Bersch N, Nakamoto JM, Scott M, Johnson NB, Golden DW. Use of *in vitro* clonogenic assays to differentiate acquired from genetic causes of insulin resistance. *Diabetes* 1991;40:28–36.
19. Hoffstein V, Rubenstein I, Mateika S, Slutsky AS. Determinants of blood pressure in snorers. *Lancet* 1988;Oct 29:992–994.
20. Waller PC, Bhopal RS. Is snoring a cause of vascular disease? An epidemiological review. *Lancet* 1989;Jan 21:143–146.
21. Redline S, Tishler PV, Browner I, Ferrette V. Risk factors for sleep apnea (SA) in a genetic–epidemiologic study: variation by age. *Am Rev Respir Dis* 1992;145:A866.
22. Shepard JW, Jr. Cardiorespiratory changes in obstructive sleep apnea. In: Kryger MH, Roth T, Dement WC, eds. *Principles and practice of sleep medicine*. Philadelphia: WB Saunders, 1989;543.
23. Young TB, Zaccaro DJ, Paulus K. Body habitus correlates of sleep-disordered breathing in a general population sample of 406 adults. *Am Rev Respir Dis* 1992;145:A866.
24. Boudoulas H, Schmidt HS, Clark RW, Geleris P, Schaal SF, Lewis RP. Anthropometric characteristics, cardiac abnormalities and adrenergic activity in patients with primary disorders of sleep. *J Med* 1983;14(3):223–238.
25. Ozaki N, Okada T, Iwata T, Ohta T, Kasahara Y, Kiuchi K, Nagatsa T. Plasma norepinephrine in sleep apnea syndrome. *Neuropsychobiology* 1986;16:88–92.
26. Krieger J, Laks L, Wilcox I. Atrial natriuretic peptide release during sleep in patients with obstructive sleep apnea before and during treatment with nasal continuous positive airway pressure. *Clin Sci* 1989;77:407–411.
27. Krieger J, Schmidt M, Sforza E, Lehr L, Imbs J-L, Coumaros G, Kurtz D. Urinary excretion of guanosine 3′:5′-cyclic monophosphate during sleep in obstructive sleep apnea patients with and without nasal continuous positive airway pressure treatment. *Clin Sci* 1989;76:31–37.
28. Grunfeld C, Baird K, Van Obberghen E, Kahn CR. Glucocorticoid-induced insulin resistance *in vitro*: evidence for both receptor and post-receptor defects. *Endocrinology* 1981;109:1723.
29. Katz I, Stradling J, Slutsky AS, Zamel N, Hoffstein V. Do patients with obstructive sleep apnea have thick necks? *Am Rev Respir Dis* 1990;141:1228–1231.
30. Czech MP, Mottola CM, Yu K-T, Oka Y. The insulin-like growth factor receptors. In: Taiti S, Tolman RA, eds. *Human growth hormone*. New York: Plenum, 1986;539–552.
31. Escouron P, Jirani A, Nedelcoux H, Duroux P, Gaultier C. Systemic hypertension in sleep apnea syndrome. *Chest* 1990;98:1362–1365.
32. DeFronzo RA, Bonadonna RC, Ferrannini E. Pathogenesis of NIDDM: a balanced overview. *Diabetes Care* 1992;15:318–368.
33. Guilleminault C, Carskadon M: Relationship between sleep disorders and daytime complaints. *Sleep* 1976, 1977;6:91–100.
34. Zorick F, Roehrs T, Koshorek G, Sicklestee J, Wittig R, Roth T. Patterns of sleepiness in various disorders of excessive daytime sleepiness. *Sleep* 1982;5:S165–S174.
35. Van den Hoed J, Kraemer H, Guilleminault C, Zarcone VP, Miles LE, Dement WC. Disorders of excessive somnolence: polygraphic and clinical data for 100 patients. *Sleep* 1981;4:23–37.
36. Reynolds CF, Coble PA, Kupfer DJ, Holzer BC. Application of the multiple sleep latency test in disorders of excessive sleepiness. *Electroencephalogr Clin Neurophysiol* 1982;65:443–452.
37. Roth T, Roehrs T, Conway W. Behavioral morbidity of apnea. *Semin Res Med* 1988;9:554–559.
38. Zorick F, Roehrs T, Conway W, Fujita S, Wittig W, Roth T. Effects of uvulopalatopharyngoplasty on the daytime sleepiness associated with sleep apnea syndrome. *Bull Eur Pathophysiol Res* 1983;19:600–603.
39. Wittig RM, Conway WA, Zorick F, Sicklesteel J, Roehrs T, Roth T. CPAP: reduction in daytime sleepiness after one night's use. *Sleep Res* 1987;16:459.
40. Bonnet MH. Performance and sleepiness as a function of the frequency and placement of sleep disruption. *Psychophysiol* 1986;23:263–271.

41. Stepanski E, Lamphere J, Roehrs T, Zorick F, Roth T. Experimental sleep fragmentation in normal subjects. *Int J Neurosci* 1987;33:207–214.
42. Levine B, Roehrs T, Stepanski E, Zorick F, Roth T. Fragmenting sleep diminishes its recuperative value. *Sleep* 1987;10:590–599.
43. Gold AR, Schwartz AR, Bleecker ER, Smith PL. The effect of nocturnal oxygen administration upon sleep apnea. *Am Rev Respir Dis* 1986;134:925–929.
44. Colt HG, Haas H, Rich GB. Hypoxemia vs sleep fragmentation as cause of excessive daytime sleepiness in obstructive sleep apnea. *Chest* 1991;100:1542–1548.
45. Kribbs NB, Redline S, Smith PL, Schwartz AR, Schubert NM, Kline LR, Delisser L, Henry JN, Pack AI, Dinges DF. Objective monitoring of nasal CPAP usage patterns in OSAS patients. *Sleep Res* 1991;20:270.
46. Bedard MA, Montplaisir J, Richer F, Rouleau I, Malo J. Obstructive sleep apnea syndrome: pathogenesis of neuropsychological deficits. *J Clin Exp Neuropsychol* 1991;13:950–964.
47. Aguirre M, Broughton R. Stuss D. Does memory impairment exist in narcolepsy-cataplexy? *J Clin Exp Neuropsychol* 1985;7:14–24.
48. Isa FG, Sullivan CE. Alcohol, snoring, and sleep apnea. *J Neurol* 1982;45:353–357.
49. Guilleminault C, Silvestri R, Mondini S. Aging and sleep apnea: action of benzodiazepines, acetazolamide, alcohol, and sleep deprivation in a healthy elderly group. *J Gerontol* 1984;39:655–661.
50. Scrima L, Broudy M, Nay KN. Increased severity of obstructive sleep apnea after bedtime alcohol ingestion: diagnostic potential and proposed mechanism of action. *Sleep* 1982;5:318–322.
51. Tassan VC, Block AJ, Poysen PG. Alcohol increases sleep apnea and oxygen desaturation in asymptomatic men. *Am J Med* 1981;71:240–245.
52. Zwyghuizen-Doorenbos A, Roehrs T, Lamphere J, Zorick F, Roth T. Increased daytime sleepiness enhances ethanol's sedative effects. *Neuropsychopharmacology* 1988;1:279–286.
53. Roehrs T, Zwyghuizen-Doorenbos A, Knox M, Moskowitz H. Roth T. Sedating effects of ethanol and time of drinking. *Am Clin Exp Res* 1992;16:553–557.
54. Cheshire K, Engleman H, Deary I, Shapiro C, Douglas NJ. Factors impairing daytime performance in patients with sleep apnea/hypopnea syndrome. *Arch Intern Med* 1992;152:538–541.
55. Redline S, Young T. *The epidemiology and natural history of sleep apnea: prevalence, incidence, morbidity, mortality, and financial burden.* Report for Congressional Committee on Sleep Disorders, 1992.
56. Findley LJ, Unverzagt ME, Suratt P. Automobile accidents involving patients with obstructive sleep apnea. *Am Rev Respir Dis* 1988;138:337–340.
57. Guilleminault C, Dement WC. Sleep apnea syndromes and related disorders. In: Williams RL, Karacan I, eds. *Sleep disorders: diagnosis and treatment.* New York: Wiley, 1978.
58. Block JA, Boysen PG, Wynne JW, Hunt LA. Sleep apnea, hypopnea and oxygen desaturation in normal subjects. *N Eng J Med* 1979;300:513–517.
59. Redline S, Millman RP, Tosteson T, Carskadon M, Tishler PV. Familial aggregation of symptoms of sleep-related disorders. *Am Rev Respir Dis* 1992;145:58–67.
60. Broughton RJ. *Sleep, arousal, and performance.* Ogilvie RD, ed. Boston: Birkhauser, 1990.
61. Pasnau RO, Naitoh P, Stier S, Koller E. The psychological effects of 205 hours of sleep deprivation. *Arch Gen Psychiatry* 1968;18:496–505.
62. Hart RP, Buchsbaum DG, Wade JB, Hamer RM, Kwentus JA. Effect of sleep deprivation on first-year resident's response times, memory, and mood. *J Med Ed* 1987;62:94–112.
63. Horne JA, Anderson NR, Wilkinson RT. Effects of sleep deprivation on signal detection measures of vigilance: implications for sleep function. *Sleep* 1983;6:347–358.
64. Jacques CHM, Lynch JC, Samtoff JS. The effects of sleep loss on cognitive performance of resident physicians. *J Fam Pract* 1990;30:223–229.
65. Nilsson L-G, Backman L, Karlsson T. Priming and cued recall in elderly, alcohol-intoxicated and sleep-deprived subjects: a case of functionally similar memory deficits. *Psychol Med* 1989;19:423–433.
66. Wilkinson RT. Effects of up to 60 hours of sleep deprivation on different types of work. *Ergonomics* 1964;7:175–186.
67. Bonnet MH. Effect of sleep disruption on sleep, performance and mood. *Sleep* 1985;8:11–19.
68. Bonnet MH. The restoration of performance following sleep deprivation in geriatric normal and insomniac subjects. *Sleep Res* 1984;13:188.
69. Pirolli A, Smith C. REM sleep deprivation in humans impairs learning of a complex task. *Sleep Res* 1989;18:375.

70. Smith C, Pirolli A. Learning deficits following REM sleep deprivation of either the first two or last two REM periods of the night. *Sleep Res* 1989;18:377.
71. Carskadon MA, Dement WC. Cumulative effects of sleep restriction on daytime sleepiness. *Psychopathology* 1981;18:107–113.
72. Carskadon MA, Brown ED, Dement WC. Sleep fragmentation in the elderly: relationship to daytime sleep tendency. *Neurobiol Aging* 1982;3:321–327.
73. Philip P, Stoohs R, Castronovo C, Guilleminault C. Sleepiness and performance under experimental sleep fragmentation. *Sleep Res* 1992;22:29.
74. Levine B, Roehrs T, Stepanski E, Zorick F, Roth T. Fragmenting sleep diminishes its recuperative value. *Sleep* 1987;10:590–599.
75. Adam K. Sleep as a restorative process and a theory to explain why. *Prog Brain Res* 1980;53:289–304.
76. Wu JC, Gillin JC, Buchsbaum MS, et al. The effect of sleep deprivation on cerebral glucose metabolic rate in normal humans assessed with PET. *Sleep* 1991;14:155–162.
77. Cohen P, Alexander S, Smith R, Reivich M, Wollman H. Effects of hypoxia and normocarbia on cerebral blood flow and metabolism in conscious man. *J Appl Physiol* 1967;23:183–189.
78. Krop HD, Block JA, Cohen E. Neuropsychological effects of continuous oxygen therapy in COPD. *Chest* 1973;64:317–322.
79. Prigatano GP, Parsons O, Wright E, Levin DC, Hawryluk G. Neuropsychological test performance in mildly hypoxemic patients with chronic obstructive pulmonary disease. *J Consult Clin Psychol* 1983;51:108–116.
80. Findley LJ, Barth JT, Powers DC, Wilhout SC, Boyd DG, Suratt PM. Cognitive impairment in patients with obstructive sleep apnea and associated hypoxemia. *Chest* 1986;90:686–690.
81. Telakivi T, Kajaste S, Partinen M, Koskenvuo M, Salmi T, Kaprio J. Cognitive function in middle-aged snorers and controls: role of excessive daytime somnolence and sleep-related hypoxic events. *Sleep* 1988;11:454–462.
82. Kales A, Caldwell AB, Cadieux RJ, Vela-Bueno A, Roch LG, Mayes SD. Severe obstructive sleep apnea. II. Associated psychopathology and psychological consequences. *J Chronic Dis* 1985;38:427–434.
83. Millman RP, Fogel BS, McNamara ME, Carlisle C. Depression as a manifestation of obstructive sleep apnea: reversal with nasal continuous positive airway pressure. *J Clin Psychiatry* 1989;50:348–351.
84. Reynolds CF, Kupfer DJ, McEachran AM, Taska LS, Sewitch DE, Coble PA. Depressive psychopathology in male sleep apneics. *J Clin Psychiatry* 1984;45:287–290.
85. Greenberg, GD, Watson RK, Deptula D. Neuropsychological dysfunction in sleep apnea. *Sleep* 1987;10:254–262.
86. Bedard M-A, Montplaisir J, Richer F, Rouleau I, Malo J. Obstructive sleep apnea syndrome: pathogenesis of neuropsychological deficits. *J Clin Exp Neuropsychol* 1991;13:950–964.
87. Charbonneau M, Tousignant P, Lamping DL, Cosio MG, Montserrat JM, Olha AE, Levy RD, Kimoff RJ. The effects of nasal continuous positive airway pressure (nCPAP) on sleepiness and psychological functioning in obstructive sleep apnea (OSA). *Am Rev Respir Dis* 1992;145:168.
88. Engleman HM, Cheshire KE, Deary IJ, Douglas NJ. Daytime sleepiness and psychometric function after CPAP for the sleep apnea/hypopnea syndrome. *Am Rev Respir Dis* 1992;135:169.
89. Klonoff H, Fleetham J, Taylor R, Clark C. Treatment outcome of obstructive sleep apnea: physiological and neuropsychological concomitants. *J Nerv Mental Dis* 1987;175:203–212.
90. Guilleminault C, Stoohs R, Duncan S. Snoring: daytime sleepiness in regular heavy snorers. *Chest* 1991;99:40–48.

Snoring and Obstructive Sleep Apnea, Second Edition,
edited by D.N.F. Fairbanks and S. Fujita.
Raven Press, Ltd., New York © 1994.

4

Disorders of Excessive Sleepiness

Samuel J. Potolicchio, Jr.

Department of Neurology, Georgetown University Hospital, Washington, D.C. 20007

Undesirable sleepiness during waking hours that is often associated with decreased cognitive and motor performance is the primary symptom of the disorders of excessive somnolence (DOES). The diagnosis of DOES applies to patients who have sleep attacks or who fall asleep quickly in the waking state when sedentary. There are various functional and organic conditions which lead to inappropriate sleepiness during waking hours (Table 1). This type of symptomatology should not be confused with the complaint of general fatigue and loss of mental alertness, more often the associative signs of insomnia, or disorders of initiating and maintaining sleep (DIMS).

Proper physiological assessment of DOES necessitates the following: overnight and daytime recording of biological functions including brain wave [electroencephalogram (EEG)], muscle activity [electromyogram (EMG)], and eye movements [electro-oculogram (EOG)] for sleep staging; monitoring of oral and nasal airflow and respiratory parameters by thermistors and inductive plethysmography; monitoring of oxygen saturation (oximetry); and recording of body movements, particularly of the legs (EMG of anterior tibial muscles). The daytime multiple sleep latency test (MSLT) is used in conjunction with overnight polysomnography to assess excessive daytime sleepiness by measurement of sleep-onset latency over several recording sessions. The presence of sleep-onset rapid eye movement (SOREM) is another important parameter detected by the MSLT.

SLEEP APNEA: CLINICAL PRESENTATION, DIAGNOSIS, AND TREATMENT

Sleep apnea syndrome is characterized by multiple obstructive or mixed apneas during sleep associated with repetitive episodes of loud snoring and microarousals. Excessive daytime sleepiness is typically the presenting complaint because nocturnal sleep is disrupted and of poor quality. The patient is usually not aware of the breathing difficulty or of the numerous microarousals and body movements associ-

TABLE 1. *Disorders of excessive sleepiness*

Sleep apnea
Narcolepsy/cataplexy syndrome
Excessive daytime sleepiness associated with psychophysiological states and psychiatric disorders
Drug-related syndromes responsible for daytime hypersomnolence
Restless legs/periodic limb movement disorder
Idiopathic CNS hypersomnolence
Toxic-metabolic conditions associated with excessive hypersomnolence
Intermittent disorders of excessive somnolence
    Klein–Levin syndrome
    Menstrual-associated syndrome
    Sleep drunkenness

ated with it. Most often reports from a sleep observer are necessary for an adequate description of the breathing pattern (1).

Although a modest degree of obesity is often associated with sleep apnea syndrome, many patients with the disorder are not significantly overweight. They may exhibit anatomical abnormalities of the upper airway or demonstrate a short, thick neck, sometimes with micro- or retrognathia. Although sleep apnea can occur at all ages, more than half of the patients are 40 years of age or older when first diagnosed. The prevalence of sleep apnea is not precisely known, but it appears in approximately 45% of loud snorers or 2–3% of the male population. Men do outnumber women by a ratio of approximately 30:1. Because a hereditary influence for snoring is strong, heredity is also suggested for most cases of sleep apnea syndrome.

Additional presenting symptoms of the sleep apnea syndrome include morning headaches, secondary depression, anxiety, irritability, and impotence or loss of libido. Hypertension is present in approximately 40% of cases. Cardiac arrhythmias are frequently observed during sleep and range from sinus arrhythmia and premature ventricular contractions to atrioventricular block and sinus arrest. The appearance of secondary cardiac failure, either right- or left-sided, may be evident in severe cases. There is an increased risk of sudden death during sleep, usually due to arrhythmia (2).

Apneic episodes during sleep are defined as cessations of airflow at nose and mouth lasting 10 sec or longer and easily documented by polysomnographic recordings (Fig. 1). The sleep-disordered breathing is associated with brief microarousals as detected by EEG just prior to resumption of breathing. Repeated K-complexes or generalized slowing of brain wave activity may occur toward the end of each non-rapid-eye-movement (NREM) sleep apneic period in sleep. Slow-wave sleep stages 3 and 4 are either absent or much reduced. Apneic episodes are preponderant in stages 1 and 2 of NREM sleep or REM sleep. Night-to-night variation in the frequency of pauses exists in many patients and is increased by supine body position, presence of upper respiratory infections, or use of certain drugs and alcohol.

Three types of sleep apnea can be distinguished by polysomnography: (a) central

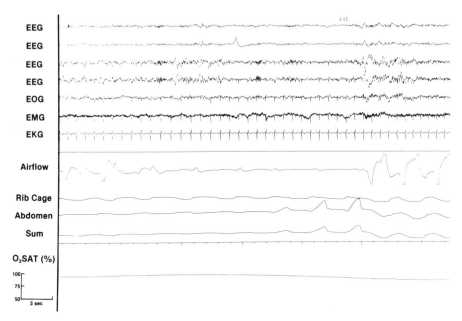

FIG. 1. Obstructive apneic period is denoted by progressive diminution in airflow, paradoxical movement of rib cage and abdominal excursions, and lowering of oxygen saturation. EEG arousal pattern occurs with resumption of normal breathing.

apnea, characterized by cessation of airflow resulting from termination of respiratory effort, (b) obstructive apnea, characterized by cessation of airflow despite persistent respiratory effort, and (c) mixed central and obstructive apnea, characterized by the occurrence of an early central phase and a late obstructive phase (3). The degree of sleep apnea can range from mild to severe, with the frequency of apneic episodes varying from 6–20/hr to several hundred per night (>40/hr). In the vast majority of patients, the obstructive type predominates. The severity of consequent hypercapnia and hypoxemia is influenced by the duration and type of apneic episode (4).

The treatment of sleep apnea syndrome includes both medical and surgical approaches. The most effective drug therapy for sleep-disordered breathing in the adult is protriptyline in daily doses of 10–40 mg. The mechanisms of action of protriptyline are probably twofold: the reduction in stage 5 REM sleep and an increase in tone of upper airway dilator muscles. Drug therapy is most effective in mild-to-moderate cases of sleep apnea (20–40/hr) in conjunction with weight loss. Side effects of dry mouth, loss of libido, and altered states of consciousness are frequently encountered and result in limited success. The most successful nonsurgical approach to sleep apnea syndrome has been the recent use of nasal continuous positive airway pressure (CPAP) introduced by Sullivan et al. (5). Compressed air delivered to the nasal passage through a tightly fitted mask at pressures of 5–15 cm of H_2O can result in complete alleviation of upper airway obstruction. In those patients who require pressures above 15 cm of H$_2$O, the use of BiPAP, or differentiated control of inspired and expired pressure devices, may help with compliance. In moderate-to-severe sleep apnea cases who are poor surgical candidates or even postsurgical failures, such therapy, on a chronic basis, is 80–85% effective.

Dental appliances such as tongue retainers and orthodontic prostheses have gained popularity in recent years, particularly in patients with milder obstructive sleep apnea who are averse to other mechanical treatments.

The ultimate surgical approach to obstructive sleep apnea is tracheostomy, a procedure most often recommended in severe cases associated with life-threatening cardiac disease.

Uvulopalatopharyngoplasty (UPPP) has been the most popular surgical intervention over the past several years. The success rate of UPPP in severe cases of obstructive sleep apnea, however, is only 50%. To date, various radiographic evaluations including cephalometrics and cineradiography have not been thoroughly successful in the selection of appropriate surgical candidates. Mandibular osteotomy and more aggressive maxillomandibular interventions have proven effective in subgroups of sleep apnea patients.

NARCOLEPSY/CATAPLEXY SYNDROME: CLINICAL FEATURES, DIAGNOSIS, AND TREATMENT

Narcolepsy is a syndrome which consists of excessive daytime sleepiness and abnormal manifestations of REM sleep, most commonly frequent SOREM periods. Excessive daytime sleepiness is usually the first of the tetrad of symptoms of narcolepsy to appear. Sleep attacks occur throughout the day, commonly after meals or in the late afternoon, even while the patient is engaging in such activities as driving a car, conversation, or active sexual relations. A history of cataplexy is a characteristic and unique feature of narcolepsy. Cataplectic attacks consist of brief periods of loss of muscle tone, giving rise to jaw drop, head droop, facial sagging, weakening of the knees or hand grip, or sudden paralysis of all skeletal muscles with complete postural collapse. Consciousness is usually preserved, though cataplexy can occur in combination with a REM sleep episode and intense sleepiness. Sleep paralysisis and hypnogogic hallucinations are two other symptoms associated with the syndrome. Sleep paralysis appears at entry or emergence from sleep. The patient is unable to move but regains use of his muscles after 1 or 2 min. Hypnogogic hallucinations are vivid, perceptual, dreamlike experiences which occur at sleep onset or on awakening. These hallucinations are often accompanied by feelings of fear (6–8).

Narcolepsy usually begins in the second decade of life. There is a 60-fold greater risk of developing the syndrome among relatives of narcoleptics. The prevalence of the disorder is estimated at 1 in 2000 with no gender dominance. Recent studies have shown a high correlation with the DR$_{15}$ (DR$_2$) antigen of the histocompatibility gene complex. Such a correlation can help in the differentiation of those cases with

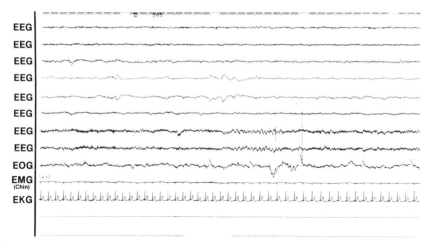

FIG. 2. Sleep-onset REM period is depicted by the presence of rapid eye movements on EOG associated with sawtooth waves in EEG channels 7 and 8.

borderline findings on polysomnographic recordings. It has been documented to be inherited in dogs (8).

The most characteristic polysomnographic feature of narcolepsy is the occurrence of SOREM periods. These are best demonstrated in multiple daytime naps (MSLT) or in nocturnal sleep recordings with or without programmed awakenings. REM sleep will occur within 10 min of sleep onset (Fig. 2).

Narcolepsy must be differentiated from all other disorders of excessive daytime sleepiness, particularly sleep apnea, drug withdrawal, alcoholism, or previous REM sleep deprivation (10). The distinction between narcolepsy and other causes of excessive daytime sleepiness can be difficult because of the variable order in which symptoms can appear. Overnight polysomnography followed by a daytime MSLT are now considered to be mandatory to make an accurate diagnosis.

The mainstay of therapy for narcolepsy includes amphetamines or amphetamine-like compounds. Recent studies have shown the beneficial effects of drugs such as codeine and propranolol. Central nervous system (CNS) stimulants are linked with numerous side effects and habituation, factors which mandate close supervision and frequent drug holidays.

EXCESSIVE DAYTIME SLEEPINESS ASSOCIATED WITH PSYCHOPHYSIOLOGICAL STATES AND PSYCHIATRIC DISORDERS

Transient and situational DOES arise particularly from participating events such as illness, death of a relative or close friend, marital separation or divorce, job demotion, or stress. There is a disruption of the normal sleep–wake pattern manifested by excessive difficulty remaining awake with prolonged periods of time spent in bed or frequent naps during the day. Individuals prone to increased sleepiness in the face of rejection or change have "passive" makeups: They tend to worry and withdraw from their own aggressive feelings (11).

Persistent psychophysiological DOES applies to patients with a chronic disposition to excessive sleeping, bed rest, and daytime napping when confronted with stress or when coping capacities are overwhelmed. The condition itself is rare but most often found in individuals who repeatedly experience a sense of fatigue and defensive tiredness when encountering challenges (12).

Excessive daytime sleepiness is often associated with major affective and other depressive syndromes. The disturbance is subjectively described as increased daytime napping and prolonged sleep at night. In the bipolar depressions, the severity of the sleep disturbance is correlated with the severity of the affective episodes. Polysomnography reveals a short REM latency (<60 min) and decreased slow-wave sleep (NREM stages 3 and 4). This pattern is most often detected in middle-aged depressed patients, but it can also be seen in childhood and adolescence. Concomitant symptoms of increased appetite, reduced concentration, and increased fatigue are common, particularly if hypersomnic conditions of metabolic or drug origin have been eliminated (13,14). Chronic fatigue syndrome, whether or not it is associated with specific clinical findings (such as viral illnesses, fibromyalgia, or drug-induced syndromes), may be associated not only with fatigue and hypersomnia but also with well-defined sleep disorders.

DRUG-RELATED SYNDROMES RESPONSIBLE FOR DAYTIME HYPERSOMNOLENCE

Tolerance to or withdrawal from CNS stimulants and sustained use of CNS depressants are the conditions most commonly associated with excessive daytime sleepiness (15,16). Daytime complications, particularly from amphetamine-like drugs, include irritability, blackouts, altered mood states, paranoid thinking, automatic behaviors, amnesia, disturbances in autonomic functioning, and weight loss. With increasing tolerance to stimulants, the confirmed addict becomes aware of the hypersomnolence that follows reduction or elimination of drugs. Excessive use of caffeine beverages could also lead to a similar condition, particularly when the daily requirement for caffeine increases with tolerance to 10 or more cups of coffee per day.

The symptoms associated with amphetamine-like agents can also be encountered with the overuse of CNS depressants, sedatives, hypnotics, tranquilizers, and alcohol. Patients are often initiated to drug-induced somnolence following prescribed treatment of insomnia or following hospitalization for medical conditions. Patients may not recognize at first the soporific actions of the drugs and how quickly they become dependent on them. Inquiry into social and marital problems or work difficulties will usually help in the differentiation of drug-related hypersomnolence from other DOES syndromes.

Overnight polysomnographic recordings in patients withdrawing from psycho-tropic agents can reveal rebound effects such as early-onset REM sleep. If CNS depressants are taken in the evening, sleep time could be excessive at night. The polysomnogram at that point in time may show a reduction in REM sleep and an increase in slow-wave sleep stages 3 and 4.

RESTLESS LEGS/PERIODIC LIMB MOVEMENT DISORDER

Sleep-related periodic limb movements consist of stereotyped abrupt contractions of extremity muscles, particularly of the legs, during sleep. The EMG of the ante-rior tibialis muscle will show repetitive muscle contractions, each lasting 0.5–10 sec and occurring at intervals of 20–40 sec (Fig. 3). The contractions will result in extension of the big toe with partial flexion of the ankle, knee, and at times the hip. These periodic movements are followed by microarousals or even awakening. The patient usually has no knowledge of the muscle twitches but will present with a history of frequent nocturnal awakenings associated with excessive daytime sleepi-ness. The condition is seen predominantly in middle-aged and elderly individuals of both sexes. The incidence of the disorder ranges from 1% to 15%, with a suggestion of familial patterns in only a few studies (17). Restless legs syndrome is a disorder of wakefulness associated with irresistible movement of the legs, related to uncom-fortable sensory symptoms such as tingling, pricking, and aching. It can compound the problem of disturbed sleep in up to 40% of familial cases.

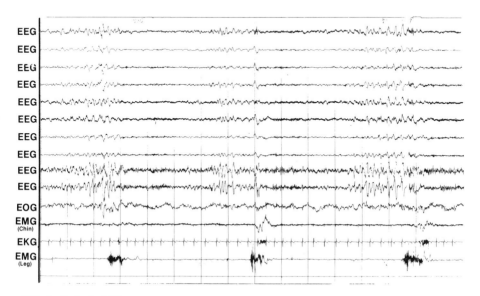

FIG. 3. Periodic EEG microarousals are time-locked to periodic leg movements (myoclonus) recorded by EMG of anterior tibialis muscle.

It is necessary that a complete polysomnogram be performed on patients suspected of having the disorder, since other conditions such as sleep apnea, narcolepsy, uremia, and drug-induced myoclonus can mimic the syndrome. Sleep-related myoclonus must also be differentiated from nocturnal myoclonic seizures and benign hypnic jerks, the latter occurring during drowsiness before the onset of stage 1 sleep or following arousals (18). The most effective therapy for periodic leg movements is either low-dose carbidopa-levodopa (25/100 mg) (19) or clonazepam (0.5–1 mg) taken at bedtime. When restless legs symptomatology is present, drugs such as carbamazepine or clonidine may be necessary during waking hours (20,21).

IDIOPATHIC CNS HYPERSOMNOLENCE

Patients with idiopathic CNS hypersomnolence complain of recurrent daytime sleepiness, the need for lengthy naps, and automatic behaviors related to microsleep. The majority of patients report that they sleep very well through the night. Daytime sleep attacks such as those seen with narcolepsy are not encountered. They do not have the frequent disruption of sleep reported by narcoleptics. The familial appearance of the disorder is observed most frequently. The syndrome could account for 12–15% of patients complaining of excessive daytime sleepiness, though the condition is relatively neglected by most physicians. Familial forms of idiopathic CNS hypersomnolence have been associated with the HLA CW2 antigen.

Polysomnography fails to demonstrate the SOREM periods of narcolepsy or sleep-disordered breathing of the sleep apnea syndrome. The MSLT does show significant daytime hypersomnolence with short, mean sleep-onset latencies.

Idiopathic CNS hypersomnolence differentiates itself from narcolepsy by its poor response to stimulants such as the amphetamines and methylphenidate. Moreover, the amphetamine-like compounds often exacerbate the associated symptoms of headache, nausea, and syncope encountered in this syndrome. Numerous drugs such as tricyclic antidepressants, monoamine oxidase (MAO) inhibitors, and methysergide have been shown to alleviate the primary symptoms of excessive daytime sleepiness, a finding which suggests that serotonin metabolism may be playing some role in the etiology of the disorder (22,23).

TOXIC-METABOLIC CONDITIONS ASSOCIATED WITH EXCESSIVE HYPERSOMNOLENCE

Many medical, toxic, and environmental conditions are associated with disorders of excessive sleepiness either as direct causes or because of daytime consequences of disrupted nocturnal sleep or sleep deprivation.

Hypersomnolent states are associated with endocrine and metabolic disorders such as hypothyroidism, diabetes, and hypoglycemia. Other metabolic disturbances such as uremia, liver failure, and hypercapnia secondary to chronic lung disease can cause DOES. Structural CNS disorders such as brain tumor, subdural hematomas, or increased intracranial pressure from various causes could lead to excessive sleepiness. Infection, degenerative disease, and trauma to the brain, the latter possibly associated with hydrocephalus, are other causes to be considered (24–27).

Complete neurological and psychiatric evaluations along with pertinent metabolic screening are often necessary to clarify the situation.

INTERMITTENT DISORDERS OF EXCESSIVE SOMNOLENCE

Kleine–Levin Syndrome

Kleine–Levin syndrome is a relatively rare condition in which a patient suffers from recurrent bouts of excessive sleepiness associated with intervals of normal sleep and alertness. During the periods of hypersomnolence, the patient will withdraw from social contacts and display apathy, confusion, voracious eating, and loss of sexual inhibitions. The disorder is thought to be related to intermittent organic dysfunction of limbic and hypothalamic structures (28,29).

In the typical patient, several attacks of hypersomnolence, each lasting a few weeks, occur on a yearly basis. The onset of attacks is usually before the end of the second decade. The disorder is often self-limiting, with remissions occurring before the age of 40. Physical and emotional stress and febrile illness can precipitate periods of hypersomnolence. The exact prevalence of the disorder is unknown but is primarily restricted to males. This disorder must be differentiated from neoplastic and inflammatory disease of the diencephalon.

Menstrual-Associated Syndrome

Menstrual-associated syndrome is defined as excessive sleepiness which occurs only during menstrual periods. It is fairly distinct from other periodic disorders of hypersomnolence, though certain behaviors noted during the sleepy period may be reminiscent of Kleine–Levin syndrome. A search for consistent endocrine changes during attacks has yet to be rewarding, though a hypothalamic disturbance is highly suspected. Polysomnography does not demonstrate any specific changes in sleep architecture (30,31).

Sleep Drunkenness

When the lack of clear sensorium in transition from sleep to full wakefulness is prolonged and exaggerated, sleep drunkenness should be suspected. Inappropriate behaviors are often associated with the sleep drunken state because the capacity to carry out less demanding motor tasks is preserved in the face of poor rational judgment and cloudy perception. The condition has been diagnosed only in adults, with a preponderance among males. There is an affinity for certain families. The condition should be differentiated from other unrelated conditions such as somnambulism, epilepsy, hysterical dissociative states, and sudden withdrawal from stimulants (32).

REFERENCES

1. Guilleminault C, Dement WC. Sleep apnea syndromes and related sleep disorders. In: Williams, RL, Karacan, I, eds. *Sleep disorders: diagnosis and treatment.* New York: John Wiley, 1978;9–28.
2. Lugaresi E. Snoring and its clinical implications. In: Guilleminault C, Dement WC, eds. *Sleep apnea syndromes.* New York: Alan R Liss, 1978;13–21.
3. Guilleminault C. Obstructive sleep apnea: electromyographic and fiberoptic studies. *Exp Neurol* 1968;62:7–16.
4. Guilleminault C, Dement W. 235 cases of excessive daytime sleepiness: diagnosis and tentative classification. *J Neurol Sci* 1977;31:13
5. Sullivan CE, Berthon-Jones M, Issa FG, Eves L. Reversal of obstructive sleep apnea by continuous positive airway pressure applied through the nares. *Lancet* 1981;1:862–865.
6. Roth B. Narcolepsy and hypersomnia. In: Williams RL, Karacan I, eds. *Sleep disorders: diagnosis and treatment.* New York: John Wiley, 1978;29–60.
7. Zarcone V. Narcolepsy. *N Engl J Med* 1973;288:1156–1166.
8. Rechtschaffen A, Wolpert EA, Dement WC, Mitchell SA, Fisher C. Nocturnal sleep of narcoleptics. *Electroencephalogr Clin Neurophysiol* 1963;15:599–609.
9. Mitler M, Boysen B, Campbell L, Dement W. Narcolepsy–cataplexy in a female dog. *Exp Neurol* 1974;45:332–340.
10. Yoss R, Daly D. Narcolepsy. *Med Clin North Am* 1960;44:953–968.
11. Hartmann EL. *The functions of sleep.* New Haven, CT: Yale University Press, 1974;123–130.
12. Murray EJ. *Sleep, dreams and arousal.* New York: Appleton–Century–Crofts, 1965;257–261.
13. Kupfer DJ, Himmelhock JM, Swartzburg M, Anderson C, Byck R, Detre TP. Hypersomnia in manic–depressive disease. *Dis Nerv Syst* 1972;33:720–724.
14. Kupfer DJ, Foster FG. The sleep of psychotic patients: does it all look alike? In: Freeman DX, ed. *Biology of the major psychoses: a comparative analysis.* New York: Raven, 1975;143–164.
15. Oswald I. Sleep and dependence on amphetamine and other druges. In: Kales A, ed. *Sleep: physiology and pathology.* Philadelphia: JB Lippincott, 1969;317–330.
16. Sutherland EW. Dependence on barbiturates and other CNS depressants. In: Pradhan SN, Dutta SN, eds. *Drug abuse: clinical and basic aspects.* St. Louis: CV Mosby, 1977;235–247.
17. Coleman RM, Pollak CP, Kokkoris CP, McGregor PA, Weitzman ED. Periodic nocturnal myoclonus in patients with sleep–wake disorders: a case series analysis. In: Chase MH, Mitzer M, Walter PL, eds. *Sleep research, vol 8.* Los Angeles: Brain Information Service/Brain Research Institute, UCLA, 1979;175.
18. Lugaresi E, Coccagra G, Gambi D, Berticeroni G, Poppi M. Symond's nocturnal myoclonus. *Electroencephalogr Clin Neurophysiol* 1967;23:289.
19. Montplaisir J, Godbout R, Poirer G, Bedard MA. Restless legs syndrome and periodic movements of sleep: physiopathology and treatment with L-DOPA. *Clin Neuropharmacol* 1986;9:456–463.
20. Telstad W, Sorensen O, Larsen S, et al. Treatment of the restless legs syndrome with carbamazepine: a double blind study. *Br Med J* 1984;89:1–7.
21. Handwerker JV, Palmer RF. Clonidine in the treatment of "restless legs" syndrome. *N Engl J Med* 1985;313:1228–1229.
22. Guilleminault C, Dement W. Pathologies of excessive sleep. In: Weitzman ED, ed. *Advances in sleep research,* vol 1. New York: Spectrum Publications, 1974;345–390.
23. Roth B, Functional hypersomnia. In: Guilleminault C, Dement WC, Passouant P, eds. *Narcolepsy. Advances in sleep research,* vol 3. New York: Spectrum Publications, 1976;333–350.
24. Freemon FR. Sleep in patients with organic diseases of the nervous system. In: Williams RL, Karacan I, eds. *Sleep disorders: diagnosis and treatment.* New York: John Wiley, 1978;261–283.
25. Kales A, Tan TL. Sleep alterations associated with medical illness. In: Kales A, eds. *Sleep physiology and pathology.* Philadelphia: JB Lippincott, 1969;148–157.
26. Walker AE, Caveness WE, Gutchley M. eds. *The late effects of head injury.* Springfield, Il: Charles C Thomas, 1969.

27. Williams RL. Sleep disturbances in various medical and surgical conditions. In: Williams, RL, Karacan, I, eds. *Sleep disorders: diagnosis* and treatment, New York: John Wiley, 1978;285–301.
28. Critchley M. Periodic hypersomnia and megaphagia in adolescent males. *Brain* 1962;85:627–656.
29. Levin M. Periodic somnolence and morbid hunger. *Brain* 1936;59:494–515.
30. Billiard M, Guilleminault C, Dement WC. A menstruation-linked periodic hypersomnia. *Neurology* 1975;25:436–443.
31. Ho A. Sex hormones and the sleep of women. In: Chase MH, Stern WC, Walter PL, eds. *Sleep research*, vol 1. Los Angeles: Brain Information Service/Brain Research Institute, UCLA, 1972; 184.
32. Roth B, Nevsimalova S, Rechtschaffen A. Hypersomnia with sleep drunkenness. *Arch Gen Psychiatry* 1972;26:456–462.

Snoring and Obstructive Sleep Apnea, Second Edition,
edited by D.N.F. Fairbanks and S. Fujita.
Raven Press, Ltd., New York © 1994.

5

Nonsurgical Management of Snoring and Obstructive Sleep Apnea

Mark H. Sanders

*Department of Medicine and Anesthesiology, University of Pittsburgh School of Medicine,
Pittsburgh, Pennsylvania 15261; Pulmonary Sleep Disorders Program, Division of
Pulmonary, Allergy and Critical Care Medicine, and Clinical Pulmonary Sleep Evaluation
Laboratory, University of Pittsburgh Medical Center, Pittsburgh, Pennsylvania 15213; and
Pulmonary Service, Veterans Affairs Medical Center, Pittsburgh, Pennsylvania 15206*

The most effective and expedient therapy for a disorder is usually that which reverses a basic element in the pathophysiologic sequence. Given the multiplicity of hypotheses regarding the pathogenesis of obstructive and "central" sleep apnea, the diversity of currently employed therapies is understandable. Some treatments for obstructive sleep apnea such as tracheostomy intervene at the culmination of the pathophysiologic sequence, whereas others may act earlier in the pathogenic chain of events (i.e., protriptyline). In general, it can be said that many therapeutic modalities work with some success in some patients but that, for a variety of reasons, no single modality succeeds in all patients. This suggests that there are several pathophysiologic processes responsible for disturbed breathing during sleep, and highlights our lack of knowledge in these regards.

Following the initial recognition of obstructive sleep apnea (OSA), tracheostomy was the therapeutic mainstay for providing a consistently patent upper airway during sleep. While providing a definitive treatment (1–3), tracheostomy has substantial medical and psychological morbidity (4–6). The problems associated with tracheostomy and the disappointing 50% response rate of uvulopalatopharyngoplasty for sleep apnea (7,8) have prompted many clinicians and investigators to search for effective, noninvasive therapies with which patients will be compliant. This chapter will provide an update on the nonsurgical treatments which are currently available for patients with OSA or are undergoing evaluation to comprehensively assess their therapeutic efficacy in this patient population. Initially, the discussion will focus on reducing or eliminating known risk factors for sleep apnea. Subsequently, those agents that are thought to alleviate sleep-disordered breathing by action at the level of the central nervous system (CNS) will be described. Lastly, there will be a discussion addressing nonsurgical interventions that act directly to reverse the final manifestation of the pathophysiologic sequence of obstructive sleep apnea, namely, upper airway occlusion.

REDUCTION OF RISK FACTORS

Obesity

While obesity is not a prerequisite for the development of obstructive sleep apnea (9), the experience of the author and others (10) suggests that there is a high prevalence of obesity in this patient population. A direct contribution of obesity to the pathogenesis of obstructive sleep apnea is supported by the improvement in sleep-disordered breathing and daytime alertness following either medical or surgical weight reduction (10–13). Although Guilleminault et al. (14) found no consistent benefit from weight loss, Smith et al. (11) observed that mild-to-moderate weight loss resulted in a significant reduction in apnea frequency and improved nocturnal oxygenation.

The mechanism(s) responsible for the relationship between obesity and obstructive sleep apnea have yet to be well defined. There are no data supporting the contention that the pharyngeal lumen is compromised by the infiltration of adipose tissue within the pharyngeal walls. Other data, however, suggest that pharyngeal cross-sectional area during wakefulness varies directly with lung volume, possibly via reflex mediation (15). Thus, increases in lung volume coincident with weight loss may impact favorably on the size of the pharyngeal lumen. The consequent reduction in pharyngeal resistance minimizes the generation of negative intra-luminal pressure and thereby mitigates the tendency towards airway collapse (16). Additionally, increases in lung volume with weight loss are associated with improved oxygenation (17,18); this, in turn, may reduce the frequency of apnea (see below). Although the concept of lung volume dependency on pharyngeal cross-sectional area is an attractive and sophisticated one, more recent information has suggested that this mechanism does not contribute to clinically significant changes in upper airway resistance (19–21). More recently, animal data have suggested that mass loading of the anterior cervical region augments upper airway resistance and therefore may mediate the relationship between obesity and sleep apnea (22,23). In addition, circumstantial data in humans have also indicated that there is a relationship between neck circumference and sleep apnea (24).

It is thus apparent that OSA and nocturnal hemoglobin oxygen desaturation in obese patients may be improved by weight reduction. Unfortunately, satisfactory dietary reduction is achieved in only a minority of patients, and recidivism is high in those who do lose weight. Best results are obtained by applying a team approach. The physician, dietician, and, perhaps of greatest importance, a support group of peers must all work in a cohesive fashion, motivating the patient to make the appropriate psychological and life-style adjustments that will permit satisfactory, long-lasting weight control.

Manipulation of Sleep Position

The earliest therapy for snoring and sleep apnea may arguably be an elbow in the ribs in order to induce a bed partner to assume a lateral recumbent position. Patients and bed partners commonly describe greater snoring and more frequent apneas during sleep in the supine position. Such anecdotal evidence is supported by the recent report by Cartwright (25), who documented a higher frequency of sleep-disordered breathing events during sleep in the supine position than during sleep in the lateral recumbent position. It was postulated that the supine position facilitated gravity-associated relapse of the tongue against the posterior pharyngeal wall. Interestingly, with increasing weight, sleep-disordered breathing was less influenced by body position such that the more obese patients tended to obstruct their upper airway with comparable frequency regardless of sleep position. Nonetheless, the possibility of position dependence of sleep-disordered breathing should be investigated during the medical interview with the patient and bed partner, as well as during the polysomnographic evaluation. Should supine position dependence be documented, efforts can be made to promote the maintenance of sleep in the lateral recumbent position. One method to accomplish this is employment of a "sleep ball" or "sleep sock." These techniques involve creating a pocket in the back of the patient's sleeping garment and placing a tennis ball within this pocket or safety pinning a sock containing a tennis ball to the back of the garment. Thus, should the patient roll onto his or her back during sleep, he or she will be promptly stimulated to resume sleeping on his or her side. In selected patients, management of the sleep position may provide an effective and noninvasive therapy for sleep-disordered breathing. Alternatively, in some patients it may permit satisfactory positive pressure therapy at lower pressures (see below).

Alcohol

The anecdotes of bed partners who describe increased snoring and increased apnea frequency following alcohol ingestion have been corroborated by recent scientific data indicating the provocative role of alcohol in sleep-disordered breathing. Taasan et al. (26) observed that 2 ml/kg body weight of 100-proof vodka increased the frequency of sleep-disordered breathing events (apneas and hypopneas) as well as the frequency of hemoglobin oxygen desaturation in asymptomatic, middle-aged men. In another study, Scrima et al. (27) found that alcohol did not precipitate significant sleep-disordered breathing in normal, young, nonobese patients but increased the frequency of hypoxic events in patients with preexisting, mild sleep-disordered breathing. Issa and Sullivan (28) and Guilleminault and Rosekind (29) also observed an increase in obstructive apnea frequency and duration, as well as a lower nadir of hemoglobin oxygen saturation during sleep after alcohol ingestion in patients with known OSA. These authors also noted that alcohol evoked obstructive apnea in heavy snorers who did not otherwise manifest apnea.

Animal studies suggest that alcohol precipitates and/or aggravates sleep-disordered breathing by depressing hypoglossal nerve activity. Phrenic nerve activity is unaffected, however (30). Phrenic nerve activity is ultimately translated into the generation of negative intrapharyngeal pressure via diaphragm contraction while the hypoglossal nerve innervates the upper airway dilator muscles stabilizing the pharynx against collapse in response to this pressure. Alcohol ingestion thus fosters upper airway closure by creating an imbalance between the forces which promote and those which resist pharyngeal collapse. Further evidence supporting this mechanism for alcohol-induced sleep-disordered breathing is provided by the work of Krol et al. (31) and of Issa and Sullivan (32). The former authors observed a decrease in genioglossus muscle activity after alcohol ingestion in normal individuals. The latter authors reported increased upper airway collapsibility during sleep following alcohol ingestion in nonsnorers and snorers. The recognition that apneas are longer and hemoglobin oxygen desaturation more severe following alcohol ingestion suggests that this agent depresses the arousal response to hypoxic and hypercapnic stimuli (33).

The combination of alcohol-induced augmentation of sleep-disordered breathing events and alcohol-induced depression of the arousal response to hypoxia provides a particularly undesirable set of circumstances. Accordingly, patients who are known to have sleep-disordered breathing and those who have a predisposition towards sleep-disordered breathing (heavy snorers and obese individuals, for example) should be encouraged to abstain from alcohol consumption.

Other Drugs as Risk Factors

Certain drugs may precipitate breathing abnormalities during sleep in individuals who do not otherwise have sleep-disordered breathing. These drugs can also exacerbate preexisting sleep-disordered breathing. One such agent is the benzodiazepine hypnotic, flurazepam. Data suggest that the administration of flurazepam may be associated with an abnormal frequency of obstructive and "central" apneas in otherwise normal or nearly normal subjects (34,35). It has further been suggested that the "hangover" effect on the day following the bedtime administration of flurazepam may, at least in part, be secondary to drug-induced sleep-disordered breathing. Flurazepam depresses the arousal response to hypoxia and hypercapnia during sleep (36) and decreases the ventilatory responses to hypoxia and hypercapnia during wakefulness (37). These actions provide possible mechanisms for the deleterious effects of this agent on breathing during sleep.

Although not all benzodiazepines have undergone evaluation of their impact on breathing during sleep, it seems prudent to view this class of agents as potentially dangerous for sleep apnea patients. In this regard, triazolam, which is a newer benzodiazepine, has not been observed to elevate the frequency of obstructive apneas in patients with central sleep apnea (38). It does appear to depress the arousal threshold to airway occlusion in normal subjects, however (39). Such a property could prolong apnea and worsen nocturnal oxyhemoglobin desaturation in patients with sleep apnea.

It seems reasonable to avoid administering these and any other known ventilatory depressants to patients with sleep-disordered breathing. In this regard, it should be remembered that the administration of sedatives and analgesics with potential ventilatory depressant properties to patients with sleep-disordered breathing in the postoperative setting may carry an increased risk of untoward consequences.

Narcotics are well-known ventilatory depressants (40–42) in normal humans. Although orally administered narcotics do not appear to precipitate sleep apnea in normal individuals (43), it is reasonable to be cautious in administering these agents to patients with sleep apnea, especially those individuals in whom consistent upper airway patency cannot be monitored.

Hypothyroidism

Hypothyroidism and the sleep apnea syndrome share many features, including somnolence, lethargy, and obesity. This, as well as the observation that awake hypothyroid patients may have abnormal ventilatory drives (44), suggests an association between the two entities. Along these lines, Rajagopal et al. (45) reported a high prevalence of OSA in a population of hypothyroid patients. These authors and others (46) have observed significant reversal of OSA after thyroid replacement independent of changes in weight and pulmonary function. These data indicate that an assessment of thyroid function should be made during the evaluation of the patient with sleep-disordered breathing. In those individuals with both hypothyroidism and sleep-disordered breathing, thyroid replacement might ameliorate both problems. It merits attention, however, that institution of thyroid replacement therapy may be associated with the development of nocturnal angina pectoris, especially in patients who do not have immediate alleviation of sleep apnea but do have metabolic augmentation with treatment (47). It is therefore suggested that hypothyroid patients with sleep apnea either be carefully monitored during the institution of replacement therapy or, more optimally, receive specific treatment for sleep apnea (e.g., positive pressure therapy) to ensure upper airway patency pending reevaluation after achieving a euthyroid state.

THERAPEUTIC AGENTS WITH POSSIBLE
NEURALLY MEDIATED ACTIVITY

Protriptyline

The current literature suggests that some patients with OSA experience a reduction in overnight apnea time and improvement in nocturnal oxygenation with the administration of protriptyline which is a nonsedating, tricyclic antidepressant (48–51). Although Smith et al. (51) noted no change in the total number of sleep-disordered breathing events during non-rapid eye movement (non-REM) sleep after the administration of protriptyline, the pattern of disordered breathing was altered such that there were fewer apneas but more hypopneas. While protriptyline did not alter the pattern and frequency of sleep-disordered breathing events during REM sleep, the administration of this agent reduced the percentage of total sleep time spent in this sleep stage. Because REM-related sleep-disordered breathing events were of greater duration and associated with lower hemoglobin oxygen saturation than those during non-REM sleep, shortening of REM sleep time during protriptyline therapy reduced the number of the more severe sleep-disordered breathing events and resulted in improved overnight oxygenation. In four of five patients, Brownell et al. (48) confirmed the overnight reduction in apnea time during protriptyline therapy and found it explicable primarily by drug-related reduction of time spent in REM sleep. While at least a large part of the beneficial effects of protriptyline are related to its suppressant effect on REM sleep, recent data suggest an additional, neurally mediated mechanism. In nonanesthetized, decerebrate cats, Bonora et al. (52) observed that protriptyline increased the output of the hypoglossal and recurrent laryngeal nerves without notable impact on phrenic nerve output. This activity was not mediated by the carotid chemoreceptors. The authors postulated that this effect of protriptyline resulted from an influence on the reticular activating system. Augmented neural output to the upper airway dilator muscles with greater pharyngeal stability may explain the shift in the pattern of sleep-disordered breathing from obstructive apnea to hypopnea during protriptyline administration (51). Of clinical importance, however, the response to protriptyline is usually inadequate in patients with moderate and severe obstructive apnea. These individuals continue to have substantially abnormal breathing and oxyhemoglobin desaturation during sleep despite protriptyline therapy. In this regard, it is of interest that while taking protriptyline, sleep apnea patients report an increase in daytime alertness that is not correlated with improved nocturnal oxygenation, decreased arousal frequency, or change in the rate of sleep-disordered breathing events (48,49,51). It has therefore been suggested that protriptyline has an "alerting" effect (48,49) independent of its effect on breathing during sleep.

Unfortunately, largely due to its anticholinergic properties, protriptyline is not without its side effects. These include varying degrees of urinary hesitancy, dry mouth, and constipation. Other side effects have included impotence, decreased libido, rash, confusion, ataxia, and hair loss (48–51). There is also potential for increased cardiac dysrhythmias in patients on protriptyline therapy. These side effects, particularly in the predominantly middle-aged to elderly male, sleep-disordered breathing population, place a severe limitation on the usefulness of this agent.

In summary, protriptyline may be effective in some patients with mild-to-moderate sleep apnea. Subjective improvement cannot be used as a reflection of improved breathing during sleep, however, and polysomnographic documentation of therapeutic benefit is necessary. Available data suggest that protriptyline is ineffective in the treatment of "central" sleep apnea (50).

A recent study compared the impact of protriptyline and fluoxetine on sleep apnea (53). It was noted that both agents reduced the amount of time spent in REM sleep. Although there was a comparable and statistically significant reduction of the apnea plus hypopnea frequency with both drugs, only 2 of the 12 patients who had a pretreatment apnea plus hypopnea frequency greater than 20 per hour of sleep experienced a reduction in this frequency to less than 10 events per hour of sleep on either drug. In addition, there was no significant reduction in the frequency of oxyhemoglobin saturation events or arousals on either agent. Thus, like protriptyline, fluoxetine probably has limited utility in the therapeutic armamentarium for sleep apnea.

Progestational Agents

On the basis of its ventilatory stimulant properties, medroxyprogesterone acetate (MPA) has been employed in the therapy of sleep-disordered breathing (54,55). In several studies, each involving small numbers of patients however, there were no significant group differences in frequency of obstructive apnea or apnea time (56–58) during sleep off and on MPA therapy. Nonetheless, certain individual patients did experience a reduction in sleep-disordered breathing during MPA therapy. Examination of the data suggests that those individuals with the greatest arterial carbon dioxide tensions and lowest arterial oxygen tensions while awake tended to have the greatest response to MPA (57,58). Skatrud et al. (46) reported amelioration of OSA in a hypothyroid patient after treatment with MPA. This report, however, is complicated by the fact that the patient was also on androgen therapy. Several years ago, Rajagopal et al. (59) examined the effect of MPA therapy in 13 nonhypercapnic OSA patients. These authors found that MPA therapy did not have a beneficial impact on OSA or nocturnal oxygenation, although hypercapnic ventilatory drive during wakefulness was augmented. Along similar lines, Kimura et al. (60) observed a statistically, but doubtfully clinically significant, reduction in sleep-disordered breathing following administration of another progestational agent, chlormadinone acetate. In nine OSA patients the apnea-plus-hypopnea index fell from 51.1 ± 5.7 to 43.6 ± 8.1 episodes per hour of sleep. In only one patient was the apnea-plus-hypopnea index reduced to below 20 episodes per hour of sleep, and there was no impact on apnea–hypopnea duration during non-REM and REM sleep. A recent investigation by Cook et al. (61) failed to demonstrate improvement in the disordered breathing event frequency, duration of disordered breathing events, or mean fall in oxyhemoglobin saturation in patients with sleep apnea after 1 week of treatment with 150 mg/day of medroxyprogesterone acetate.

In summary, MPA is not uniformly successful in the treatment of OSA. Although it is possible that progestational therapy may benefit the subpopulation of sleep apnea patients who are hypercapnic while awake at rest, there is recent evidence suggesting that the premise underlying the rationale for progestational therapy may be flawed. It has been reasoned that because sleep apnea is more prevalent in men and perhaps in postmenopausal women, relative androgen excess directly contributes to the pathogenesis of the disorder. Stewart et al. (62), however, recently observed that short-term androgen blockade with flutamide failed to improve breathing during sleep in men with sleep apnea. While it is possible that a longer duration of androgen blockade might have had a different impact, these and the other studies cited above significantly reduce confidence in the therapeutic utility of progestational agents in the treatment of OSA.

The administration of MPA may be of benefit in treating patients with "central" sleep apnea and primary alveolar hypoventilation (63,64). There are no published systemic evaluations of this agent or others in its class in these patient populations, however.

Tryptophan

Animal studies have suggested that serotoninergic systems can influence ventilation (65,66). L-Tryptophan is a serotonin precursor which has previously been employed in the treatment of sleep apnea (67). The limited available data suggest that administration of this agent results in little, if any, clinically significant improvement in sleep apnea. More importantly, however, L-tryptophan has been implicated as the etiology of the serious and potentially life-threatening eosinophilic–myalgia syndrome, and its administration is to be avoided (68–70).

Supplemental Oxygen

While the precise role of supplemental oxygen in the treatment of sleep-disordered breathing remains to be determined, data collected in the last decade suggest that this therapy may provide certain benefits in selected patients (71,72). In nonhypercapnic individuals with sleep apnea, Martin et al. (72) observed initial prolongation of apnea duration following supplemental oxygen delivery, although the mean duration of events shortened over the ensuing therapeutic period. In addition, there was a reduction in the number of apneas during oxygen administration. The net result was a significant reduction in the percent apnea time during oxygen therapy. In addition, oxyhemoglobin saturation during sleep was improved during oxygen administration, and apnea-related changes in heart rate were minimized. These results were substantiated in a subsequent study by Smith et al. (71). Martin et al. (72) also demonstrated that those sleep apnea patients who experienced a reduction in the percent apnea time during a 30-minute trial of oxygen therapy sustained this improvement during chronic nocturnal therapy. The mechanism(s) by which supplemental oxygen administration improves breathing during sleep remains to be defined, although several hypotheses have been proposed (72): (a) Maintenance of normal or supernormal hemoglobin oxygen saturation may prevent hypoxia-induced ventilatory depression; (b) sustained hyperoxia may augment ventilation by reducing cerebral blood flow, thus increasing cerebral carbon dioxide tension; (c) the administration of supplemental oxygen during sleep may prevent CNS dysfunction arising as a result of apnea-related hypoxia. Such CNS dysfunction could amplify the severity of sleep-disordered breathing, thereby creating a vicious cycle. The administration of supplemental oxygen may interrupt this cycle and reduce the severity of sleep-disordered breathing. This hypothesis is supported by the observation that oxygen therapy did not benefit a sleep apnea patient who maintained hemoglobin oxygen saturation above 90% during sleep without supplemental oxygen (72); and (d) A final possible mechanism is that oxygen therapy in some fashion stabilizes the ventilatory control system. Indeed, several authors have speculated that excessive oscillation of the ventilatory control system leads to exaggerated periodicity of breathing and sleep apnea (73,74). The observation that supplemental oxygen administration eliminates hypoxemia-related periodic breathing at high altitude (75) supports the hypothesis that oxygen ameliorates sleep-disordered breathing by virtue of a stabilizing effect on the neural mechanisms controlling ventilation.

Despite these favorable studies, patients with sleep-disordered breathing should *not* be indiscriminately sent home on oxygen therapy. Several studies have indicated that certain patients may experience worsening of apnea with consequent hypercapnia and acidosis during the administration of oxygen during sleep (76). Given these considerations, it is prudent to evaluate the effects of oxygen administration by polysomnography and document a beneficial effect before sending an individual with sleep-disordered breathing home on it. Finally, it is unlikely that oxygen therapy alone will sufficiently ameliorate the frequency of sleep-disordered breathing events and improve sleep continuity to provide adequate treatment for the typical sleep apnea patient. Its use as a single therapeutic intervention remains to be defined but perhaps should be reserved for those patients who are truly asymptomatic and in whom other, more comprehensive therapies for sleep apnea (those that maintain continuous upper airway patency during sleep and therefore favorably impact on both oxygenation and sleep quality) are not viable but in whom it is desirable to at least avoid oxyhemoglobin desaturation.

DEVICES WHICH ACT DIRECTLY TO MAINTAIN UPPER AIRWAY PATENCY

Nasopharyngeal Airway

Afzelius et al. (77) and more recently Nahmias and Karetzky (78) have reported the successful use of a nasopharyngeal airway during sleep to maintain upper airway patency in OSA patients. The rubber nasopharyngeal tube was fluoroscopically documented to extend below the base of the tongue, or its position was alternatively confirmed by fiberoptic visualization. In the study of Nahmias and Karetzky, 11 of 24 patients either were intolerant of the nasopharyngeal tube or had unsuccessful tube placement. Although there was a significant reduction in the frequency of disordered breathing events with the nasopharyngeal tube in place, there was only a marginal improvement in sleep architecture. The effect of this treatment on sleep fragmentation was not reported. In our laboratory, this modality has not been successful due to the inability of most patients to tolerate insertion of the airway for prolonged periods each night. This complaint persisted even when alternating nostrils. In other patients, sleep-related upper airway occlusion was not relieved until the nasopharyngeal airway was passed down to a level which evoked gagging. A similar experience has also been reported by Martin (79).

Oral Appliances

In 1982, a pilot study was published describing an investigational device, the tongue-retaining device (TRD), in the treatment of sleep apnea (80). The rationale for using the TRD is that pharyngeal patency is increased by pulling the superior aspect of the tongue forward, away from the posterior wall of the pharynx. This is accomplished by maintaining protrusive traction on the tongue with a negative pressure within the lingual portion of the device. During a half-night TRD trial, Cartwright et al. (80) observed a substantial reduction in apnea frequency in 8 of 12 patients with moderate-to-severe sleep apnea. Despite the reduction in apnea frequency, two of these eight individuals continued to have substantial degrees of apnea. Of 10 patients who underwent two additional half-night sleep studies with the TRD after having the device at home for 4–6 months, clinical relief of apnea (apnea frequency less than 7 per hour of sleep) was observed in 6 and 5 individuals on each study, respectively. This suggests that the TRD will ameliorate sleep apnea in 50–60% of patients.

In the investigation by Cartwright and Samelson (80), compliance with TRD was assessed by questionnaire at 6-month intervals. Preliminary data indicated that 61% of patients use the TRD "regularly." Unfortunately, the term "regularly" was not defined. The authors speculated that the TRD may be employed to provide immediate relief of sleep apnea symptoms, thereby facilitating and "buying time" for meaningful weight reduction. Accordingly, in a subsequent study, Cartwright et al. (81) observed that the TRD was more efficacious in patients who were less than 150% of ideal body weight and in those who experienced an ameliorative impact of sleeping in the lateral recumbent position.

In recent years there has been progressively greater interest in the therapeutic application of oral devices in sleep apnea patients. A detailed description of the wide variety of these devices is beyond the scope of this review, especially in view of the paucity of large controlled trials. However, the existing literature suggests that this type of intervention may have a beneficial impact in selected patients. Schmidt-Nowara et al. (82) recently observed that application of a mandibular repositioning appliance, adjusted such that there was incisor-to-incisor apposition, had a beneficial effect in patients with less severe elevation of sleep-disordered breathing event frequency. In addition, patients with snoring reported improvement in this regard as well. In a smaller study, Bonham et al. (83) found similar qualified success. While the initial studies appear to offer limited promise, more work is required to define the optimal type of dental orthosis, the patient population(s) most likely to benefit, the long-term compliance, and the potential adverse effects (i.e., temporomandibular joint degeneration, risk of aspiration, and dental occlusion problems) before this therapy becomes a routine part of our therapeutic armamentarium.

Electrical Stimulation of the Upper Airway

Although electrical stimulation has not as yet been proven to be an effective treatment of patients with OSA, it is worth mentioning as a reflection of the innovative efforts that are currently ongoing to develop better therapies for this disorder. Miki et al. (84) demonstrated that it is possible to reduce airway resistance in anesthetized dogs by electrical stimulation of the genioglossus muscle. Subsequently, these investigators observed that application of submental electrical stimulation of the genioglossus muscle using surface electrodes and electrical pulses of 0.5 msec (repetition rate, 50 Hz) at 15–40 volts reduced apnea frequency, percentage of apnea time, frequency of oxyhemoglobin desaturation, and apnea duration in a group of six sleep apnea patients compared with values obtained during a control night without stimulation. Because the electroencephalogram was not recorded during submental stimulation (due to electrical interference), the possibility exits that apnea frequency and duration as well as frequency of desaturations were reduced on the basis of submental stimulation-induced arousal of the patients rather than by the direct dilating effect of upper airway stimulation. Indeed, enthusiasm for this form of therapy was dampened by a recent report indicating that transcutaneous electrical stimulation failed to augment upper airway size as evidenced on fast computerized tomographic scanning of awake patients with OSA and that it did not improve sleep-disordered breathing in these patients during sleep, independent of the arousal effect of the stimulation (85). Although these data are disappointing, there are many variables that must be considered in approaching electrical stimulation of the upper airway, including stimulating the most relevant muscles, the timing of the stimulus, stimulus intensity, and the method by which the stimulating electrodes are placed. All of these factors may influence the impact of this intervention on sleep and sleep continuity as well as the effectiveness in maintaining satisfactory upper airway patency during sleep. Thus, clinicians can probably look forward to further developments and more studies addressing this potential therapeutic approach.

Positive Airway Pressure by Mask

Nasal continuous positive airway pressure (CPAP) has been increasingly recognized as an important therapeutic modality for sleep apnea. Sullivan et al. (86) initially described the relief of OSA by the administration of air under 4.5–10 cm H_2O pressure via nasal prongs sealed within the nares. Shortly thereafter, Sanders (87) and Rapoport et al. (88) described the use of a self-sealing nasal mask through

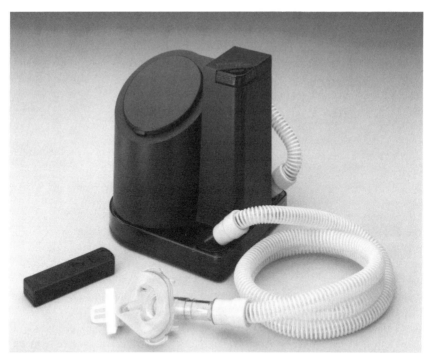

FIG. 1. Nasal continuous positive airway pressure (CPAP) apparatus with self-sealting nasal mask: one example of several designs.

which air under pressure was delivered (see Fig. 1). The application of CPAP via nasal mask has been shown by Sanders (89) to provide significant amelioration of mixed as well as occlusive apnea with improvement in nocturnal oxygenation. Interestingly, in that study nasal CPAP was found to be effective in eliminating both the "central" and obstructive portions of mixed apnea and tended to be effective in reducing central apneas. Subsequently, Issa and Sullivan (90) confirmed the effectiveness of nasal CPAP in reversing central apneas that occur in patients with primarily OSA. Other authors (88,91) have shown that patients who have cor pulmonale associated with occlusive sleep apnea and awake hypoxemia and hypercapnia experience improved cardiac function and awake arterial blood gases, as well as increased daytime alertness after a short period of nocturnal nasal CPAP therapy (92). It should be noted however, that it may be several weeks following initiation of CPAP therapy until maximal reversal of daytime sleepiness is achieved (93). The clinical implication of this observation is that patients who lack sufficient alertness for safe operation of machinery and motor vehicles or who engage in work that requires vigilance for safety and effectiveness should not return to full activities for a period of time after beginning CPAP therapy.

Nasal CPAP is generally, but not universally, well-tolerated by sleep apnea patients. Sanders (89) found that 81% of the patients in whom nasal CPAP ameliorated sleep apnea during a one-night trial wanted to use the device chronically at home. Several investigators using patient-reported data have documented good compliance with home nasal CPAP by sleep apnea patients (94–99). At present, the minimal degree and duration of nocturnal hemoglobin oxygen unsaturation which results in significant physiologic derangements is not known (100). Sanders et al. (94) therefore revaluated patient compliance with nasal CPAP in terms of both (a) the fraction of nightly sleep time during which the device was worn and (b) the frequency of nightly use (94). Nightly use of nasal CPAP for all but 1 hour of sleep time constituted the minimal requirements for good compliance. Given this defini-tion, 75% of long-term nasal CPAP users (10.3 ± 8 months, mean $\pm$ SD) were com-pliant with therapy. The potential inaccuracy of assessing patient compliance using patient-reported data is obvious. Recently, studies have been conducted which em-ployed timers on the CPAP units to measure the machine run time which ostensibly reflects the duration of patient use. With such a device, Fletcher and Luckett (101) determined that patients used nasal CPAP an average of 6.1 hours per night over 6 months. Similar results were recently presented in a preliminary report from a mul-ticenter European trial (102). Thus, in aggregate, the literature suggests that the long-term compliance of patients with nasal CPAP ranges from 55% to 85%.

In general, the problems associated with nasal CPAP therapy have not been se-vere. They include rhinitis, morning nasal congestion, conjunctivitis, dry mouth and nose, discomfort from the nasal mask, and chest wall discomfort (94,98,99, 103,104). The latter is presumably due to nasal CPAP-related increases in lung volume. The other problems can usually be mitigated by maintaining the cleanliness of the mask and tubing, placing a vaporizer in front of the nasal CPAP blower intake, and appropriately placing cotton padding on the nasal mask, respectively. Improvement in nasal mask design has also had a favorable impact on this problem. Although nasal CPAP system pressures up to 15 cm H_2O are commonly employed, the author is not aware of any published reports of pneumothorax attributable to this modality. Nonetheless, this potential complication and the risk–benefit ratio must be kept in mind when considering the use of nasal CPAP in any patient.

It is noteworthy that the relationship between these side effects and long-term therapeutic compliance is not clear. Several studies have indicated either that the prevalence of side effects is no different in compliant and noncompliant individuals or that there is no linear relation between compliance, symptoms, and side effects of therapy (101,104). It may be inappropriate, however, to examine the relationship between compliance and side effects of therapy by comparing the prevalence of the latter in the compliant and noncompliant patients. The more relevant issue is the individual patient's perception of a given side effect, rather than simply the pres-ence of the side effect with respect to the potential impact on compliance. In addi-tion, some investigators observed greater compliance in patients with more severe excessive daytime sleepiness prior to the institution of therapy (98,103), and pa-tients who complained of more side effects had worse compliance (98,99). Thus, while it appears that the exact determinants of compliance are unclear, it is prudent to make every attempt to minimize side effects of therapy.

The primary mechanism by which nasal CPAP maintains upper airway patency is by providing a pneumatic splint for the upper airway with only minimal contribution from any increased lung volume associated with its application (19,20). Earlier work has shown that in some sleep apnea patients, genioglossus muscle electromyogram activity decreases during application of nasal CPAP (105,106), supporting a non-reflex-mediated mechanism of action. Regardless of the mechanism, the most clinically relevant fact is that nasal CPAP is an effective, well-tolerated, nonsurgical therapy for obstructive and mixed apnea.

Recently, a new modality became available for delivering positive airway pressure in the treatment of sleep apnea, namely, bilevel positive airway pressure (see Fig. 2). This device allows independent adjustment of the positive pressure delivered during inspiration [inspiratory positive airway pressure (IPAP)] and expiration [expiratory positive airway pressure (EPAP)] (107), permitting specific titration of the pressures required to keep the upper airway patent during inspiration and expiration. By definition, delivered pressures are the same during both phases of the

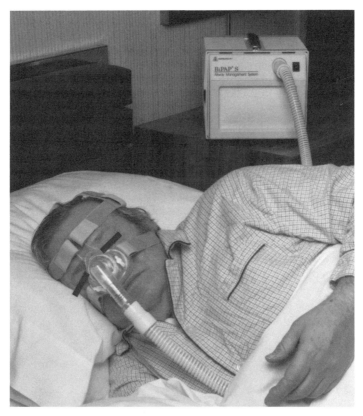

FIG. 2. Apnea patient asleep with assisted breathing from bilevel positive airway pressure (BiPAP®) delivered by nasal mask.

breathing cycle during CPAP administration; the pressure during expiration must equal that during inspiration. The use of bilevel positive airway pressure for sleep apnea is based on the reasoning that it requires less pressure to maintain upper airway patency during expiration, when airway collapse was related to the inherent instability of the airway, than during inspiration, when collapse is related to inherent airway instability and the collapsing influence of negative intrapharyngeal pressure (108,109). Furthermore, it was postulated that expiratory upper airway occlusion was an important, if not integral, element of the pathogenesis of sleep apnea (107). This hypothesis was tested and found to be clinically valid in that it has been demonstrated that sleep apnea patients can be effectively treated with expiratory pressures that are lower than those delivered during inspiration (107,110). Thus, when using bilevel positive airway pressure, patients are not required to have the expiratory pressure as high as the inspiratory pressure. The expiratory pressure need only be as high as required to maintain upper airway patency. This tends to mitigate side effects related to pressure delivery especially during expiration, including chest discomfort, smothering due to the need to exhale against high pressure, and sinus discomfort. The greater comfort with bilevel positive airway pressure may lead to patient acceptance of positive pressure therapy when CPAP is intolerable. In addition, establishing a pressure differential between inspiration and expiration provides an inspiratory pressure support that can assist or augment the patient's ventilation. This can be particularly advantageous in those individuals with complex, mixed sleep apnea hypoventilation syndromes.

SUMMARY

In summary, the multiplicity of nonsurgical therapies currently used to treat sleep apnea reflects the uncertainty regarding the pathophysiology of this disorder. The diversity of risk factors and the observation that, with the exception of those modalities that directly reverse the upper airway obstruction, no single therapy works for all patients suggests heterogeneity of the pathogenesis of this disorder. In the last several years, additional insights have been gained regarding the pathophysiology of sleep apnea. Furthermore, refinements and further innovations of existing modalities as well as the availability of new therapies provide patients and clinicians with medical options that were unavailable as of the first writing of this chapter.

ACKNOWLEDGMENT

This work was supported, in part, by the Veterans Administration.

REFERENCES

1. Weitzman ED, Kahn E, Pollak CP. Quantitative analysis of sleep and sleep apnea before and after tracheostomy in patients with the hypersomnia–sleep apnea syndrome. *Sleep* 1980;3:407–423.
2. Lugaresi E, Coccagna G, Mantovani M, Brignani F. Effects of tracheostomy in two cases of hypersomnia with periodic breathing. *J Neurol Neurosurg Psychiatry* 1973;36:15–26.

3. Guilleminault C, Cummiskey J. Progressive improvement of apnea index and ventilatory response to CO_2 after tracheostomy in obstructive sleep apnea syndrome. *Am Rev Respir Dis* 1982;126:14–20.
4. Buckwalter JA, Sasaki CT. Effect of tracheotomy on laryngeal function. *Otolaryngol Clin North Am* 1984;17:41–48.
5. Conway WA, Victor LD, Magilligan DJ Jr, Fujita S, Zorick FJ, Roth T. Adverse effects of tracheostomy for sleep apnea. *JAMA* 1981;246:347–350.
6. Kenan PD. Complications associated with tracheostomy: prevention and treatment. *Otolaryngol Clin NA* 1979;12:807–816.
7. Simmons FB, Guilleminault C, Miles LE. The palatopharyngoplasty operation for snoring and sleep apnea: an interim report. *Otolaryngol Head Neck Surg* 1984;92:375–380.
8. Fujita S, Conway WA, Sticklesteel JM, et al. Evaluation of the effectiveness of uvulopalatopharyngoplasty. *Laryngoscope* 1985;95:70–74.
9. Guilleminault C, Van den Hoed J, Mitler MM. Clinical overview of sleep apnea syndromes. In: Guilleminault CDW, ed. *Sleep apnea syndromes*, vol II. New York: Alan R Liss, 1978;1–12.
10. Peiser J, Lavie P, Ovnat A, Charuzi I. Sleep apnea syndrome in the morbidly obese. *Ann Surg* 1984;199:112–115.
11. Smith PL, Gold AR, Meyers DA, Haponik EF, Bleecker ER. Weight loss in mildly to moderately obese patients with obstructive sleep apnea. *Ann Intern Med* 1985;103:850–855.
12. Browman CP, Sampson MG, Yolles SF, et al. Obstructive sleep apnea and body weight. *Chest* 1984;85:435–436.
13. Harman EM, Wynne JW, Block AJ. The effect of weight loss on sleep-disordered breathing and oxygen desaturation in morbidly obese men. *Chest* 1982;82:291–294.
14. Guilleminault C, Eldridge FL, Tilkian A, Simmons FB, Dement WC. Sleep apnea due to upper airway obstruction. *Arch Intern Med* 1977;137:296–300.
15. Hoffstein V, Zamel N, Phillipson EA. Lung volume dependence of pharyngeal cross-sectional area in patients with obstructive sleep apnea. *Am Rev Respir Dis* 1984;130:175–178.
16. Remmers JE, De Groot WJ, Sauerland EK, Anch AM. Pathogenesis of upper airway occlusion during sleep. *J Appl Physiol* 1978;44:931–938.
17. Suratt PM, McTier RF, Findley LJ, Pohl SL, Wilhoit SC. Changes in breathing and the pharynx after weight loss in obstructive sleep apnea. *Chest* 1987;92:631–637.
18. Findley LJ, Ries AL, Tisi GM, Wagner PD. Hypoxemia during apnea in normal subjects: mechanisms and impact of lung volume. *J Appl Physiol* 1983;55:1777–1783.
19. Series F, Cormier Y, Desmueles M. Influence of passive changes of lung volume on the upper airways. *J Appl Physiol* 1990;68:2159–2164.
20. Series F, Cormier Y, Couture J, Desmueles M. Changes in upper airway resistance with lung inflation and positive pressure. *J Appl Physiol* 1990;68:1075–1079.
21. Abbey NC, Cooper KR, Kwentus JA. Benefit of nasal CPAP in obstructive sleep apnea is due to positive pharyngeal pressure. *Sleep* 1989;12:420–422.
22. Wolin AD, Strohl KP, Acree BN, Fouke JM. Responses to negative pressure surrounding the neck in anesthetized animals. *J Appl Physiol* 1990;68:154–160.
23. Koenig JS, Thach BT. Effects of mass loading on the upper airway. *J Appl Physiol* 1988;64:2294–2299.
24. Katz I, Stradling J, Slutsky AS, Zamel N, Hoffstein V. Do patients with obstructive sleep apnea have thick necks? *Am Rev Respir Dis* 1990;141:1228–1231.
25. Cartwright RD. Effect of position on sleep apnea therapy. *Sleep* 1984;7:110–114.
26. Taasan VC, Block AJ, Boysen PG, Wynne JW. Alcohol increases sleep apnea and oxygen desaturation in asymptomatic men. *Am J Med* 1981;71:240–245.
27. Scrima L, Broudy M, Nay KN, Cohn MA. Increased severity of obstructive sleep apnea after bedtime alcohol ingestion: diagnostic potential and mechanism of action. *Sleep* 1982;15:318–328.
28. Issa FG, Sullivan CE. Alcohol, snoring and sleep apnea. *J Neurol Neurosurg Psychiatry* 1982;45:353–359.
29. Guilleminault C, Rosekind M. The arousal threshold: sleep deprivation, sleep fragmentation, and obstructive sleep apnea syndrome. *Bull Eur Physiopathol Respir* 1981;17:341–349.
30. Bonora M, Shields GI, Knuth SL, Bartlett D Jr, St. John WM. Selective depression by ethanol of upper airway respiratory motor activity in cats. *Am Rev Respir Dis* 1984;130:156–161.
31. Krol RC, Knuth SL, Bartlett D Jr. Selective reduction of genioglossal activity by alcohol in normal human subjects. *Am Rev Respir Dis* 1984;129:247–250.

32. Issa FG, Sullivan CE. Upper airway closing pressures in snorers. *J Appl Physiol* 1984;57:528–535.
33. Remmers JE. Obstructive sleep apnea. A common disorder exacerbated by alcohol. *Am Rev Respir Dis* 1984;130:153–155.
34. Dolly FR, Block AJ. Effect of flurazepam on sleep-disordered breathing and nocturnal oxygen desaturation in asymptomatic subjects. *Am J Med* 1982;73:239–243.
35. Mendelson WB, Garnett D, Gillin JC. Flurazepam-induced sleep apnea syndrome in a patient with insomnia and mild sleep-related respiratory changes. *J Nerv Mental Dis* 1981;169:261–264.
36. Hedemark LL, Kronenberg RS. Flurazepam attenuates the arousal response to sleep in normal subjects. *Am Rev Respir Dis* 1983;128:980–983.
37. Hedemark L, Kronenberg R. Ventilatory responses to hypoxia and CO_2 during natural and flurazepam-induced sleep in normal adults. *Chest* 1981;80:366.
38. Berry RB, McCasland CR, Light RW. The effect of triazolam on the arousal response to airway occlusion during sleep in normal subjects. *Am Rev Respir Dis* 1992;146:1256–1260.
39. Bonnet MH, Dexter JR, Arand DL. The effect of triazolam on arousal and respiration in central sleep apnea patients. *Sleep* 1990;13:31–41.
40. Kryger MH, Yacoub O, Dosman J, Macklem PT, Anthonisen NR. Effect of meperidine on occlusion pressure responses to hypercapnia and hypoxia with and without external inspiratory resistance. *Am Rev Respir Dis* 1976;114:333–340.
41. Santiago TV, Pugliese AC, Edelman NH. Control of breathing during methadone addiction. *Am J Med* 1977; 1977:347–354.
42. Weil JV, McCullough RE, Kline JS, Sodal IE. Diminished ventilatory response to hypoxia and hypercapnia after morphine in normal man. *N Engl J Med* 1975;292:1103–1106.
43. Robinson RW, Zwillich CW, Bixler EO, Cadieux RJ, Kales A, White DP. Effects of oral narcotics on sleep-disordered breathing in healthy adults. *Chest* 1987;91:197–203.
44. Zwillich CW, Pierson DJ, Hofeldt FD, Lufkin EG, Weil JV. Ventilatory control in myxedema and hypothyroidism. *N Engl J Med* 1975;292:662–665.
45. Rajagopal KR, Abbrecht PH, Derderian SS, et al. Obstructive sleep apnea and hypothyroidism. *Ann Intern Med* 1984;101:491–494.
46. Skatrud JB, Iber C, Ewart R, Thomas G, Rasmussen E, Schultze B. Disordered breathing during sleep in hypothyroidism. *Am Rev Respir Dis* 1981;124:325–329.
47. Grunstein RR, Sullivan CE. Sleep apnea and hypothyroidism: mechanisms and management. *Am J Med* 1988;85:775–779.
48. Brownell LG, Perez-Padilla R, West P, Kryger MH. The role of protriptyline in obstructive sleep apnea. *Bull Eur Physiopathol Respir* 1983;19:621–624.
49. Brownell LG, West P, Sweatman P, Acres JC, Kryger MH. Protriptyline in sleep-disordered breathing. *N Eng J Med* 1982;307:1037–1042.
50. Conway WA, Zorick F, Piccione P, Roth T. Protriptyline in the treatment of sleep apnoea. *Thorax* 1982;37:49–53.
51. Smith PL, Haponik EF, Allen RP, Bleecker ER. The effects of protriptyline in sleep-disordered breathing. *Am Rev Respir Dis* 1983;127:8–13.
52. Bonora M, St. John WM, Bledsoe TA. Differential elevation by protriptyline and depression by diazepam of upper airway respiratory motor activity. *Am Rev Respir Dis* 1985;131:41–45.
53. Hanzel DA, Proia NG, Hudgel DW. Response of obstructive sleep apnea to fluoxetine and protriptyline. *Chest* 1991;100:416–421.
54. Skatrud JB, Dempsey JA, Bhansali P, Irvin P. Determinants of carbon dioxide retention and its correction in humans. *J Clin Invest* 1980;65:813–821.
55. Skatrud JB, Dempsey JA, Kaiser DG. Ventilatory response to medroxyprogesterone acetate in normal subjects: time course and mechanisms. *J Appl Physiol* 1978;44:939–944.
56. Orr WC, Imes NK, Martin RJ. Progesterone therapy in obese patients with sleep apnea. *Arch Intern Med* 1979;139:109–111.
57. Hensley MJ, Saunders NA, Strohl KP. Medroxyprogesterone treatment of obstructive sleep apnea. *Sleep* 1980;3:441–446.
58. Strohl KP, Hensley MJ, Saunders NA, Scharf SM, Brown R, Ingram RH Jr. Progesterone administration and progressive sleep apneas. *JAMA* 1981;245:1230–1232.
59. Rajagopal KR, Abbrecht PH, Jabbari B. Effects of medroxyprogesterone acetate in obstructive sleep apnea. *Chest* 1986;90:815–821.
60. Kimura H, Tatsumi K, Kunitomo F, et al. Progesterone therapy for sleep apnea syndrome evaluated by occlusion pressure responses to exogenous loading. *Am Rev Respir Dis* 1989;139:1198–1206.

61. Cook WR, Benich J, Wooten SA. Indices of severity of obstructive sleep apnea syndrome do not change during medroxyprogesterone acetate therapy. *Chest* 1989;96:262–266.
62. Stewart DA, Grunstein RR, Berthon-Jones M, Handelsman DJ, Sullivan CE. Androgen blockade does not affect sleep-disordered breathing or chemosensitivity in men with obstructive sleep apnea. *Am Rev Respir Dis* 1992;146:1389–1393.
63. Skatrud JB, Dempsey JA. Relative effectiveness of acetazolamide versus medroxyprogesterone acetate in correction of carbon dioxide retention. *Am Rev Respir Dis* 1983;127:405–412.
64. Lyons HA, Huang CT. Therapeutic use of progesterone in alveolar hypoventilation. *Am J Med* 1968;44:881–888.
65. Quilligan EJ, Clewlow F, Johnston BM, Walker DW. Effect of 5-hydroxytryptophan on electrocortical activity and breathing movements of fetal sleep. *Am J Obstet Gynecol* 1981;141:271–275.
66. Lundberg DBA, Mueller RA, Breeses GT. An evaluation of the mechanism by which serotonergic activation depresses respiration. *J Pharmacol Exp Ther* 1980;212:397–404.
67. Schmidt HS. L-Tryptophan in the treatment of impaired respiration during sleep. *Bull Eur Physiopathol Respir* 1983;19:625–629.
68. Strumpf IJ, Drucker RD, Anders KH, Cohen S, Fajolu O. Acute eosinophilic pulmonary disease associated with the ingestion of L-tryptophan-containing products. *Chest* 1991;99:8–13.
69. Slutsker L, Hoesly FC, Miller L, Williams LP, Watson JC, Fleming DW. Eosinophilia–myalgia syndrome associated with exposure to tryptophan from a single manufacturer. *JAMA* 1990;264: 213–217.
70. Hertzman PA, Blevins WL, Mayer J, Greenfield B, Ting M, Gleich GJ. Association of the eosinophilia–myalgia syndrome with the ingestion of tryptophan. *N Engl J Med* 1990;322:869–873.
71. Smith PL, Haponik EF, Bleecker ER. The effects of oxygen in patients with sleep apnea. *Am Rev Respir Dis* 1984;130:958–963.
72. Martin RJ, Sanders MH, Gray BA, Pennock BE. Acute and long-term ventilatory effects of hyperoxia in the adult sleep apnea syndrome. *Am Rev Respir Dis* 1982;125:175–180.
73. Longobardo GS, Gothe B, Goldman MD, Cherniack NS. Sleep apnea considered as a control system instability. *Respir Physiol* 1982;50:311–333.
74. Onal E, Lopata M. Periodic breathing and the pathogenesis of occlusive sleep apneas. *Am Rev Respir Dis* 1982;126:676–680.
75. Reite M, Jackson D, Cahoon RL, Weil JV. Sleep physiology at high altitude. *Electroencephalogr Clin Neurophysiol* 1975;38:463–471.
76. Motta J, Guilleminault C. Effects of oxygen administration in sleep-induced apneas. In: Guilleminault C, ed. *Sleep apnea syndromes*. Kroc Foundation Series, vol II. New York: Alan R Liss, 1978;137–144.
77. Afzelius L-E, Elmqvist D, Hougaard K, Laurin S, Nilsson B, Risberg AM. Sleep apnea syndrome—an alternative treatment to tracheotomy. *Laryngoscope* 1981;91:285–291.
78. Nahmias JS, Karetzky MS. Treatment of the obstructive sleep apnea syndrome using a nasopharyngeal tube. *Chest* 1988;94:1142–1147.
79. Martin RJ. Sleep-related respiratory disorders associated with daytime somnolence and hypoventilation syndromes. In: Martin RJ, ed. *Cardiorespiratory disorders during sleep*. Mt. Kisco, NY: Futura, 1984;65–117.
80. Cartwright RD, Samelson CF. The effects of a nonsurgical treatment for obstructive sleep apnea. The tongue-retaining device. *JAMA* 1982;248:705–709.
81. Cartwright R, Stefoski D, Caldarelli D, et al. Toward a treatment logic for sleep apnea: the place of the tongue retaining device. *Behav Res Ther* 1988;26:121–126.
82. Schmidt-Nowara WW, Meade TE, Hays MB. Treatment of snoring and obstructive sleep apnea with a dental orthosis. *Chest* 1991;99:1378–1385.
83. Bonham PE, Currier GF, Orr WC, Othman J, Nanda RS. The effect of a modified functional appliance on obstructive sleep apnea. *Am J Orthod Dentofac Orthop* 1988;94:384–392.
84. Miki H, Hida W, Shindu C, et al. Effects of electrical stimulation of the genioglossus on upper airway resistance in anesthetized dogs. *Am Rev Respir Dis* 1989;140:1279–1284.
85. Edmonds LC, Daniels BK, Stanson AW, Sheedy PF III, Shepard JW Jr. The effects of transcutaneous electrical stimulation during wakefulness and sleep in patients with obstructive sleep apnea. *Am Rev Respir Dis* 1992;146:1030–1036.
86. Sullivan CE, Berthon-Jones M, Issa FG, Eves L. Reversal of obstructive sleep apnoea by continuous positive airway pressure applied through the nares. *Lancet* 1981;1:862–865.
87. Sanders MH. CPAP via nasal mask: a treatment for sleep apnea. *Chest* 1983;83:144–145.

88. Rapoport DM, Sorkin B, Garay SM, Goldring RM. Reversal of the "Pickwickian syndrome" by long-term use of nocturnal nasal airway pressure. *N Engl J Med* 1982;307:931–933.

89. Sanders MH. Nasal CPAP effect on patterns of sleep apnea. *Chest* 1984;86:839–844.

90. Issa FG, Sullivan CE. Reversal of central sleep apnea using nasal CPAP. *Chest* 1986;90:165–171.

91. Sullivan CE, Berthon-Jones M, Issa FG. Remission of severe obesity–hypoventilation syndrome after short-term treatment during sleep with nasal continuous positive airway pressure. *Am Rev Respir Dis* 1983;128:177–181.

92. Rajagopal KR, Bennett LL, Dillard TA, Tellis CJ, Tenholder MF. Overnight nasal CPAP improves hypersomnolence in sleep apnea. *Chest* 1986;90:172–176.

93. Lamphere J, Roehrs T, Wittig R, Zorick F, Conway WA, Roth T. Recovery of alertness after CPAP in sleep apnea. *Chest* 1989;96:1364–1367.

94. Sanders MH, Gruendl C, Rogers RM. Patient compliance with nasal CPAP therapy for sleep apnea. *Chest* 1986;90:330–333.

95. McEvoy RD, Thornton AT. Treatment of obstructive sleep apnea syndrome with nasal continuous positive airway pressure. *Sleep* 1984;7:313–325.

96. Frith RW, Cant BR. Severe obstructive sleep apnoea treated with long term nasal continuous positive airway pressure. *Thorax* 1985;40:45–50.

97. Sullivan CE, Issa FG, Berthon-Jones M, McCauley VB, Costas LJV. Home treatment of obstructive sleep apnoea with continuous positive airway pressure applied through a nose mask. *Bull Eur Physiopathol Respir* 1984;20:49–54.

98. Rolfe I, Olson LG, Saunders NA. Long-term acceptance of continuous positive airway pressure in obstructive sleep apnea. *Am Rev Respir Dis* 1991;144:1130–1135.

99. Hoffstein V, Viner S, Mateika S, Conway J. Treatment of obstructive sleep apnea with nasal continuous positive airway pressure. Patient compliance, perception of benefits, and side effects. *Am Rev Respir Dis* 1992;145:841–845.

100. Sanders MH, Rogers RM. Sleep apnea: when does better become benefit? *Chest* 1985;88:320–321.

101. Fletcher EC, Luckett RA. The effect of positive reinforcement on hourly compliance in nasal continuous positive airway pressure users with obstructive sleep apnea. *Am Rev Respir Dis* 1991;143:936–941.

102. Idatna R. A multicentric survey of long term compliance with nasal CPAP treatment in patients with obstructive sleep apnea syndrome. *Am Rev Respir Dis* 1990;141:A863.

103. Rauscher H, Popp W, Wanke T, Zwick H. Acceptance of CPAP therapy for sleep apnea. *Chest* 1991;100:1019–1023.

104. Waldhorn RE, Herrick TW, Nguyen MC, O'Donnell AE, Sodero J, Potolicchio SJ. Long-term compliance with nasal continuous positive airway pressure therapy of obstructive sleep apnea. *Chest* 1990;97:33–38.

105. Strohl KP, Redline S. Nasal CPAP therapy, upper airway activation, and obstructive sleep apnea. *Am Rev Respir Dis* 1986;134:555–558.

106. Rapoport DM, Garay SM, Goldring RM. Nasal CPAP in obstructive sleep apnea: mechanisms of action. *Bull Eur Physiopathol Respir* 1983;19:616–620.

107. Sanders MH, Kern N. Obstructive sleep apnea treated by independently adjusted inspiratory and expiratory positive airway pressures via mask. Physiologic and clinical implications. *Chest* 1990;98:317–324.

108. Sanders MH, Rogers RM, Pennock BE. Prolonged expiratory phase in sleep apnea: a unifying hypothesis. *Am Rev Respir Dis* 1985;131:401–408.

109. Sanders MH, Moore SE. Inspiratory and expiratory partitioning of airway resistance during sleep in patients with sleep apnea. *Am Rev Respir Dis* 1983;127:554–558.

110. Sanders MH, Black J, Stiller RA, Donohoe MP. Nocturnal ventilatory assistance with bi-level positive airway pressure. *Op Tech Otolaryngol Head Neck Surg* 1991;2:56–62.

Snoring and Obstructive Sleep Apnea, Second Edition,
edited by D.N.F. Fairbanks and S. Fujita.
Raven Press, Ltd., New York © 1994.

6

Pharyngeal Surgery for Obstructive Sleep Apnea and Snoring

Shiro Fujita*

Department of Otolaryngology—Head and Neck Surgery, Henry Ford Hospital, Detroit, Michigan 48202

HISTORICAL BACKGROUND

Surgery for snoring began in 1952 in Japan with Ikematsu, when he saw a 23-year-old woman whose obnoxious snoring had caused her marriage to fail. On examination, he found only a redundant posterior pillar of the soft palate with oropharyngeal web formation and an elogated uvula. Removal of this seemingly excessive tissue eliminated the loud snoring. Encouraged by this initial success, he treated more patients whose snoring had seriously disrupted their lives, and he expanded his investigations into snoring (1).

In 1964, he reported the results of his surgical treatment of 152 habitual snorers. His procedure consisted of palatectomy—excision of redundant posterior pillar mucosa—and partial uvulectomy under local anesthesia. The treatment was considered successful by 81.6% of his patients (2). He then studied the oropharyngeal anatomy of 300 habitual snorers whose snoring had been tape-recorded, and he correlated the sound with the anatomy. Based on measurements of oropharyngeal dimensions of snorers and nonsnorers, he concluded that 91% of habitual snorers had relatively narrower oropharynges, characterized by redundant pillar mucosa with longer soft palates and elongated uvulas.

In 1979, I began to explore the treatment of patients with severe obstructive sleep apnea syndrome (OSAS), almost all of whom are heavy snorers, in search of surgical alternatives to tracheostomy.

In 1980, I introduced a new operation to correct the anatomic abnormalities of obstructive sleep apnea patients by uvulopalatopharyngoplasty (UPPP), a procedure designed to enlarge the potential airspace in the oropharynx. Initially, I performed this operation on 12 patients with OSAS. Nine of the 12 experienced symptomatic relief; and in 8, nocturnal respiration and sleep architecture objectively improved

---

*Shiro Fujita (1929–1993).

(3). The report of our results generated great enthusiasm and interest in this new operation among otolaryngologists associated with major sleep disorder centers throughout the nation. This procedure was further developed through the efforts of Simmons et al. (4) at Stanford and Hernandez (5) at Mt. Sinai Hospital (Miami).

In 1985, we published the results of an efficacy study of UPPP for the treatment of OSAS in a series of 66 consecutive unselected patients (6). Although 76% claimed significant subjective response in daytime sleepiness and 94% thought their snoring was much improved, only 50% were considered to have had an appreciable reduction in the frequency of their sleep apnea. To classify a patient as a UPPP responder, we required at least a 50% reduction in the apnea index as determined by polysomnographic study 6 weeks after surgery, compared to the preoperative diagnostic study. Even in the group judged to be nonresponders by this criterion, hypoxemia significantly improved, although the apnea index showed little change.

After retrospective anatomic analysis, we concluded that UPPP significantly reduced the apnea index only in those patients whose airway obstruction was primarily oropharyngeal. If airway obstruction extended into the hypopharynx, UPPP was much less likely to produce a significant reduction in the apnea index. Based on the collective experience of six medical centers (Stanford University, University of Mississippi, Mt. Sinai Hospital in Miami, Deaconess Hospital in St. Louis, Presbyterian Hospital in Oklahoma City, and Henry Ford Hospital in Detroit), Roth investigated the overall response rate to UPPP (T. Roth, *personal communication*). Pre- and postoperative polysomnographic studies in the sleep centers of these six institutions documented the change attributable to UPPP. From a total of 314 patients, the overall reduction of the sleep apnea index was 49%, with a range of 36% to 85% (7). Variability of the data was thought to be related to differences in the surgical techniques at the various centers and to different criteria for selecting patients.

Thus, UPPP significantly reduced the frequency of sleep-related apnea in approximately half of the patients who were operated on during the first few years of experience with this procedure. Recent efforts have attempted to improve the success rate by using more refined patient selection criteria.

As a result of our earlier experiences with UPPP, we have been developing new surgical procedures in an attempt to correct hypopharyngeal obstruction for obstructive sleep apnea. Over the past 6 years, our approach to snoring and sleep apnea syndrome has evolved to the point where we can identify the specific anatomic narrowing contributing to the patient's problem, whether it is snoring or the sleep apnea syndrome. This chapter describes the evolution of our surgical concepts and explains my current approach to patients with these problems.

RATIONALE OF SURGICAL TREATMENT

Surgical treatment of obstructive sleep apnea is basically aimed at either bypassing the obstructive area by tracheostomy or eliminating the obstructive lesion in order to prevent soft tissue collapse in the upper airway during an apneic episode.

In order to develop a surgical approach to OSAS, it is essential to understand the upper airway anatomic abnormalities commonly seen in these patients and their relation to upper airway collapse during apneic episodes. Although specific pathologic conditions or overt obstructive lesions may occasionally be identified in adult apneics (such as hypertrophic tonsils, tumors, or cystic masses in the various parts of the pharynx), most adult sleep apnea patients show only subtle upper airway anatomical findings. In evaluating 200 patients with OSAS, Rojewski et al. (8) found only three who had a single, surgically correctable pathologic lesion. Almost all (98%) had more subtle malproportioned anatomic relationships in their otherwise normal upper airways. They usually had smaller pharyngeal inlets than did normal (nonapneic) individuals. Our experience is similar (9).

Anatomic Abnormalities of OSAS Patients

The anatomic abnormalities or variations to look for in these patients during routine otolaryngological examination are as follows:

Redundant Oropharyngeal Tissues

Excessive oropharyngeal tissues are often found in OSAS patients. These may include the following:

1. Large edematous uvula, which may act as an obstructing mass when the patient assumes a recumbent sleeping position (Fig. 1).

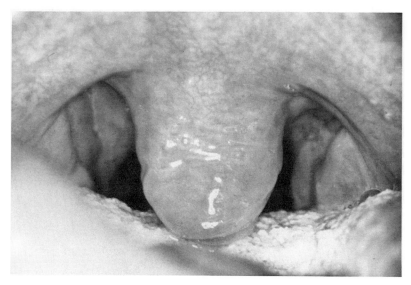

FIG. 1. Large uvula.

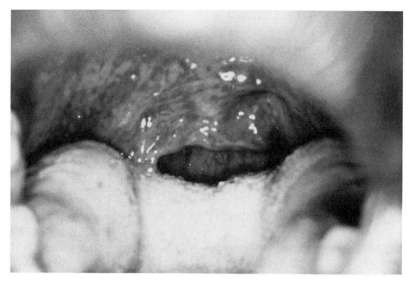

FIG. 2. Webbing of posterior pillar.

2. Wide posterior pillar mucosa (web formation) (Fig. 2).

3. Redundant mucosal folds of the lateral and posterior pharyngeal wall which may extend from the nasopharynx to the hypopharynx (Fig. 3). Excessive mucosal folds may be the result of heavy snoring for many years. The pharyngeal mucosa may have been stretched by continuous inspiratory force or negative airway pressure (suction) necessary to maintain constant airflow in a patient with partial airway obstruction. This process may explain the progression from heavy snoring at a pre-

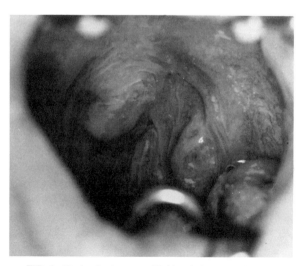

FIG. 3. Redundant mucosal folds of pharyngeal wall.

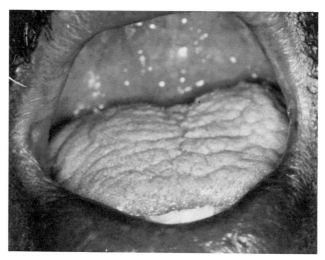

FIG. 4. Trailing edge of soft palate lies below the horizontal plane of the tongue.

clinical stage of sleep apnea to varying degrees of obstructive apnea in many individuals.

Low Palatal Arch with Long Low-Hanging Soft Palate

The soft palate is excessively long when its free margin cannot be seen in the open mouth without forceful use of a tongue depressor. It may not be seen even on phonation, which usually will lift the soft palate. This anatomical variant may contribute to the narrowing of the pharynx and facilitate airway collapse because of a flap valve mechanism during inspiration that occurs with simultaneous hypnogenic hypotonia of the pharyngeal dilator muscle (Figs. 4 and 5).

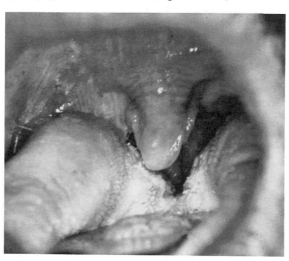

FIG. 5. Free margin of soft palate seen only when tongue is forcibly depressed.

Large Tongue

The tongue may be large relative to the oral cavity—either the dorsum of the tongue, with a relatively patent lower supraglottic area, or the base of the tongue. In the latter case, the posteriorly positioned tongue may make it difficult or impossible for the larynx to be seen with a mirror. This condition may be associated with mandibular retrognathia or micrognathia. When this is combined with an extremely shallow but not narrow oropharynx, maxillomandibular retrognathia should be suspected.

Floppy Epiglottis

An omega-shaped or floppy epiglottis with redundant aryepiglottic folds is occasionally seen in severe obstructive apneics, probably as the result of heavy snoring for many years (Fig. 6).

Hypertrophic Tonsils

Hypertrophic lingual tonsils are not uncommon in adult apneics, often reaching the vallecula and displacing the epiglottis posteriorly. As a result, the anteroposterior dimension of the hypopharynx is reduced (Figs. 7 and 8). Hypertrophic palatine (faucial) tonsils reduce the lateral dimension of the oropharyngeal airway (Fig. 9).

Redundant Lateral Pharyngeal Walls

Redundant lateral pharyngeal walls, secondary to excessive submocosal fat infiltration or hypertrophied musculature, are seen in some obese patients. This anatom-

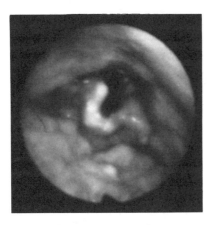

FIG. 6. Omega-shaped epiglottis.

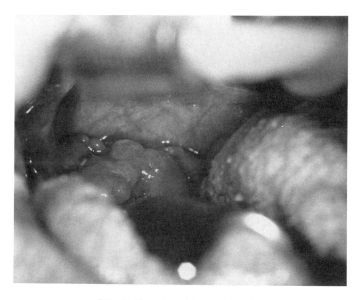

FIG. 7. Hypertrophic lingual tonsils.

ical variant reduces the lateral dimension of the pharynx and predisposes the airway to inspiratory collapse.

Pathogenesis of Obstructive Sleep Apnea

The formula in Fig. 10 represents upper airway dynamics in respiration and may help to explain the upper airway collapse mechanism associated with obstructive sleep apnea. V_A represents the amount of airflow during the inspiratory cycle of

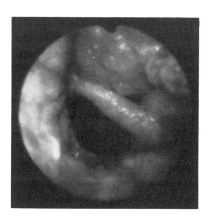

FIG. 8. Lingual tonsils reaching vallecula with epiglottis displaced posteriorly.

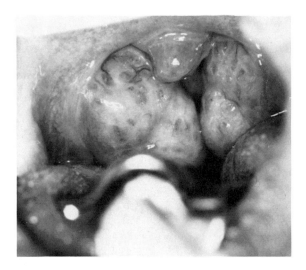

FIG. 9. Large tonsils occupying airway space.

respiration (tidal volume). It is directly related to the pressure difference between atmospheric and intrathoracic (inspiratory) pressures and inversely related to respiratory resistance. Lower atmospheric pressure, or any lesion increasing resistance to airflow, whether in the upper or lower airway, would increase the respiratory effort needed to maintain airflow. When inspiratory airflow accelerates, intraluminal pressure suddenly drops in the area of narrowing due to the Venturi effect, and the airway is further compromised. At some point, turbulence develops in the airstream, and soft tissue vibrations are produced, usually in the soft palate, hence "snoring."

To maintain airway patency during inspiration, a physiological mechanism increases the tone of pharyngeal dilator muscles (genioglossus, tensor palatini, ge-

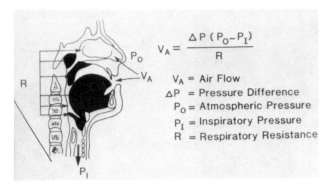

FIG. 10. Formula illustrating upper airway dynamics in respiration.

niohyoid, stylohyoid) coordinated with diaphragmatic activity. In sleep apnea patients, these muscular activities diminish or disappear during the inspiratory cycle of breathing as they begin to fall asleep (10).

When the intraluminal negative pressure of the airway reaches a critical point, the combination of redundant tissues and the loss of pharyngeal muscle tone causes airway collapse (obstructive apnea) during inspiration. This process continues with repetitive inspiratory effort for the duration of the apnea until it ends with a brief awakening (arousal). With immediate restoration of normal pharyngeal muscle tone, the airway opens and airflow resumes. This sequence is repeated cyclically throughout the night. If airway occlusion is incomplete and airflow is significantly reduced, arousal still can result, but the event would be classified as a hypopnea. Hypopneas may have the same effect as apneas in disrupting sleep, but they usually produce less hypoxemia.

Rational surgical treatments should therefore be aimed at eliminating any collapsible tissue in the airway and reducing airway resistance without creating functional impairment of the upper airway structures. The obstructive lesion may occur anywhere along the upper airway from the nose down to the level of the epiglottis.

The level of obstruction responsible for apnea should be determined by careful upper airway anatomical assessment before surgery is planned. Often, more than one site of anatomical narrowing is involved.

Surgically correctable upper airway lesions include:

1. *Nasal cavity*: deviated septum, hypertrophic turbinates, polyps, tumor (papilloma), and so on
2. *Nasopharynx*: adenoids, cyst, stenosis
3. *Oropharynx*: large tonsils, elongated uvula, redundant mucosal folds of the pharyngeal wall, wide tonsillar pillar (webbing), or low-hanging soft palate
4. *Hypopharynx*: large lingual tonsils, vallecular cyst, tumor, floppy epiglottis with redundant aryepiglottic folds, or large tongue base.

INDICATIONS FOR SURGICAL TREATMENT

The need for surgical treatment of obstructive sleep apnea and/or snoring is determined basically by three factors: (a) the severity of medical complications, (b) socioeconomic compromise due to disabling daytime sleepiness, or (c) socially disturbing (debilitating) loud snoring.

The patient should also be informed of the nonsurgical options. Appropriate management decisions are most effectively achieved by a multidisciplinary team that includes a sleep specialist (polysomnographer), a pulmonary physician, and an otolaryngologist. Oral surgeons, cardiologists, neurologists, and psychiatrists may be consulted for additional advice about the most effective treatment for individual patients.

The following guidelines for making management decisions may be helpful. The disease is considered life-threatening if any one of the following conditions is met:

TABLE 1. *Multiple sleep latency test (nap test)*

Degree of sleepiness	Average sleep latency
Marked	3 min or less
Moderate	3–5 min
Mild	5–7 min
Normal	7 min or longer

1. Significant bradycardia (below 40/min) with apnea
2. Asystole
3. Ventricular tachycardia
4. So_2 falling frequently below 50%
5. Severe hypercarbia (Pco_2 greater than 50 mm)
6. Cor pulmonale
7. Extreme hypersomnolence as measured objectively by the multiple sleep latency test (MSLT) (Table 1), because of the danger of causing an accident while driving

Three degrees of hypersomnolence are considered (Table 2):

1. *Marked*: The patient cannot stay awake even when motivated.
2. *Moderate*: The patient frequently falls asleep whenever sedentary; thus job performance suffers, and driving is usually a significant concern.
3. *Mild*: The patient can stay awake to work satisfactorily and can drive short distances (up to 30 min).

If the patient has great difficulty in staying awake on the job, is worried about the loss of employment or has already lost his or her job, and is falling asleep at inappropriate times, such as driving or during conversation with clients or customers, he or she is certainly a candidate for treatment even though cardiopulmonary complications are absent or mild. Patients with socially disturbing, obnoxious loud snoring may be considered surgical candidates if they are highly motivated to solve these serious social problems. Heavy snoring can be disruptive in family or marital life, frequently causing sleepless nights for bed partners and disastrous social consequences such as divorce. These patients also become unwelcome guests, which creates social stress and embarrassment for them.

TABLE 2. *Severity of obstructive sleep apnea (polysomnography)*

Severity	Apnea index/hour of sleep	So_2 below 85% (fraction of total sleep time)
Marked	>50	25% or more (frequently below 50%)
Moderate	50–30	25%–15%
Mild	30–15	<15%

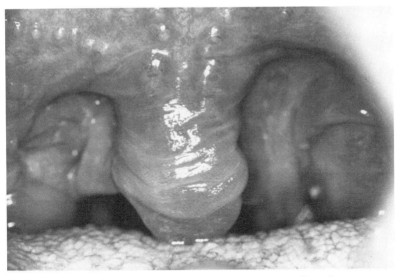

FIG. 11. Large uvula and redundant pillar mucosa (Type I).

CLASSIFICATION OF UPPER AIRWAY ANATOMY
IN OBSTRUCTIVE SLEEP APNEA

Patients with OSAS may be classified into three types based on upper airway anatomical findings:

Type I represents a group in which the airway narrowing predominantly involves the oropharynx but the palatal arch is in a normal position. The patients in this group are characterized by large tonsils, enlarged uvula, and webbing of pillar mucosa (Figs. 9 and 11).

Type II represents a group in which the palatal arch is in a low position and the tongue is relatively large. This group is divided into two subgroups, depending on the level of predominant airway narrowing: *IIa* predominantly involves the oropharynx, but the larynx and hypopharynx are easily seen with a mirror; *IIb* involves both the oro- and hypopharynx, and it is often difficult to see the hypopharynx or larynx with a mirror.

Type III represents a group in which the oropharynx is normal; airway compromise is limited to the hypopharyngeal airway. This compromise may include a large or posteriorly positioned tongue base (retrognathia), lateral wall bulge extending to the hypopharynx, hypertrophic lingual tonsils, and/or floppy epiglottis with redundant aryepiglottic folds.

When significant nasal obstruction is present (i.e., the patient has significant nasal obstruction to be treated), N (+) is added to each type, but N (−) is added if there is no nasal obstruction to be treated (Table 3). This classification is helpful in

TABLE 3. *Upper airway anatomy classification of Mueller's maneuver*[a]

	Site of obstruction	Oropharynx	Hypopharynx
Type I	Normal palatal position		
N(+,−)	Oropharyngeal	3+, 4+	0, 1+
Type II	Low palatal position		
N(+,−)	Predominantly oropharynx	3+, 4+	1+, 2+
	Orohypopharynx involved	3+, 4+	3+, 4+
Type III	Normal oropharynx		
	Hypopharyngeal obstruction		
	(retrognathia, micrognathia)	0, 1+	3+, 4+

[a]The degree of pharyngeal obstruction at each level is determined by the reduction of pharyngeal lumen and is recorded as follows: 1+, less than 25% (minimal movement); 2+, 50%; 3+, 75%; 4+, 100% (total airway collapse).

planning the total surgical management of upper airway obstruction associated with OSAS. For example, patients of type I or type IIa would likely respond to oropharyngeal surgery (UPPP ± tonsillectomy) alone, whereas type IIb patients would probably need staging procedures involving both the oro- and hypopharynx. Type III patients require only hypopharyngeal surgery.

Because upper airway patency changes during the respiratory cycle, the dynamic range of the airway must be observed during different phases of the respiratory cycles. Fiberoptic nasopharyngolaryngoscopy is a useful diagnostic tool for evaluating the airway dynamics of sleep apnea patients. During this examination, the patient can be asked to perform a Mueller's maneuver, which consists of a forced inspiratory effort with the mouth and nose closed. It should be performed with the patient in both upright and supine positions. The fiberoptic endoscope is passed transnasally to observe upper airway patency at two different levels, the oropharyngeal level (soft palate and the junction of the nasopharynx) and the hypopharyngeal level (just above the epiglottis) (Figs. 12 and 13). The degree of airway

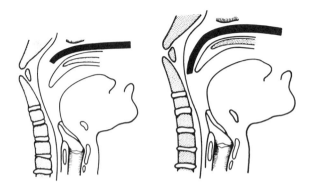

FIG. 12. Mueller's maneuver: Fiberoptic endoscope positioned just above (L) and below (R) oropharyngeal inlet. (From ref. 12.)

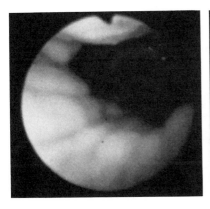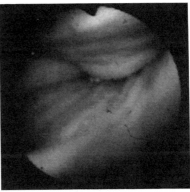

FIG. 13. **Left:** *Arrow* indicates soft palate. Numerous mucosal folds seen in the posterior pharyngeal wall. **Right:** Airway collapse seen at the oropharynx during forced inspiration (Mueller's maneuver).

collapse should be noted, with particular attention to the posterior movement of soft palate, uvula, and tongue and to the medial movement of the lateral walls of the hypopharynx.

Table 3 and Fig. 14A and 14B illustrate the relation of the three types to Mueller's maneuver findings.

Cephalometric analysis is another useful tool to identify the hypopharyngeal obstructive lesion of OSAS if associated with skeletal II and/or soft tissue abnormalities. Riley et al. (11), in a study of palatopharyngoplasty (PPP) failures, reported a small posterior airspace (4–5 mm; control, 11.6 mm) as the only consistent cephalometric finding in all nine patients evaluated. The posterior airspace is the linear measurement between the base of the tongue and posterior pharyngeal wall on cephalometric x-ray. Inferiorly positioned hyoid and shorter palatal length on cephalometry (Fig. 15) are also characteristic features of PPP failures. An abnormal mandibular position was present in only 50% of PPP failures.

Upper airway soft tissue roentgenograms (lateral view) taken in upright and supine positions help to determine the degree of posterior shift of soft palate and/or tongue base due to change of posture from upright to supine position (Fig. 16A and 16B).

SURGICAL PLANNING INCLUDING PREOPERATIVE UPPER AIRWAY ASSESSMENT

Once the decision has been made that the individual patient needs surgical treatment, the best procedure or set of procedures must be selected. This process depends on the major site and extent of upper airway compromise or anatomic abnormalities. If several corrective operations are necessary, they are staged accordingly. It is mandatory to evaluate thoroughly the patient's entire upper airway anatomy to

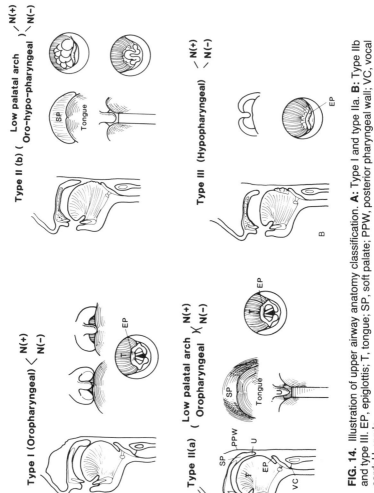

FIG. 14. Illustration of upper airway anatomy classification. **A:** Type I and type IIa. **B:** Type IIb and type III. EP, epiglottis; T, tongue; SP, soft palate; PPW, posterior pharyngeal wall; VC, vocal cord; U, uvula.

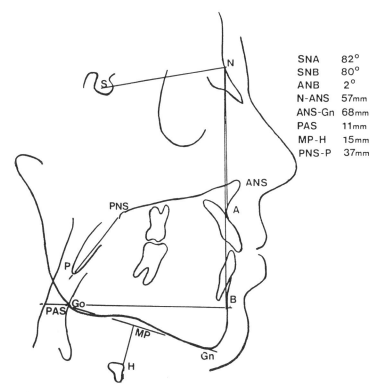

SNA	82°
SNB	80°
ANB	2°
N-ANS	57mm
ANS-Gn	68mm
PAS	11mm
MP-H	15mm
PNS-P	37mm

FIG. 15. Cephalometric analysis. S, sella; N, nasion; A, subspinale; B, supramentale; ANS, anterior nasal spine; PNS, posterior nasal spine; Go, gonion; Gn, gnathion; H, hyoid; PAS, posterior air space; P, palate. (From ref. 18.)

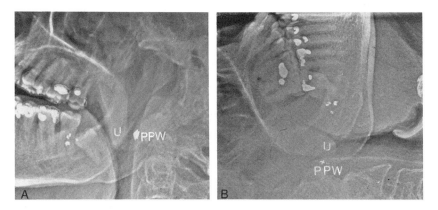

FIG. 16. Upper airway soft tissue xerogram of OSAS patient. **A:** Oropharynx in upright position. Note air column between uvula (U) and posterior pharyngeal wall (PPW). **B:** In supine position. Note compromised air column.

TABLE 4. *Pharyngeal surgical procedures*

Location of obstruction	Surgical procedures
Nasopharynx	Adenoidectomy
	Excision of cyst
Oropharynx	Tonsillectomy
	Uvulopalatopharyngoplasty
Hypopharynx	
Nonskeletal	Lingual tonsillectomy
	Midline partial glossectomy (reduction surgery)
	Excision of redundant aryepiglottic folds and partial epiglottectomy
	Excision of vallecular cyst
Skeletal	Mandibular advancement with sagittal splitting osteotomy (mandibular retrognathia or micrognathia)
	Maxillomandibular advancement with vertical osteotomy (maxillo-mandibular retrognathia)
	Inferosagittal osteotomy of the mandible with hyoid myotomy suspension (Riley–Powell)

assess potential sites of airway compromise. This evaluation must include (a) careful otorhinolaryngological examination, (b) fiberoptic nasopharyngolaryngoscopy with Mueller's maneuver, (c) upper airway soft tissue x-ray in the upright and supine positions, and (d) cephalometric measurement. Computerized tomography or magnetic resonance imaging may be useful in selected unusual cases.

Currently available pharyngeal surgical procedures are listed in Table 4.

Because most patients with sleep apnea syndrome are thought to have oropharyngeal airway compromise, UPPP has become the most commonly used procedure to treat obstructive sleep apnea and snoring. This operation is designed to enlarge the potential oropharyngeal airway lumen in an attempt to reduce airway collapse during sleep. It consists of excising redundant oropharyngeal tissues from the free margin of the soft palate, tonsillar pillars, and uvula. After excision, the noncollapsible oropharyngeal space is reconstructed by stretching the posterolateral pharyngeal wall and approximating the two palatal arch muscles. Current experience among otolaryngologists affiliated with sleep disorder centers is that UPPP eliminates the loud snoring of most patients undergoing the operation. However, it is effective for approximately 50% in curing or considerably improving sleep apnea when patients are selected only for the sleep syndrome and do not undergo any more detailed anatomic analysis.

The obvious question is how to predict preoperatively who will have a good response to UPPP and who will not respond. Several efforts have been made to establish better patient selection criteria to improve the success rate of this procedure. Mueller's maneuver with fiberoptic nasopharyngoscopy and cephalometric measurement are presently the key diagnostic tools used to identify the location of airway narrowing that is primarily causing the apneic episode. Sher et al. (12) reported the predictive value of Mueller's maneuver in selecting patients for UPPP. Of 30 patients considered suitable candidates for UPPP (marked airway collapse seen predominantly at the level of the soft palate during the Mueller's maneuver),

TABLE 5. *UPPP results of 30 OSAS patients selected by Mueller's maneuver (mean values)*[a]

	Presurgery	Postsurgery	P value
Apnea index	61.4 ± 27.2 SD	16.6 ± 22.8 SD	<0.001
Obstructive apnea index	53.4 ± 35.9 SD	12.9 ± 21.6 SD	<0.001
Apnea-hypopnea index	82.1 ± 40.5 SD	32.5 ± 30.5 SD	<0.001
Lowest So_2	59.4 ± 24.1 SD	79.7 ± 14.4 SD	<0.001
Percent ideal weight (pounds)	153.0 ± 38.5 SD	148.0 ± 32.3 SD	<0.01

[a]Courtesy of Dr. A. E. Sher (12), Montefiore Hospital, Bronx, New York.

87% had a greater than 50% decrease in the apnea–hypopnea index, and 40% of patients had a postoperative apnea index of less than 5. Thus, in carefully selected patients, a much higher success rate can be achieved than the 50% reported in unselected patients (Table 5).

Katsantonis and Walsh (13) have used somnofluoroscopy, a combination of cineradiography and polysomnography, for evaluating the dynamic function of the airway as well as the level of occlusion during sleep. They were able to identify patients as good candidates for UPPP if they demonstrated the oropharynx as the narrowest level of the upper airway while awake and the first point of airway collapse during apneic episodes. Those showing at least 50% improvement in the apnea–hypopnea index and 90% improvement in the severity index were classified as good responders. In this study, 12 of 16 patients had a good response to this operation.

Riley et al. (11) reported on nine patients with OSAS who underwent unsuccessful PPP and had abnormal cephalometric roentgenogram measurements. Their findings indicated that a small posterior airway space and inferiorly placed hyoid bone were responsible for these PPP failures. They concluded that cephalometric findings are a helpful guide in deciding whether PPP alone or PPP in combination with other surgical procedures will be more efficacious. DeBerry-Borowiecki and Sassin (14), on the other hand, utilized both fiberoptic nasopharyngoscopy (Mueller's maneuver) and cephalometric studies (tongue-space index, mandible-hyoid angle) to identify potentially successful candidates for PPP.

In patients who have extensive airway narrowing, hypopharyngeal surgery is indicated as the second-stage procedure following UPPP (type IIb) or as the primary procedure for hypopharyngeal obstruction (type III).

Basically, there are two surgical approaches. The first approach is to reduce the bulk of excessive soft tissue mass or eliminate collapsible redundant mucosa in the hypopharynx (nonskeletal). This approach includes lingual tonsillectomy, partial midline glossectomy, excision of cystic mass or redundant aryepiglottic folds, or partial epiglottectomy.

The second approach is the advancement of the mandible in order to enlarge the hypopharyngeal airspace. This is indicated when significant retrognathia is identified by cephalometric analysis. When maxillary retrognathia is also present, the maxilla should be advanced in order to maintain a normal occlusive relationship. This requires sagittal split osteotomy and intermaxillary fixation for 6–8 weeks.

In order to reduce surgical intervention, Riley et al. (15) designed an inferosagittal osteotomy on the mandible, which advances the geniotubercle with hyoid myotomy suspension. This procedure has the advantage of avoiding intermaxillary fixation. In their report of the results of this procedure for five patients, all improved clinically and apnea was reduced.

Our experience with maxillomandibular advancement (16) and a recent series of soft tissue reduction surgery of the hypopharynx have been encouraging (17).

POSTOPERATIVE EVALUATIONS AND FOLLOW-UP

Technical aspects of UPPP, surgical results, and complications will be discussed in the next chapter.

Our patients undergoing pharyngeal surgery are evaluated 6 weeks after surgery for subjective response and undergo objective measures of sleep pattern, nocturnal respiratory parameters (apnea and hypopnea), cardiac rhythm, and oxygen saturation, as well as the sleep latency test by polysomnography. In those who had tracheostomy with UPPP, the tracheostomy tube remains capped for 1 week before the sleep study.

SUMMARY

Habitual loud snoring is not only a social problem but also a potential health risk because it is often associated with OSAS. Abnormalities or variations of the upper airway anatomy commonly seen in OSAS and their relation to the airway collapse mechanism (pathogenesis) have been discussed.

Appropriate selection of patients for pharyngeal surgical procedures based on careful upper airway evaluation in individual cases has successfully eliminated the need for tracheostomy for many patients with OSAS.

REFERENCES

1. Ikematsu T. Clinical study of snoring for the past 30 years. In: Meyer E, ed. *New dimensions in otorhinolaryngology—head and neck surgery*, vol 1. Amsterdam: Elsevier Science Publishers, B.V. (Excerpta Medica), 1985;199–202.
2. Ikematsu T. Study of snoring. 4th report. Therapy [in Japanese]. *J Jpn Otol Rhinol Laryngol Soc* 1964;64:434–435.
3. Fujita S, Conway W, Zorick F, Roth T. Surgical correction of anatomic abnormalities in obstructive sleep apnea syndrome: uvulopalatopharyngoplasty. *Otolaryngol Head Neck Surg* 1981;89:923–927.
4. Simmons FB, Guilleminault C, Silvestri R. Snoring, and some obstructive sleep apnea, can be cured by oropharyngeal surgery. *Arch Otolaryngol* 1983;109:503–507.
5. Hernandez SF. Palatopharyngoplasty for obstructive sleep apnea syndrome: technique and preliminary report of results in ten patients. *Am J Otolaryngol* 1982;3:229–234.
6. Fujita S, Conway WA, Sicklesteel JM, Wittig RM, Zorick FJ, Roehrs TA, Roth T. Evaluation of the effectiveness of uvulopalatopharyngoplasty. *Laryngoscope* 1985;95:70–74.
7. Roth T. UPPP update. Presented at the annual meeting of American College of Chest Physicians, San Antonio, Texas, October 1984.

8. Rojewski TE, Schuller DE, Clark RW, Schmidt HS, Potts RE. Videoendoscopic determination of the mechanism of obstruction in obstructive sleep apnea. *Otolaryngol Head Neck Surg* 1984;92: 127–131.
9. Wilms D, Popovich J, Fujita S, Conway W, Zorick F. Anatomical abnormalities in obstructive sleep apnea. *Ann Otol Rhinol Laryngol* 91:595–596.
10. Hill NW, Guilleminault C, Simmons FB. Fiberoptic and EMG studies in hypersomnia–sleep apnea syndrome. In: Guilleminault C, Dement WC, eds. *Sleep apnea syndromes*. New York: Alan R Liss, 1978;249–258.
11. Riley RW, Guilleminault C, Powell N, Simmons FB. Palatopharyngoplasty failure, cephalometric roentgenograms, and obstructive sleep apnea. *Otolaryngol Head Neck Surg* 1985;93:240–243.
12. Sher AE, Thorpey MJ, Shprintzen RJ, Spielman AJ, McGregor PA. Predictive value of Mueller's maneuver in selection of patients with UPPP. *Laryngoscope* 1985;95:1483–1487.
13. Katsantonis GP, Walsh JK. Cinefluoroscopy, its role in selection of candidates for UPPP. Presented at the meeting of the American Academy of Otolaryngology, Las Vegas, October 1984.
14. DeBerry-Borowiecki B, Sassin, JF. Surgical treatment of sleep apnea. *Arch Otolaryngol* 1985; 109:508–512.
15. Riley RW, Powell NB, Guilleminault C. Inferior sagittal osteotomy of the mandible with hyoid myotomy-suspension. A new procedure for obstructive sleep apnea. Presented at the meeting of the American Academy of Otolaryngology, Las Vegas, October 1984.
16. Fujita S. Sleep apnea. In: *Current therapy in otolaryngology/head and neck surgery. 1984–1985.* St. Louis: CV Mosby 1984;373–381.
17. Fujita S. Midline laser glossectomy with linguloplasty: operative techniques in otolaryngology— head and neck surgery. In: Friedman M, ed. *Sleep apnea surgery*, vol 2, no 2. 1991.
18. Riley, RW, Guilleminault C. Cephalometric analysis and flow-volume loops in obstructive sleep apnea patients. *Sleep* 1983;6(4):301–311.

Snoring and Obstructive Sleep Apnea, Second Edition,
edited by D.N.F. Fairbanks and S. Fujita.
Raven Press, Ltd., New York © 1994.

7

Uvulopalatopharyngoplasty: Variations

A. Palatopharyngoplasty and Partial Uvulectomy Method of
Ikematsu: A 30-Year Clinical Study of Snoring
Takenosuke Ikematsu (1913–1990)
Ikematsu Clinic of Otorhinolaryngology, Noda City, Japan

B. Method of Fujita
Shiro Fujita (1929–1993)
*Department of Otolaryngology—Head and Neck Surgery, Henry Ford Hospital,
Detroit, Michigan 48202*

C. Palatopharyngoplasty: Method of Simmons
F. Blair Simmons
*Division of Otolaryngology—Head and Neck Surgery, Stanford University Medical
Center, Stanford, California 94305*

D. Method of Fairbanks
David N. F. Fairbanks
*Department of Otolaryngology, George Washington University School of Medicine,
Washington, D.C. 20037*

E. Method of Dickson:
How Much Palate to Resect
Robert I. Dickson
*Division of Otolaryngology—Head and Neck Surgery, University of British Columbia,
Vancouver, British Columbia, V6J 4G7 Canada*

F. Modification of Woodson: Transpalatal Advancement
Pharyngoplasty
B. Tucker Woodson
*Department of Otolaryngology and Human Communication, Medical College of
Wisconsin, Milwaukee, Wisconsin 53226*

G. Method of Coleman: Laser-Assisted Uvulopalatoplasty
Jack A. Coleman
*Department of Otolaryngology, Vanderbilt University Medical Center, Nashville,
Tennessee 37232*

A. Palatopharyngoplasty and Partial Uvulectomy Method of Ikematsu: A 30-Year Clinical Study of Snoring

This portion of the chapter presents my clinical experience in evaluation and treatment of more than 4000 habitual snorers in Japan during the past 30 years. The data in this study are based on 1979 patients seen in my clinic from 1970 through 1983.

CONTRIBUTING FACTORS AND/OR PHYSICAL SIGNS ASSOCIATED WITH HABITUAL SNORING

My initial approach in this endeavor was to study tape-recorded snoring of 300 patients collected in 5 years between 1952 and 1956. These tapes were correlated to oropharyngeal anatomy, facial appearance, or any other contributing factors such as sex difference, physical condition, sleeping posture, and so on.

The following is a list of underlying conditions, contributing factors, or physical signs frequently seen in heavy habitual snorers:

1. Obesity
2. Upper airway abnormality or obstruction
   a. Nasal obstruction—sleeping with mouth open
   b. Excessive secretion or dryness in the upper airway tract
   c. Oro- or hypopharyngeal mass (enlarged tonsils, lingual tonsils, cyst)
   d. Nasopharyngeal mass or stenosis
3. Upper airway anatomical deviation
   a. Enlarged or elongated uvula
   b. Redundant pillar mucosa (soft palatal arch)
   c. Micro- or retrognathia (bird-face, pigeon-jaw)
   d. Macroglossia
4. Sleeping posture
5. Physical fatigue
6. Idiopathic (unknown cause)

ANATOMICAL VARIATIONS OF SOFT PALATE AND UVULA IN SNORING PATIENTS

From 1970 through 1983, 1979 patients were evaluated for snoring at my clinic. Of that figure, 694 were males (35%) and 1285 were females (65%).

The following observations were made in snoring patients with regard to the dimension of oropharyngeal structures. These were classified basically according to six types (A, B, C, D, E, F) based on the shape and size of the soft palate or the uvula. The combination of more than two types is frequently seen.

1. Type A (long soft palate). The anteroposterior dimension of the soft palate is greater than 50 mm.
2. Type B (elongated uvula). The length of uvula is greater than 11 mm.
3. Type C (enlarged uvula). The width of the uvula is greater than 10 mm.
4. Type D (redundant posterior pillar mucosa or posterior palatal arch). The width of the pillar mucosa is greater than 5 mm. Type D is subdivided into four groups (Fig. 1):
   a. Type DI (parallel type). The anterior palatal arch curves parallel with the posterior palatal arch.
   b. Type DII (webbing type). The posterior palatal arch forms a web-like appearance.
   c. Type DIII (embedded type). The uvula is imbedded in the posterior palatal arch.
   d. Type DIV (emerging type). The uvula emerges from the posterior palatal arch.
5. Type E (narrowing of the oropharynx) (Fig. 2)
   a. Type EI (anterior arch narrowing). The distance between the anterior palatal arches is less than 20 mm.
   b. Type EII (posterior arch narrowing). The distance between the posterior arches is less than 15 mm.
   c. Type EIII (shallow oropharynx). The distance between the posterior surface of the uvula and the posterior pharyngeal wall is less than 5 mm.
6. Type F (large dorsum tongue). The oropharyngeal space cannot be visualized at phonating "A" sound.

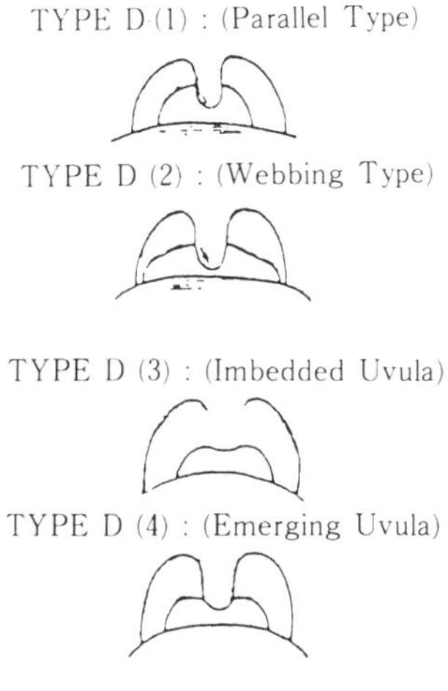

TYPE D (1) : (Parallel Type)

TYPE D (2) : (Webbing Type)

TYPE D (3) : (Imbedded Uvula)

TYPE D (4) : (Emerging Uvula)

FIG. 1. Anatomical variations of the soft palate, uvula, and palatal arches (tonsillar pillars) typical for snoring patients.

TYPE E (1)   TYPE E (3)
(Ant-PA-Nar)   (Shallow O-P)

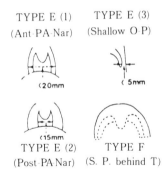

<20mm   < 5mm

<15mm
TYPE E (2)   TYPE F
(Post-PA-Nar) (S. P. behind T)

FIG. 2. Narrowing of the oropharynx in snoring patients. **Top left** shows distance between anterior palatal arches (Ant-PA) narrowed (Nar) to 20 mm or less. **Bottom left** shows distance between posterior palatal arches (Post-PA) narrowed (Nar) to 15 mm or less. **Top right** shows side view of uvula with distance to posterior pharyngeal wall of 5 mm or less, resulting in a shallow oronaso-pharynx (O-P). **Bottom right** depicts the soft palate (S.P.), arches, and uvula as being obscured from view behind the dorsum of a large tongue (T).

PLASTIC SURGERY OF SOFT PALATE AND UVULA FOR SNORING (PALATOPHARYNGOPLASTY AND PARTIAL UVULECTOMY)

The technique of this surgery (1) is illustrated in Fig. 3. A wedge section is made in the posterior pillar mucosa adjacent to the root of the uvula. The mucosa of the pillar between the palatal arches is removed. The mucosal edges of the anterior and posterior palatal arches are approximated by interrupted sutures. A small partial resection of mucosa and submucosal tissues from the root of the uvula would cause anterior displacement of the uvula (Fig. 3).

RESULTS

A total of 152 patients underwent this surgery in 1963 through 1967 (Table 1). Of this number, 81.6% reported improvement of snoring after the surgery (46.1%—marked, 35.5%—moderate). No significant complications were noted.

Between 1970 and 1983, 1979 patients were seen for snoring evaluation and treatment at Ikematsu ENT Clinic (Table 2). Of this total, 1690 cases were considered as surgical candidates, and 1646 underwent the surgery. However, 1007 cases were lost for follow-up (61.2%), since the majority of these patients came from various parts of Japan far from Noda City. Of those who were followed, 584 (35.5%) reported an improvement, while 55 (3.3%) indicated no positive effect.

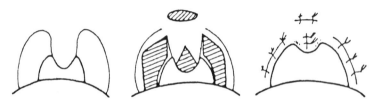

FIG. 3. Technique for palatopharyngoplasty and partial uvulectomy. **Left:** Preoperative anatomy. **Center:** *Shaded areas* represent wedge resection of uvula and resection of tissues between palatal arches (pillars) and at root of uvula. **Right:** Appearance after suture closure.

TABLE 1. *Results of UPPP (1963–1967)[a]*

Subjective response[b]	Number of cases
Snoring markedly improved	70 (46.1%)
Snoring moderately improved	54 (35.5%)
Snoring unimproved	8 (5.3%)
Snoring unknown	20 (13.1%)

[a]Total of 152 cases (49 males, 103 females).
[b]81.6% reported improvement.

TABLE 2. *Treatment of snoring at Ikematsu ENT Clinic, Noda City, Chiba Prefecture (1970–1983)[a]*

Counseling for snoring control alone	204 cases
Palatopharyngoplasty and partial uvulectomy	1646 cases
Surgery cancelled	44 cases
Those who reported improvement by surgery	584 (35.5%)
Those who reported no improvement by surgery	55 (3.3%)
Those lost for followup	1007 (61.2%)

[a]Total cases: 1979; males 694; females 1285.

REFERENCE

1. Ikematsu T. Study of snoring, 4th report. Therapy [in Japanese]. *J Jpn Otol Rhinol Laryngol Soc* 1964;64:434–435.

B. Method of Fujita

Indications for uvulopalatopharyngoplasty (UPPP) and patient selection criteria have been discussed in my chapter on pharyngeal surgery (Chapter 6, *this volume*). In this chapter, the surgical techniques, complications, and results of UPPP will be described. Since my original technique was described in a 1981 article (1), some modification has been made to improve the technique.

UPPP is performed under general anesthesia with the patient in the Rose's position (supine with head hanging). This is supplemented by local infiltration of 0.5–1.0% percent lidocaine with epinephrine (1:200,000 or 1:100,000) for hemostasis. After orotracheal intubation is performed, a self-retaining mouth gag (Crowe–Davis) is inserted to maintain adequate exposure of the surgical field. The dental arch is covered with dental wax to protect the teeth and tongue from the pressure of the mouth gag. Particularly when a large tongue is present in a small oral cavity, the teeth may lacerate the undersurface of the tongue after prolonged use of the mouth gag. Intermittent decompression of the tongue may reduce postoperative edema.

UPPP can be performed safely without tracheostomy in patients who have less severe sleep apnea. However, precautionary tracheostomy is recommended if the patient has significant cardiopulmonary complications. This will prevent immediate postoperative respiratory embarrassment due to oropharyngeal edema or inadequate respiratory drive.

My guidelines for selecting patients for UPPP without tracheostomy are as follows:

1. Apnea index less than 50 per hour of sleep
2. Lowest So$_2$ above 50%
3. No significant abnormalities on electrocardiogram
4. No significant cardiopulmonary complications

Those who require multiply staged procedures (type IIb) or hypopharyngeal surgery (type III) need tracheostomy before pharyngeal surgery.

For those who require long-term care, I prefer to perform a tracheoplasty. In this procedure, advanced cervical skin flaps are developed and sutured to the mucosal edge of tracheal flaps (reversed U-shaped) to create a tracheostoma, as originally described by Fee and Ward (2). Combined with cervical defatting for obese patients, this procedure will significantly reduce postoperative complications and facilitate long-term tracheostoma care.

SURGICAL STEPS

Step 1. The oropharyngeal structures are closely inspected to determine the dimension of the oropharyngeal inlet; the size of uvula, posterior pillar, and tongue; and the length of the soft palate. The uvula and soft palatal arch are frequently in direct contact or in apposition with the posterior pharyngeal wall. Measurement of the oropharyngeal dimension may be helpful for a comparison between pre- and postoperative data.

Step 2. At the outset, 2-0 silk suture is passed through the distal third of the uvula and held by a hemostat attached to the end of the string. When the string is pulled upward, the soft palate is pulled away from the pharyngeal wall, and redundant posterolateral pharyngeal wall mucosae are stretched, expanding the oropharyngeal space (Fig. 1, steps 1 and 2). In this way, we can estimate the potential airspace to be acquired and the amount of excessive tissue to be removed. This maneuver also makes surgical resection of the palatal tissue easier because it increases tension of the surgical field. Tonsillectomy is performed if not previously done.

Step 3. A mucosal incision is made on the oral side of the soft palate, starting at the midline, just above the base of the uvula along the crease created by lifting the uvula. The incision is extended bilaterally in a curvilinear fashion as far as the base

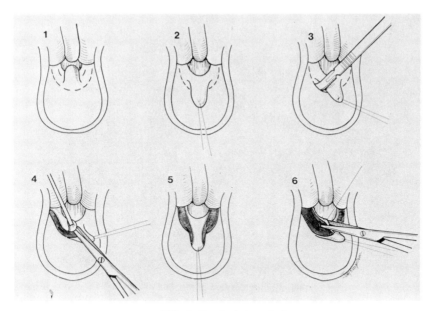

FIG. 1. Surgical steps 1–6.

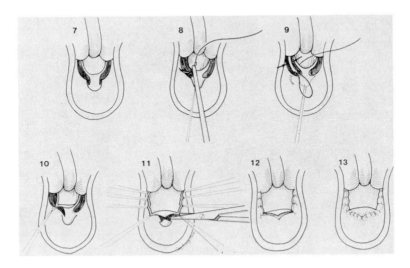

FIG. 2. Surgical steps 7–13.

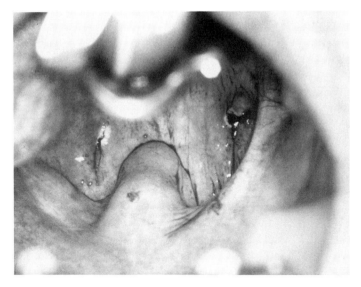

FIG. 3. Surgical view of oropharynx.

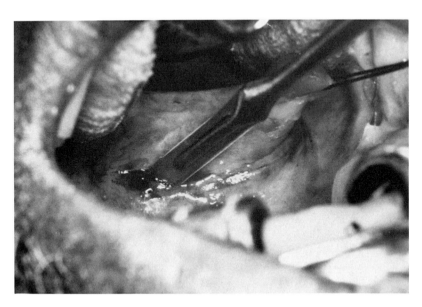

FIG. 4. Mucosal incision on the soft palate.

of the tongue. The line of the incision is 1–2 cm from the free margin of the soft palate. The mucosa and submucosal tissues are sharply dissected away between the anterior and posterior arches of the tonsillar fossa with sharp trimming scissors. Bleeding is controlled with electrocoagulation (Fig. 1, steps 3–5; Figs. 3 and 4).

Step 4. Next, redundant mucosa is removed from the rim of the posterior pillar. The mucosal edge is pulled medially with hook or forceps to stretch the lateral wall mucosa separating from the palatopharyngeal muscle. Excessive mucosa is then sharply excised, as much as necessary, along the posterior arch, but the underlying musculature is spared (Fig. 1, steps 1–6; Figs. 5 and 6).

Step 5. The palatopharyngeal muscle is grasped with forceps at its medial third and pulled anterolaterally as far as possible before it is sutured into the palatoglossal muscle with 3-0 Vicryl (Fig. 7). Several interrupted sutures are likewise placed through the muscles between the corresponding portions of the two palatal arches. In this manner, the tonsillar fossae are closed, and the redundant pharyngeal mucosa is eliminated so as to make the mucosal surface smooth and taut (Fig. 2, steps 7–10; Figs. 6 and 8).

Step 6. The uvula is amputated at the base; however, the uvula should be clamped before amputation to prevent troublesome bleeding from the uvular artery. A V-shaped incision is made on the palatal mucosa at the base of the uvula, leaving adequate mucosal flap to rotate forward to approximate the mucosal edges of the soft palate on the oral side with interrupted 4-0 Vicryl sutures (Fig. 2, steps 11–13; Figs. 9 and 10).

Step 7. When mucosal redundancy extends to the hypopharynx, it can be reduced

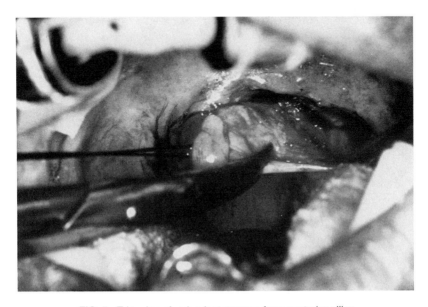

FIG. 5. Trimming of redundant mucosa from posterior pillar.

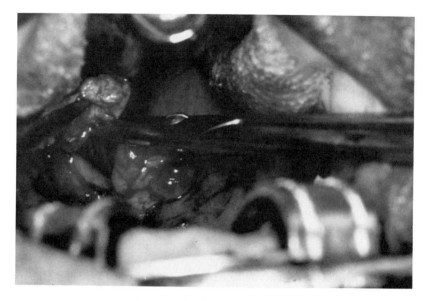

FIG. 6. Excision of redundant mucosa from posterior pillar.

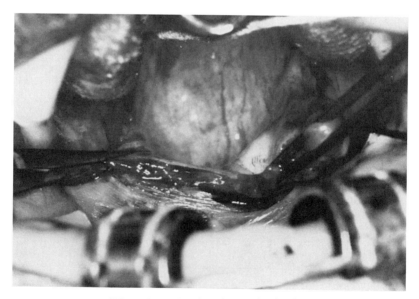

FIG. 7. Approximation of two palatal arches.

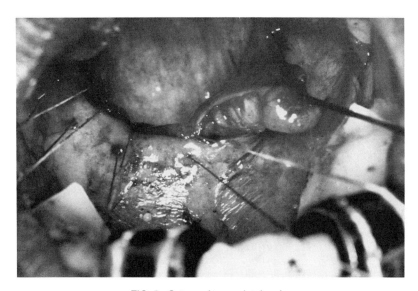

FIG. 8. Suture of two palatal arches.

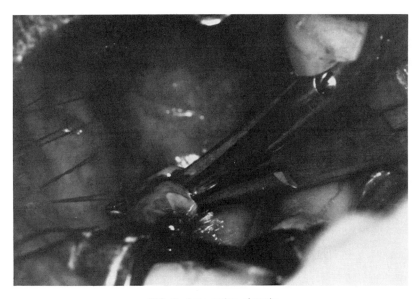

FIG. 9. Amputation of uvula.

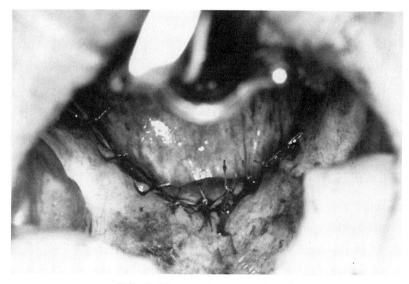

FIG. 10. Mucosal closure of soft palate.

by pulling the inferior edge of the posterior pillar upward and laterally. When excessive hypopharyngeal mucosa is drawn upward, a horizontal mucosal ridge is produced on the posterior pharyngeal wall. This is corrected by making a midline vertical incision on the posterior pharyngeal wall with an electric knife to relax mucosal tension laterally. In patients who have extensive scarring in the tonsillar

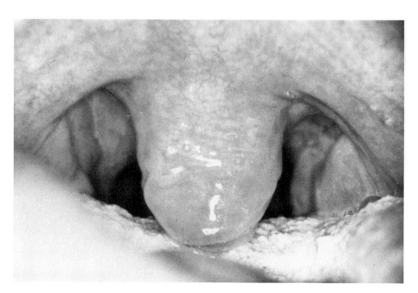

FIG. 11. Preoperative oropharynx with large uvula: apnea index $= 76/hr$, lowest $So_2 = 58\%$.

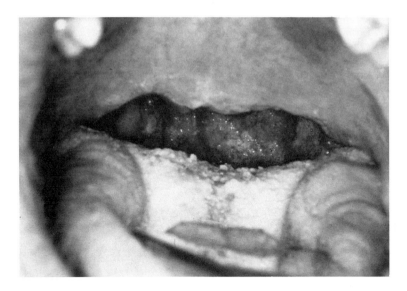

FIG. 12. Postoperative oropharynx: apnea index = 6.7/hr, lowest So_2 above 90%.

fossa from an earlier tonsillectomy, redundant mucosa may not be reduced by stretching the posterior pillar. In such cases, additional excision of the mucosa and submucosal tissues of the posterior pharyngeal wall may be necessary.

Figures 11 through 14 illustrate the presurgical and postsurgical appearance of the oropharynx, and they demonstrate a significant enlargement of oropharyngeal space

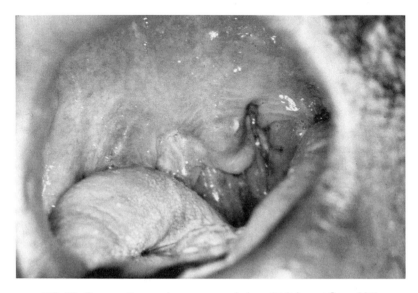

FIG. 13. Preoperative oropharynx: apnea index = 87.3, lowest So_2 = 33%.

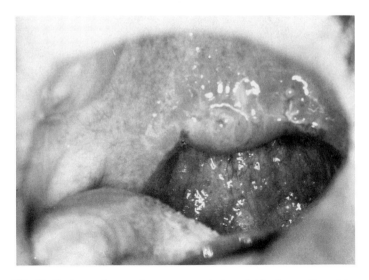

FIG. 14. Postoperative oropharynx: apnea index = 2.3/hr, lowest So_2 = 88%.

by means of UPPP, which was performed on patients with obstructive sleep apnea syndrome (OSAS).

COMPLICATIONS

Postoperative complications directly related to UPPP are minimal. No significant bleeding or local infections are noted in most of our patients who have undergone UPPP. Postoperatively, each patient receives prophylactic antibiotics, usually cephalosporin, 1 g intravenously every 6 hr for 48 hr.

Postoperative odynophagia does not significantly differ from what might be expected after tonsillectomy. Temporary nasal regurgitation may occur during the early recovery period, although it usually resolves within a week as postsurgical edema subsides. In our series, no patients have complained of persistent nasal regurgitation, voice or speech change, or persistent dysphagia. Velopharyngeal insufficiency has been reported elsewhere in a few patients (5–10%) (3), although it was not considered a major problem once all learned to swallow more cautiously (4). Its incidence is most likely related to the surgical technique. Other minor complaints include dryness or tightness of the mouth, increased gag reflex, and change in taste. However, these seem to resolve with time. No nasopharyngeal stenosis has occurred in our series, but it has been reported as a potential, if rare, complication (4). It is more likely to occur when the surgery is combined with simultaneous adenoidectomy or if extensive resection of the soft palatal arch is performed in the shallow oropharynx. This complication should be prevented by careful and appropriate surgical management during the primary operation, since it is a difficult problem to correct after it has occurred.

TABLE 1. *Subjective response to UPPP in 66 patients*

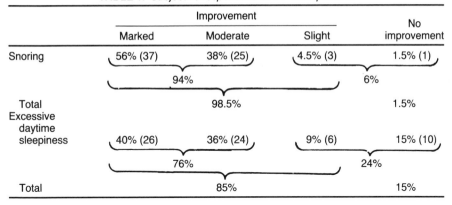

	Improvement			No improvement
	Marked	Moderate	Slight	
Snoring	56% (37)	38% (25)	4.5% (3)	1.5% (1)
	94%			6%
Total	98.5%			1.5%
Excessive daytime sleepiness	40% (26)	36% (24)	9% (6)	15% (10)
	76%			24%
Total	85%			15%

RESULTS

Our patients who undergo UPPP are evaluated 6 weeks after surgery for their subjective response as well as for objective measures of sleep patterns, nocturnal respiratory parameters (apnea and hypopnea), cardiac rhythm, oxygen saturation, and the sleep latency test by polysomnography. Those who had a tracheostomy along with UPPP keep the tracheostomy tube capped for 1 week before the sleep study. From our earlier series of 66 consecutive, unselected patients undergoing UPPP, the subjective response is shown in Table 1.

After surgical recovery, 85% of patients subjectively experienced an improvement in their excessive daytime sleepiness: 40% rated their improvement marked (appreciable), 36% rated it moderate, and 9% rated it slight. Almost all patients (98.5%) noted improvement in their snoring; 94% felt it was marked or moderate.

OBJECTIVE RESPONSE

Despite these high percentages, the subjective response to UPPP has not always been substantiated by objective measures of sleep-related respiratory impairment (apnea and hypopnea index), nocturnal oxygenation (lowest So_2 or number or duration of So_2 below 85% per hour of sleep), and sleep architecture (percent of sleep stage 1). While statistically significant post-UPPP improvements were found in the total group, there was great variability in the degree to which individual patients responded.

To better assess individual response to UPPP, we divided the patients into responders and nonresponders on the basis of the degree of postoperative changes in the number of apneas per hour of sleep (apnea index). Patients who showed a 50% or more reduction in the apnea index were placed in the responder group, whereas

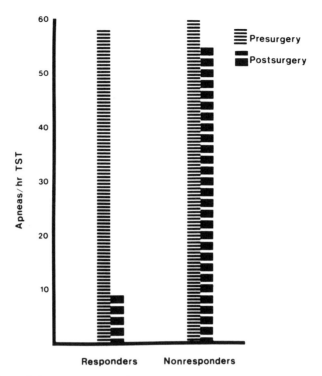

FIG. 15. Apnea index: presurgery and postsurgery responders versus nonresponders.

all others were placed in the nonresponder group. About 50% of these patients were considered as responders. The reduction from 58.3 to 9.5 in apnea index was shown for the responder group (Fig. 15), whereas no appreciable change was seen in the nonresponder group. In the responder group, there was almost total remission after surgery of the signs and symptoms of obstructive sleep apnea. Likewise, nocturnal oxygenation and sleep architecture improved dramatically. In the nonresponder group, while no significant reduction of apnea index was noted, nocturnal oxygenation improved significantly (Figs. 16 and 17) (5). The multiple sleep latency test (MSLT) is an objective measure of excessive daytime sleepiness. In the responder group, mean latency to sleep stage 1 on the MSLT increased from 3.4 to 9.6 min, which is within normal limits. In nonresponders, sleep latency on the MSLT did not change (4.4 versus 3.7 min) (Fig. 18) (6).

Simmons et al. (3) reported similar results with modified palatopharyngoplasty (PPP) performed on 155 patients with the sleep apnea syndrome. They indicated that about 50% of patients were effectively cured or considerably improved according to polysomnographic criteria, although symptomatic results in these patients again suggested a much higher success rate.

The success rate of UPPP appears to depend primarily on the patient selection

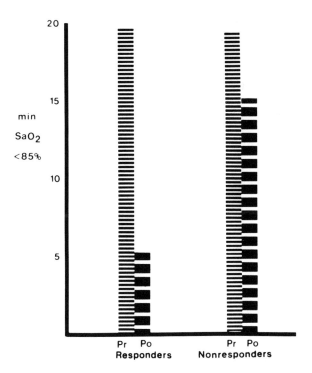

FIG. 16. SaO_2 <85% duration (min) per hour of sleep: presurgery (Pr) and postsurgery (Po), responders versus nonresponders.

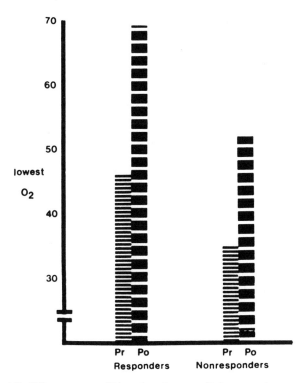

FIG. 17. Lowest O_2 (%): presurgery (Pr) and postsurgery (Po), responders versus nonresponders.

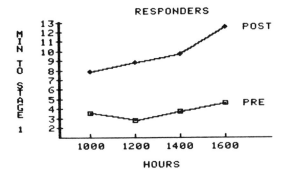

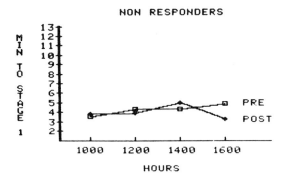

FIG. 18. Multiple sleep latency test. Latency to stage 1 (min): presurgery and postsurgery, responders versus nonresponders.

criteria, as discussed in my chapter on pharyngeal surgery (Chapter 6, *this volume*). UPPP is effective for the patient whose major airway compromise is limited to the oropharynx or velopharyngeal inlet, judged by the anatomical findings obtained from careful otolaryngological examination, fiberoptic nasopharyngolaryngoscopy with Mueller's maneuver, and cephalometric analysis (type I, type IIa).

FOLLOW-UP EVALUATION

An important question is, How long does the beneficial effect achieved with UPPP or a related procedure last after surgery? May redundant oropharyngeal tissues return over time after surgery? Does further weight gain cause its recurrence, since excessive body weight is a contributing etiologic factor? In this context, long-term follow-up evaluations on UPPP are vitally important.

One-year follow-up polysomnographic data are available in 20 of 33 responders to UPPP (7). Apnea index and nocturnal oxygenation measures did not differ significantly from the 6-week postsurgical evaluation data and remained better than pre-

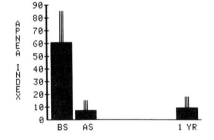

FIG. 19. One-year follow-up data (UPPP). Apnea index before surgery (BS) and after surgery (AS) at 6 weeks and 1 year.

surgical data (Figs. 19 and 20). Body weight remained stable over the entire period. Thus, 1 year after UPPP, patients maintained the improvement seen at the 6-week postoperative study.

However, three of the patients not included in the 1-year follow-up became symptomatic about 2 years after surgery and were investigated. Apnea returned to and above the presurgical levels in these patients whose body weight had increased dramatically above presurgical levels. Our impression is that as long as body weight is stable, apnea is less likely to recur.

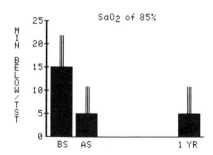

FIG. 20. One-year follow-up data (UPPP). So_2 <85% duration (min) per hour of sleep before surgery (BS) and after surgery (AS) at 6 weeks and 1 year.

REFERENCES

1. Fujita S, Conway W, Zorick F, et al. Surgical correction of anatomic abnormalities of obstructive sleep apnea syndrome: uvulopalatopharyngoplasty. *Otolaryngol Head Neck Surg* 1981;89:923–934.
2. Fee WE, Ward PH. Permanent tracheostomy: a new surgical technique. *Ann Otol Rhinol Laryngol* 1977;86:635–638.
3. Simmons FB, Guilleminault C, Miles LE. The palatopharyngoplasty operation for snoring and sleep apnea: an interim report. *Otolaryngol Head Neck Surg* 1984;92:375–380.
4. Thawley SE. Surgical treatment of obstructive sleep apnea. Symposium on sleep apnea disorder. *Med Clin North Am* 1985;69:1337–1358.
5. Fujita A, Conway WA, Zorick FJ, et al. Evaluation of the effectiveness of uvulopalatopharyngoplasty. *Laryngoscope* 1985;95:70–74.
6. Zorick F, Roehrs T, Conway W, et al. Effects of uvulopalatopharyngoplasty on the daytime sleepiness associated with sleep apnea syndrome. *Bull Eur Physiopathol Respir* 1983;19:600–603.
7. Conway W, Fujita S, Zorick F, et al. Uvulopalatopharyngoplasty. One-year followup. *Chest* 1985; 88:385–387.

C. Method of Simmons

The palatopharyngoplasty (PPP) operation is an excellent solution for chronic heroic snoring and for some patients with obstructive sleep apnea.

The technique of the PPP is illustrated in Fig. 1 (1). It is similar both in concept and execution to the technique of UPPP of Fujita et al. (2).

However, we made no attempt to recontour the uvula but resected it along with the entire posterior border of the soft palate. Preserving the uvula is unimportant. (We believe we remove more palate than Fujita et al. report that they remove in their article.)

The entire thickness of the posterior margin of the soft palate is resected along with about half of the anterior tonsillar pillar (Fig. 1A). The amount of palate resected is usually about 1.5 cm at the midline, not including the length of the uvula. Palate lengths vary, and so does the amount removed. The goal is to remove as much as possible without causing permanent nasal regurgitation. Remove too little palate, and the operation will not work. The resection should stop just short of the thick muscular part of the palate—the bulk of the levator muscles. This can be determined by palpation. The cut edge remaining will usually be about 1 cm thick. (There is an understandable tendency for most surgeons to take too little rather than

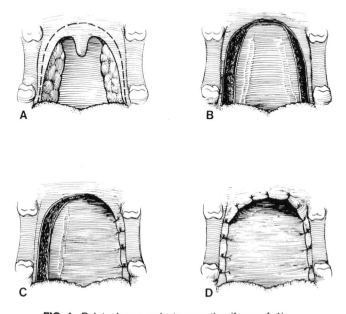

FIG. 1. Palatopharyngoplasty operation (from ref. 1).

too much palate.) Remove all of the anterior tonsillar pillar except for a 0.5-cm margin, leaving just enough tissue for suturing later on.

The tonsils, or the mucosa (with some underlying muscle) of the tonsil fossa, are removed next (Fig. 1B). The remaining posterior tonsillar pillar (pharyngopalatine arch) is then pulled forward to meet the resected edge of the anterior pillar (Fig. 1C). This stretching should eliminate all the redundant mucosa on the posterolateral pharyngeal wall. If the tissue is still redundant, resect a segment of the posterior pillar sufficient to create a smooth posterior pharynx when this tissue meets the anterior pillar. This posterior margin is then sutured to the anterior pillar, using generous bites of tissue. (Small bites will tear through, either immediately or later on. We use polyglactin suture because catgut dissolves too quickly and does not hold tissues in place long enough.) The edge of the soft palate is then sutured as an extension medially of the lateral closure (Fig. 1D). A mucosa-to-mucosa closure of the palate is done laterally, but this is usually not practical near the midline.

It is probably important to get a good mucosa-to-mucosa closure of the upper two-thirds of the tonsil–posterior pharynx excisions and the lateral half of the palate. As Fujita et al. (2) mention, there is a tendency for lateral narrowing of the oronasal aperture in the months following. Whether this narrowing is caused by muscle hypertrophy (as they suggest) or by the classic problem of scar contracture in a semicircular wound is debatable. By whatever means, the possibility for palatal stenosis is definitely a risk with this operation.

The postoperative management is similar to that of a tonsillectomy. There is considerable pain afterwards, and medication for this pain should be titrated against the known tendency of patients with sleep apnea to become obtunded by sedation. The length of the hospital stay is dictated by the patient's ability to maintain oral hydration.

There have been no serious complications. Wound infections resolve with antibiotics. About one-third of the patients have had transient and infrequent episodes of nasal regurgitation of fluids lasting up to 3 months. A few patients have some regurgitation after 6 months that will probably be permanent. None consider it a real problem. When offered the possibility of a surgical revision, they were all unwilling to risk a return to their former symptoms. None have had hypernasal speech, even though the palatal defect in some clearly does not allow for complete closure of the nasopharynx. Some patients do notice that their hypopharynx seems drier.

REFERENCES

1. Simmons FB, Guilleminault C, Silvestri R. Snoring and some obstructive sleep apnea can be cured by oropharyngeal surgery: palatopharyngoplasty. *Arch Otolaryngol* 1983;109:503–507.
2. Fujita S, Conway W, Zorick F, et al. Surgical corrections of anatomic abnormalities in obstructive sleep apnea syndrome: uvulopalatopharyngoplasty. *Otolaryngol Head Neck Surg* 1981;89:923–934.

D. Method of Fairbanks

OPERATIVE TECHNIQUE

The technique I utilize resembles Ikematsu's and Fujita's original descriptions (1,2) (see also T. Ikematsu's and S. Fujita's sections of this chapter), but it is modified to achieve what seem to be some desirable objectives: (a) to maximize the lateralization of the posterior pharyngeal pillars including submucosal musculature, which would increase the lateral dimension of the oropharyngeal airway, (b) to interrupt some of the sphincteric action of the palatal–nasopharyngeal musculature, which would increase the patency of the nasopharyngeal airway, and (c) to maximize soft palatal shortening of the soft palate in the lateral ports, while sparing midline musculature (resulting in a "squared off" soft palate appearance). This objective is important to the prevention of tethering and nasopharyngeal stenosis and to preserve mobility and function of the palate to achieve purposeful closure.

TECHNIQUE

Prophylactic antimicrobials are initiated 1 hr before surgery with intravenous ampicillin/sulbactam (Unasyn 3 g) or clindamycin 600 mg if the patient is penicillin allergic. The orally intubated and anesthetized patient is placed in the head-extended position with the Crowe–Davis tonsillectomy mouth gag and the Ring tongue blade in place.

The areas to be surgically excised are injected with small amounts of epinephrine 1:100,000 solution (usually provided in 1% lidocaine). This is to promote hemo-

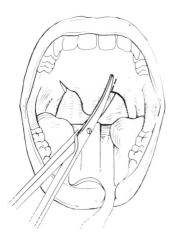

FIG. 1. Apnea patient with absent tonsils, redundant pharyngeal mucosa with longitudinal folds, and drooping soft palate with webbing between uvula and pillars. Begin procedure by severing the uvulopalatal webs. This mobilizes the posterior tonsillar pillars, releases the contracture, and prevents palatal tethering.

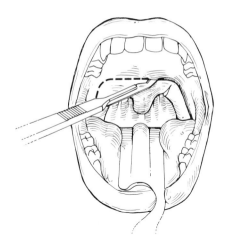

FIG. 2. Box-shaped incision through mucosa only. The incision begins at tongue base, ascends in sulcus between anterior pillar and mandible, and then turns medially to cross soft palate about midway between trailing edges of soft and hard palates.

stasis, and it is done by prior agreement with the anesthesiologist, who selects an appropriate inhalation agent (e.g., not halothane).

The mucosa on either side of the uvula is clamped with hemostats and then incised in an oblique direction as in Fig. 1. This severs the drooping mucosal web between the uvula and the posterior pillar, increases the mobility of the pillar, prevents soft palatal scar contraction (with "tethering"), and incises some of the lowermost fibers of the nasopharyngeal sphincter.

The palatopharyngeal incision is designed as three sides of a rectangle (see Fig. 2). It begins at the base of the tongue lateral to the inferior tonsillar pole and extends cephalad in the sulcus or angle formed between the internal surface of the mandible and the anterior tonsillar pillar. At about 1 cm above the level of the trailing edge of the soft palate, the incision makes a 90° angle, transverses the soft palate horizontally, then angles 90° downward again in a symmetrical fashion compared to the opposite side.

The soft palatal mucosa and submucosa with glands and fat are then stripped away from the muscular layers beginning at the horizontal palatal incision and moving downward, toward the trailing edge of the soft palate and uvula. One or two brisk bleeders will often be encountered near the corners of the incision, and they must be suture-ligated with ō plain catgut (cautery is inadequate). The uvula is amputated at the level of the trailing edge of the soft palatal muscle fibers (Fig. 3). A tiny bleeder on each of the uvula requires electrocoagulation.

Tonsils (present in one-third of snoring and apnea patients) are excised, and other soft tissues between the posterior tonsillar pillars and the lateral incisions are all stripped out, down to the muscular layers. The plane of dissection is readily apparent when a tonsillectomy is done. However, if a previous tonsillectomy was done, dense fibrous scar tissue will be encountered, which will inhibit mobilization of the posterior pillars. This fibrous scar should be carefully stripped away from the muscle fibers of the tonsillar fossa (superior pharyngeal constrictor), and the dissection

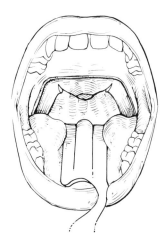

FIG. 3. Mucosa, glands, fat, and fibrous tissue removed down to—but not through—muscular layers. Uvula amputated at trailing edge of soft palatal muscle fibers.

should avoid damage to the underlying musculature and also avoid penetration of the muscle into the structures of the carotid sheath.

Bleeders are clamped and suture-ligated (which is less traumatic to the musculature than heavy electrocoagulation); good hemostasis is essential. Dissection below (inferior to) the lower pole of the tonsil is carried as far as visibility and safety allows, at which point lymphoid aggregations there and on the base of the tongue (lingual tonsils) may be reduced with gentle electrocoagulation.

The posterior tonsillar pillar is then advanced in a lateral-cephalad direction toward the corner of the palatopharyngeal incision (Fig. 4). Contiguous submucosal muscle fibers should be included in this advancement because that will increase the lateralizing effect and expand the lateral dimension of the pharyngeal airway. This maneuver should flatten out the vertical fold's redundancy of the posterior pharyngeal mucosa and smooth it out. If this does not occur, then more of the posterior pillar mucosa should be trimmed.

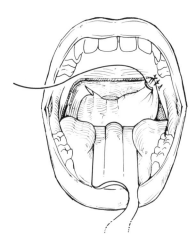

FIG. 4. Posterior pillar is trimmed and advanced in upward-outward direction to increase lateral dimension of oropharyngeal airway. Note how this tightening maneuver removes redundant pharyngeal folds.

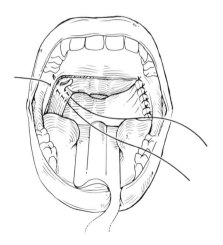

FIG. 5. Sutures pass through mucosal edges and through superficial muscular layers to (a) prevent hematoma, (b) maximize lateralization of posterior pillar, and (c) provide mucosal coverage of surgical defect.

Note, however, that the best results are obtained from anterior pillar resection, rather than posterior pillar. This is because when the intact posterior pillar is pulled forward (to cover the tonsillar fossa and meet the incision of the resected anterior pillar) the soft palate will move along forward with it, thus *enlarging* the anterior–posterior dimension of the nasopharynx. Conversely (and adversely), if the posterior pillar were to be resected, the closure would pull the anterior pillar and soft palate posteriorly, thus *narrowing* the nasopharynx (3).

The pillar is advanced and fixated into its new lateralized position with multiple sutures of 3-0 polyglycolic acid (Dexon "S") or polyglactin 910 (Vicryl). The sutures pass through the mucosa into superficial muscular layers so as to lateralize the muscular elements of the pillar as well as the mucosal. Furthermore, it eliminates "dead space" where hematoma might accumulate. I prefer to put in the second stitch before I tie the first so that the positioning is more visible (Fig. 5). Suturing then progresses downward to the tongue base where a small opening is left unsutured to allow for spontaneous drainage.

The dissection and closure on the opposite side is identical.

Then the palatal closure is accomplished as the nasal surface of the mucosa is advanced to meet the incision on the oral surface (Fig. 6). Redundant or flabby mucosa is trimmed, and the sutures are put in place, including a small amount of muscle fiber in the mucosal closure.

POSTOPERATIVE MANAGEMENT

Intravenous antimicrobial prophylaxis is maintained for 48 hr (i.e., Unasyn 3 g every 8 hr). During surgery a single dose of a corticosteroid is given (e.g., Solu-Cortef 100 mg), and if swelling/edema or excess pain begins to be apparent early in the postoperative period, a short course of steroids is given (i.e., Solu-Medrol 125 mg, up to every 4 hr for four doses, then every 8 hr for four doses).

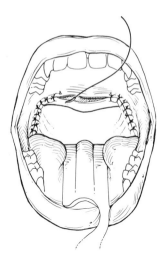

FIG. 6. Nasal surface of soft palate is advanced forward to meet cut edge on oral surface. This covers the surgical defect on oral surface and minimizes risk of stenosis. It also expands the anterior–posterior dimension of the nasopharyngeal airway. Note squared-off appearance, designed to minimize nasopharyngeal regurgitation.

Many apneic patients are already hypertensive before surgery, or they are hypertensive immediately afterwards. Salt overloading with intravenous fluids contributes to this problem, and antihypertensive therapy is often required.

Postoperative care in simple snoring patients is the same as that in adult tonsillectomy patients. However, in obstructive sleep apnea patients, pain medication is given more conservatively (i.e., low-dose parenteral morphine or oral elixir of acetaminophen with added codeine 30 mg/tsp), with the recognition that apnea is aggravated by narcotics and life-threatening loss of airway can be precipitated, especially in the postanesthetic period or the period of postoperative edema of the airway.

Similarly, antiemetics, sleeping medications, and sedative-tranquilizers can precipitate an apneic crisis; therefore, my nurses are instructed never to accept a telephone order for any of these medications by a physician who is not personally acquainted with my particular patient and his disease.

AVOIDING A TRACHEOSTOMY

Any patient with significant apnea preoperatively will need vigilant postoperative monitoring of respirations. The intensive care unit is frequently the ideal place for the first 24 hr after surgery.

Severe apnea cases who do not quite meet criteria for tracheostomy but who are, nevertheless, worrisome to the surgeon and anesthesiologist can be managed with 24–48 hr of endotracheal intubation. The oral endotracheal tube is simply left in place with 40% oxygen and mist running over its opening (a bypass connector) and frequent suctioning for secretions. The cough reflex is obtunded with occasional instillations of 2 ml of 4% lidocaine into the tube as necessary. Fortunately, narcotics and hypnotics can be administered more liberally for pain relief in such an intubated patient.

NASAL SURGERY

Some patients with combined etiologies for their obstructive sleep breathing disorders will require not only pharyngeal surgery (i.e., UPPP) but also nasal surgery, such as nasal septoplasty and submucous resection of turbinates (4,5).

While it might be safe and cost-effective to combine these procedures into a single operation for a simpler snorer, it is more risky in an apnea patient. Nasal packing itself can precipitate obstructive sleep apnea (6), and the combined effect of nasal obstruction (packing), pharyngeal edema, and postoperative sedation could cause significant airway compromise. Nasal surgery would be better done a few weeks later under local anesthesia.

REFERENCES

1. Ikematsu T. Study of snoring, 4th report. Therapy [in Japanese]. *J Jpn Otol Rhinol Laryngol* 1964; 64:434–435.
2. Fujita S, Conway W, Zorick F, et al. Surgical corrections of anatomic abnormalities in obstructive sleep apnea syndrome: uvulopalatopharyngoplasty. *Otolaryngol Head Neck Surg* 1981;89:923–934.
3. Fairbanks DNF. Uvulopalatopharyngoplasty complications and avoidance strategies. *Otolaryngol Head Neck Surg* 1990;102:239–245.
4. Fairbanks DNF. Effect of nasal surgery on snoring. *South Med J* 1985;78:268–270.
5. Fairbanks DNF. Snoring: surgical vs. nonsurgical management. *Laryngoscope* 1984;94:1188–1192.
6. Fairbanks DNF. Risks of nasal packing for epistaxis. *Otolaryngol Head Neck Surg* 1986;94:412–415.

E. Method of Dickson: How Much Palate to Resect

Uvulopalatopharyngoplasty (UPPP) is the operation recommended for snoring and obstructive sleep apnea when the major site of airway obstruction is at the soft palate level. The objective of the palatal component of the surgery is to remove as much excessive soft palatal tissue as possible without jeopardizing function.

Figure 1 is a posterior view of the palatal anatomy, demonstrating the main muscles used in palate contraction and velopharyngeal closure. The musculus uvulae provides central mounding needed for adequate palatal closure.

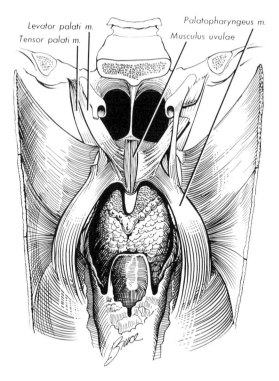

FIG. 1. Soft palatal musculature viewed from posterior (mucosa and submucosa absent).

The levator palati muscle is the main elevator of the palate. Contraction of it produces the palatal dimpling seen on the oral surface of the palate (Figs. 2 and 3). Preservation of this muscle is most important to maintain normal speech and protection of the nose from pharyngeal liquids.

Most of the palate posterior and inferior to this levator attachment—including part of the palatopharyngeus, palatoglossus, tensor palati, and the musculus uvulae—can be removed without jeopardizing the valve function of the palate (1).

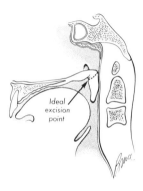

FIG. 2. Lateral view of the dimple point where the soft palate approximates the posterior pharyngeal wall for closure.

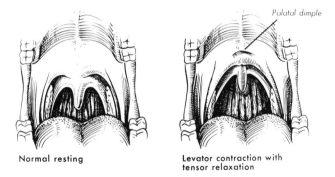

Normal resting   Levator contraction with
tensor relaxation

FIG. 3. Intraoral view of the soft palate at rest (**left**) and during nasopharyngeal closure (**right**), demonstrating dimple point.

Ideally, excision should begin just posterior and inferior to the palatal dimpling point, but it should never be above it (Figs. 2 and 4).

The dimple occurs universally 2 cm posterior to the edge of the hard palate. It should be checked preoperatively as the patient gags. If the palate lies very far anteriorly at rest, 0.5 cm more soft palate should be preserved to avoid postoperative insufficiency. The incision should be curved into the edge of the anterior pillar on both sides. As the incision is deepened in the midline, more length of the posterior part of the musculus uvulae should be saved to facilitate the central mounding on contraction.

This method, based on the underlying anatomy, will prevent reflux which is the most frequent complication of this procedure.

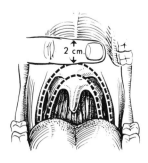

FIG. 4. Surgical incision begins immediately below the dimple point, approximately 2 cm below posterior margin of the hard palate.

REFERENCE

1. Dickson R, Blokmanis A. Treatment of obstructive sleep apnea by uvulopalatopharyngoplasty. *Laryngoscope* 1987;97:1054–1058.

F. Modification of Woodson: Transpalatal Advancement Pharyngoplasty

Uvulopalatopharyngoplasty (UPPP), the most commonly performed surgical procedure for obstructive sleep apnea (OSA), has had inconsistent success. It is highly effective in the treatment of snoring (1) and moderately effective for mild apnea. Yet, in severe apnea, using criteria of a respiratory disturbance index (RDI) of less than 20 events/hour, UPPP demonstrates a response rate in the range of 0–50% (2–4). Attempts at prospectively improving patient selection and making technical modifications have not markedly improved these rates. With the advent of nasal continuous positive airway pressure (nasal CPAP), UPPP is currently performed infrequently as an isolated procedure for severe apnea. However, expanding the surgical treatment to include other upper airway segments, in addition to the palate, has resulted in significantly improved results. Such surgery may be an alternative to nasal CPAP in selected patients with severe OSA (5,6). However, in some patients, surgical failure occurs from inadequate enlargement of the retropalatal airway. Because of these persistent abnormalities at the palatal level, transpalatal advancement pharyngoplasty was developed.

The upper airway pathology in OSA frequently involves the palate. Endoscopy, manometry, fluoroscopy, and computerized tomography (CT) have all demonstrated that in 50–80% of cases the primary site of sleeping airway obstruction is at the level of the palate (6,7). Even in nonobstructed breathing, the upper oropharynx is frequently the primary site of abnormally increased airway resistance in sleep (8). This obstruction and collapse continues after UPPP failure when observed with both manometric and endoscopic techniques (9,10).

CT scanning has demonstrated that the most collapsible upper airway segment in OSA patients in response to increasing negative pressure is the retropalatal segment. Furthermore, this segment is smaller in apneic than in nonapneic patients, with up to 70% of OSA patients during wakefulness having the retropalatal area measured at less that 1 cm^2 (11).

Following UPPP, both CT and acoustic reflection have demonstrated increases in oropharyngeal size and decreases in oropharyngeal collapsibility. Larger size and decreased collapsibility are associated with a more successful clinical response (12,13). Smaller changes in volume and compliance occur in UPPP failures. These findings suggest that retropalatal size is crucial in OSA, and UPPP failure may occur due to inadequate enlargement of the palatal segment.

Although the clinical results of UPPP on sleep and breathing have been extensively studied, the actual mechanical effects of the procedure are often speculative. Several features of UPPP may produce the desired result of increasing airway volume and decreasing compliance, including (a) removal of redundant and obstructive tissues and tonsils, (b) approximation of the posterior to anterior pillars after excising lateral wall tissues, and (c) shortening of the soft palate. Ultimately, the surgical result of UPPP may be determined by the individual anatomy of the patient and therefore be much less affected by surgical technique. For example, redundant tissue and tonsils, once removed, cannot be further excised to enlarge the airway. Approximating the tonsillar pillars and advancing soft tissues and enlarging the retropalatal airway may initially be successful, but only temporarily because of tension placed on thin tissues. Volume effects produced by palatal shortening are determined by the inherent original shape and position of the palate and may not be altered by varying surgical techniques.

Various modifications of UPPP have been proposed. Fujita et al. (14) initially conservatively excised the tonsils, redundant tissue, and uvula. Simmons et al. (15) proposed a more aggressive excision of palatal mucosa and muscle. The level of palatal excision in which complications were minimal subsequently was defined as the "dimple point," and palatal excision was extended more laterally to produce a more rectangular defect with improved results (16,17). Later, modifications included (a) a "Z-plasty" technique to prevent scar contracture of the pharynx and (b) a complete excision of the palatopharyngeus muscle, but the results are unknown (18,19).

Most proposed modifications to the UPPP may be postulated to increase oropharyngeal volume by more aggressive resection of distal soft palate and pharyngeal tissues. Such an approach is eventually limited by the potential of velopharyngeal incompetence. In the traditional UPPP, the risk of clinical velopharyngeal injury and incompetence is low, but symptomatic nasal regurgitation or speech changes are a devastating consequence of this overaggressive tissue resection. Therefore, traditional UPPP techniques are unable to compensate for collapse above the margin of the palatal excision.

Because prior modifications of UPPP may be limited by the inherent characteristics of the velopharynx, a palatopharyngoplasty was developed to increase the size of the upper oropharynx by advancing the soft palate anteriorly. This approach avoids aggressive velopharyngeal soft tissue excision, but provides a strong anterior support for advanced tissues.

PATIENT SELECTION

Patients selected for transpalatal advancement pharyngoplasty are selected on the basis of anatomic abnormalities of the palate and upper oropharynx. This includes a narrow or obstructed oropharyngeal depth and a narrow nasopharyngeal airway superior to the proposed line of resection with traditional UPPP. Initial patients selected for this procedure also were UPPP failures or had severely obstructed anatomy of both the upper and lower oropharynx which made the likelihood of UPPP success low (20). All surgical patients have a trial of nasal CPAP in an established sleep laboratory as the initial treatment. If not successful, the patient is considered for surgery. Preoperative evaluation includes complete medical work-up, clinical upper airway evaluation, endoscopic Mueller's maneuver, and cephalometry.

SURGICAL TECHNIQUE

The procedure is performed under general anesthesia delivered either oro-endo-tracheally or via tracheotomy, if present. Patients were placed supine in the Rose position, and operative exposure is obtained with a Dingman mouth gag (Pilling Instrument Co., Philadelphia, PA). All patients were administered perioperative antibiotics and dexamethasone, 10 mg. One percent lidocaine with 1:100,000 epinephrine was infiltrated into the greater palatine foramen and the planned incision sites prior to the procedure for hemostasis. Four percent cocaine-soaked pledgets were placed along the floor of the nose. The procedure is divided into three stages. The first stage involves a conservative UPPP, the second advances the soft palate, and the third advances the lateral soft palate and closes the wound.

In the first stage, the UPPP is performed in a conservative manner, excising only tonsils, redundant mucosal tissues, and the free portion of the uvula. Care is taken to preserve normal pharyngeal structures which may provide additional blood supply to the palatal flap.

In the second stage, a palatal incision is outlined beginning at the central hard palate just posterior to the alveolus and carried posteriorly, in a curvilinear "gothic arch" fashion, immediately medial to the greater palatine foramen. The incision is then flared laterally over the palpable process of the hamulus to the buccal mucosa (Fig. 1A). Residual bleeding can be controlled with further infiltration of anesthetic into the mucosal margins and a judicious electrocautery. A mucoperiosteal flap is elevated, thereby exposing the hard palate and the proximal soft palate (Fig. 1B). Centrally the mucosa is quite thin, and care must be taken to avoid laceration. More laterally there is thick fibroadipose tissue. The elevation is carried superficial to the tensor aponeurosis until the muscular palate is reached. Then, using electrocautery, the soft palate is separated from the hard palate and the nasopharynx is exposed (Fig. 1C). Frequently the septal mucoperiosteum can be left intact in the midline. Using a mastoid curette, the tensor tendon is exposed. In the initial cases the tendon was carefully elevated off the hamulus, and the hamulus was then fractured using a heavy hemostat. This allowed mobilization of the central soft palate. Subsequent experience indicated that mobilization does not always require fracturing the hamulus, and mobilization may be achieved with digital traction on the soft palate. In order to provide a space to move the soft palate, a Kerrison rongeur is then used to remove a posterior 1- to 2-cm margin of the hard palate (palatine bone). This includes the central palate exposing the posterior nasal septum (Fig. 1D). The cocaine pledgets, placed on the floor of the nose earlier, are then removed. Palatal drill holes are placed at a 45° angle to the palate, extending from the oral surface of the palate into the nasal cavity (Fig. 2). A solid segment of bone must be left between these drill holes and the excised bony margin. A large tapered free needle is then

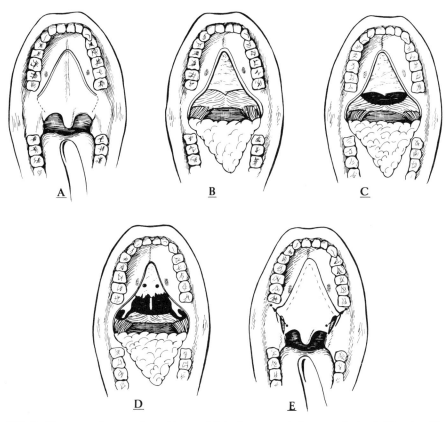

FIG. 1. Diagrammatic procedure of transpalatal advancement pharyngoplasty. **A:** Site of gothic arch incision outlined beginning posterior to alveolus and continued toward palatoglossal fold. **B:** Flap elevated. **C:** Soft and hard palate separated, thereby exposing nasopharynx. **D:** Hamulus exposed and fractured and posterior hard palate removed. **E:** Redundancy of palate mucosa shown and lateral flaps advanced and sutured to alveolar mucoperiosteum. (From ref. 21, with permission.)

used to pass a doubled single 2-0 proline suture through the drill holes into the nasopharynx. After the suture is grasped in the nasopharynx, it is withdrawn from the mouth and the free needle is cut off. This results in two strands of suture through each palatal drill hole. The sutures are then secured medially in the tensor aponeurosis and laterally in the tensor tendon in a figure-of-eight fashion (Fig. 2). The Dingman gag is helpful at this point in organizing sutures. Care must be taken in passing the sutures so they do not cut or tear the tensor tendon.

In the third stage, palatal incisions are continued laterally along the margin of the soft palate to just above the superior aspect of the palatoglossal folds. These incisions are carried down through mucosa and fibroadipose tissue, but are superficial to the muscular soft palate. This is to preserve the blood supply to the palatal mucosa which is derived from the underlying muscle. A limited undermining of the

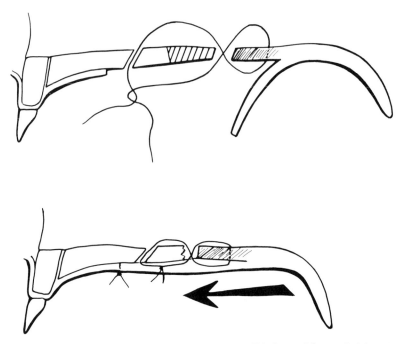

FIG. 2. Midsagittal diagram of palate demonstrating palatal drill holes and figure-of-eight suture placement. Drill holes are at a 45° angle and should be medially placed to avoid the inferior turbinate of the nose with suture placement.

flaps is then performed. The medial soft palate mucosa and muscle are then pulled forward until adequate position is obtained (Fig. 1E). A "corner" suture, using 3-0 vicryl, firmly secures this to the posterior alveolar periosteum (Fig. 3). Subsequently, the tension in this suture line is distributed through multiple simple sutures that are placed to support the flap laterally. Following the second and third stages, redundancy of palatal mucosa is present. This is carefully trimmed, and a tension-free closure is performed with fine absorbable sutures. The final closure is assisted with several millimeters of back undermining of the proximal palatal mucosa. A regular diet may begin on the first day. The use of an upper denture is avoided for at least 4 weeks, or until healing is completed.

Initial experience with transpalatal advancement pharyngoplasty noted to significant reductions in respiratory disturbance index (RDI) and apnea index (AI) is shown in Table 1. A 67% successful response rate with an RDI of less than 20 events/hour was observed in patients who only underwent transpalatal advancement. Respiratory disturbance index in the responder group decreased from 52.8 to 12.3 events/hour. Seven of 11 patients (64%) had RDI reduced to less than 20 events/hour. Supine endoscopic evaluation during quiet tidal ventilation demonstrated significant postoperative enlargement in the retropalatal space (Fig. 4). The

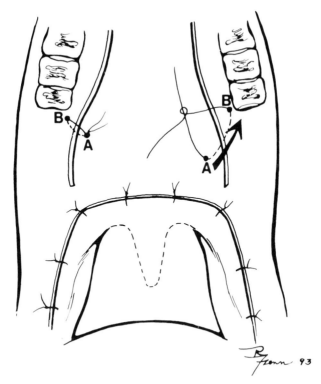

FIG. 3. Soft palate lateral advancement is performed by simple flap advancement techniques. Corner sutures are anchored in the alveolar periosteum (point B). Sutures are placed distally at the desired point of the soft palate (point A) and advanced (*arrow*).

velopharynx increased in size in an anterior posterior dimension following the procedure. With this increase in the retropalatal area, there is characteristic flattening in the configuration of the palate.

Postoperatively, all patients had complete velopharyngeal closure. Complications have been minor. Similar to experience with UPPP, transient symptoms of mild nasopharyngeal reflux may occur immediately postoperatively. Mild intermittent vallecular pooling that required multiple swallows to clear occurred in one patient. This also occurred in a second patient with both pharyngoplasty and hyoid suspension. A hyoid release procedure was performed. Symptoms resolved in both patients, and swallow studies were subsequently normal. In both cases, the potentially increased pharyngeal volume may have decreased transpharyngeal bolus pressures and contributed to delayed pharyngeal clearance. One patient developed partial palatal flap necrosis and a subsequent oronasal fistula. This occurred following the resumption of denture-wearing at 10 days postoperatively. The fistula closed spontaneously with conservative treatment. In all patients, a small area of wound breakdown occurred along the anterior palatal flap which epithelialized without treat-

TABLE 1. Respiratory results[a]

Patient number	Sex	Age	BMI (kg/m²)	Pre RDI	Post RDI	Pre AI	Post AI	Pre $O_2\%$[b]	Post $O_2\%$[b]	Status	Procedure
1	M	67	37.3	55.8	14	49.4	2	80	81	R	TAP
2	F	44	49.5	57.8	15	35.1	1	<50	—	R	TAP
3	M	36	34.3	129	73.9	127	58.3	73	76	NR	TAP
4	M	67	34.8	35	9	22	0	82	84	R	TAP
5	M	24	35.1	75.4	37	18.9	3	64	62	NR	TAP
6	M	46	43.6	62.6	11	49.6	6.1	76	66	R	TAP
7	M	56	25.5	55.4	2	15	0	72	88	R	TAP/lingualplasty
8	F	27	47	117	3	117	1.5	<50	66	R	TAP/lingualplasty
9	M	28	44.2	83.2	81.6	83.2	81.6	73	65	NR	TAP/genioplasty
10	M	34	36.4	90	27	83	25	47	66	NR	TAP/hyoid suspension
11	M	60	32.7	44.6	2.5	29.6	1	83	82	R	TAP/lingualplasty
Mean		44.5 ± 15.3	38.2 ± 6.8	73.3 ± 28.1	25.1 ± 26.9	57.3 ± 37.7	16.3 ± 26.6	68.2 ± 12.8	73.6 ± 9.1		

[a]Transpalatal advancement pharyngoplasty (TAP) as an isolated procedure ($N = 6$) and combined with other procedures ($N = 5$). All patients had clinical tongue base abnormalities on physical exam. Overall successful response (R) was 67%, and nonresponder rate (NR) was 33%. There are no differences in age or body mass index (BMI) between groups.

[b]Lowest recorded O_2 saturation by pulse oxymetry.

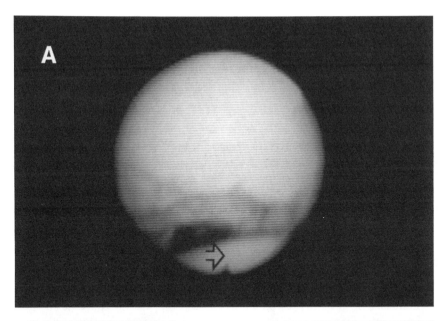

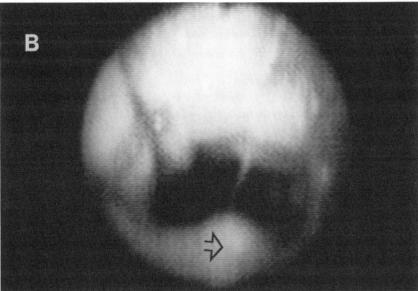

FIG. 4. In a patient with previous UPPP, preoperative (**A**) and postoperative (**B**) endoscopic views of the nasopharynx and retropalatal airway show enlargement of the retropalatal space (palate at *arrow*). Resting airway volume during quiet nonoccluded nasal respiration with the patient supine is shown.

ment. One patient who developed serious otitis media was treated with myringotomy and tube placement.

Transpalatal advancement pharyngoplasty offers a potential alternative to aggressive UPPP in an attempt to enlarge the upper oropharyngeal airway and improve respiratory function. With this procedure the soft palate, although mobilized, is not extensively distally excised. The enlargement of the airway occurs with advancement of the tensor aponeurosis which primarily moves the central palate and with lateral palatal flaps which move the lateral tissues. The bony hard palate and alveolar periosteum provide a strong structural framework to suspend tissues anteriorly. This is in contrast to the thin mucosa and musculature of the palatoglossal fold, which is the primary anterior support in UPPP. In this procedure, the lesser palatine vessels are disrupted, and vascularity is maintained through lateral and posterior pharyngeal muscles and vessels. Therefore, aggressive dissection or resection of lateral pharyngeal tissues is avoided.

An oronasal fistula may potentially occur, especially with hemorrhage or infection that would impair healing. Gentle tissue technique, careful hemostasis, perioperative antibiotics, and placement of the site of incision to minimally overlap the bone removal are recommended.

Transpalatal advancement is only a part of the surgical procedure for the treatment of OSA. All segments of the airway—nasal, palatal, tongue base, and hypopharyngeal—need to be enlarged if necessary. Transpalatal advancement should only be applied to carefully selected patients who have failed, or who are poor candidates for, alternative procedures. Because the soft palate provides blood supply to the maxillary segment if greater palatine vessel are disrupted during bimaxillary advancement surgery, transecting the palate may increase the risk of this procedure. Patients who are likely candidates for bimaxillary advancement should be considered for a more traditional palatopharyngoplasty.

The conceptual basis of transpalatal advancement pharyngoplasty is based on the observation that some patients have persistent abnormalities at the palate and retropalatal airway which may contribute to abnormal collapse, increased resistance, and subsequent obstruction during sleep, leading to failure of UPPP. Although the respiratory effects of this procedure demonstrate dramatic postoperative improvements in some patients with severe OSA, the ultimate effect will require further study.

REFERENCES

1. Pelausa EQ, Tarshis LM. Surgery for snoring. *Laryngoscope* 1989;99:1006–1010.
2. Wetmore SJ, Schima L, Snyderman NL, Hiller FC. Postoperative evaluation of sleep apnea after uvulopalatopharyngoplasty. *Laryngoscope* 1986;96:738–741.
3. Macaluso RA, Reams SC, Gibson WS, Vrabec DP, Matragrano A. Uvulopalatopharyngoplasty: postoperative management and evaluation of results. *Ann Otol Rhinol Laryngol* 1989;98:502–507.
4. Riley RW, Powell NB, Guilleminault C. Obstructive sleep apnea syndrome: a review of 306 consecutively treated surgical patients. *Otolaryngol Head Neck Surg* 1993;108:117–126.
5. Woodson BT, Fujita S. Clinical experience with lingualplasty as part of the treatment of severe obstructive sleep apnea. *Otol Head Neck Surg* 1992;107:40–47.

6. Shepard JW, Gefter WB, Guilleminault C, Hoffman EA, Hoffstein V, Hudgel DW, Suratt PM, White DP. Evaluation of the upper airway in patients with obstructive sleep apnea. *Sleep* 1991; 14:361–371.
7. Hudgel DW, Hendrick C. Palate and hypopharynx-sites of inspiratory narrowing of the upper airway during sleep. *Am Rev Respir Dis* 1988;138:1542–1547.
8. Hudgel DW. Variable site of airway narrowing among obstructive sleep apnea patients. *J Appl Phys* 1986;61:1403–1409.
9. Metes A, Hoffstein V, Mateika S, Cole P, Haight JS. Site of airway obstruction in patients with obstructive sleep apnea before and after uvulopalatopharyngoplasty. *Laryngoscope* 1991;101:1102–1108.
10. Woodson BT, Wooten MR. A multisensor solid state pressure manometer to identify the level of collapse in obstructive sleep apnea. *Otol Head Neck Surg* 1992;107:651–656.
11. Shepard JW, Garrison M, Uas W. Upper airway distensibility and collapsibility in patients with obstructive sleep apnea. *Chest* 1990;98:84–91.
12. Shepard JW, Thawley SE. Localization of upper airway collapse during sleep in patients with obstructive sleep apnea. *Am Rev Respir Dis* 1990;141:1350–1355.
13. Wright S, Haight J, Zamel N, Hoffstein, V. Changes in pharyngeal properties after uvulopalatopharyngoplasty. *Laryngoscope* 1989;99:62–65.
14. Fujita S, Conway W, Zorick F, Roth T. Surgical correction of anatomic abnormalities in obstructive sleep apnea syndrome: uvulopalatopharyngoplasty. *Otolaryngol Head Neck Surg* 1981;89:923–934.
15. Simmons FB, Guilleminault C, Silvestri R. Snoring, and some obstructive sleep apnea, can be cured by oropharyngeal surgery. *Arch Otolaryngol* 1983;109:503–507.
16. Dickson RI, Blockmanis A. Treatment of obstructive sleep apnea by uvulopalatopharyngoplasty. *Laryngoscope* 1987;97:1054–1058.
17. Moran WB, Orr WC. Diagnosis and management of obstructive sleep apnea, part II. *Arch Otolaryngol* 1985;111:650–658.
18. Koopman CF, Moran WB. Surgical management of obstructive sleep apnea. *Otolaryngol Clin North Am* 1990;23:787–808.
19. O'Leary MJ, Millman RP. Technical modification of uvulopalatopharyngoplasty: the role of the palatopharyngeus. *Laryngoscope* 1991;101:1332–1335.
20. Wittig R, Fujita S, Fortier J, Zorick F, Potts G, Roth T. Results of uvulopalatopharyngoplasty (UPPP) in patients with both oropharyngeal and hypopharyngeal collapse on Mueller's maneuver. *Sleep Res* 1988;17:269.
21. Woodson BT, Toohill RJ. Transpalatal advancement pharyngoplasty for obstructive sleep apnea. *Laryngoscope* 1993;103:269–276.

G. Method of Coleman: Laser-Assisted Uvulopalatoplasty

The laser-assisted uvulopalatoplasty (LAUP) is a technique that was developed by Dr. Yves-Victor Kamami in Paris, France in the late 1980s (1); it was introduced to the United States in 1992 as a treatment for snoring *without apnea.*

The procedure is designed to correct breathing abnormalities during sleep caused by airway obstruction and soft tissue vibration at the level of the soft palate by reducing the amount of tissue in the velum and uvula.

A very select group of patients who have obstruction at only the level of the soft palate are responsive to this treatment. However, in the majority of apnea patients the obstruction occurs at several levels in the airway (2), and this procedure directs attention to only one anatomic portion of the airway.

DESCRIPTION OF PROCEDURE

The procedure is performed with the patient sitting in an exam chair in the upright position. Prior to treatment, the patient is given certain instructions. The patient is requested to relax the tongue. This is for a couple of reasons. First, the patient (in attempts to be cooperative) will very often lower the anterior portion of the tongue, intending to give better visualization to the oropharynx. In reality, lowering the anterior tongue raises the posterior tongue, and the surgeon will find it a constant struggle to push the posterior tongue down. Also, if the patient is actively moving his or her tongue, the tendency is for the palate to move as well, and the surgeon winds up chasing a moving target.

The patient then is given breathing instructions. The patient may either take a deep breath and very slowly let it out, or the patient may take a deep breath and hold it. The palate is more stable during breath-holding than during slow exhalation, and the forced exhalation at the end of the breath-holding blows any smoke and laser plume out of the oral cavity so it will not be inhaled or swallowed. The laser plume is very irritating and can result in respiratory irritation or coughing and/or nausea if inhaled or swallowed.

The patient is also informed that as the posterior palate and pharynx become numb, he or she will lose the sensation of swallowing and breathing. The loss of this tactile feedback can cause concern in some patients, and the patient must be reassured that he or she is able to swallow and breathe without obstruction.

Once the patient understands these instructions, the anesthetic can be administered. Our choice for anesthetic is a 10% lidocaine spray in a metered dose form. Three to four sprays, each one administering approximately 10 mg of lidocaine, are placed along the posterior palate and uvula (Fig. 1). After giving adequate time for this spray to take effect, a solution of 1% lidocaine with 1:100,000 epinephrine is infiltrated at the base of the uvula on both sides, with a 27-gauge needle and 1-c.c. syringe. Between 0.5 and 1 c.c. are infiltrated on each side (Fig. 2).

Other anesthetic options can be used. If gagging is a problem, 10 mg of diazepam orally 1 hr before the procedure is beneficial, along with a nose spray of 1:1 solution of tetracaine hydrochloride 0.5% and phenylephrine hydrochloride 0.5%. In patients who travel a long distance or in whom long-term anesthetic is desired, bupivacaine hydrochloride 0.25% can also be mixed in with the anesthetic solution as well. Adequate time is allowed for the anesthetic to take effect and for vasoconstriction to occur.

It is important not to inject too superficially, creating a bleb of anesthetic in the

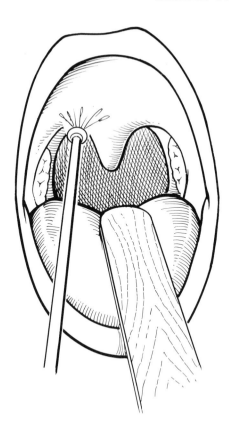

FIG. 1. Diagram of topical anesthetic being applied to the posterior palate and uvula.

tissue, nor is it desirable to go through and through the palate and spray the posterior pharyngeal wall with the anesthetic solution and not infiltrate the tissue itself.

The procedure is performed with a carbon dioxide laser. The carbon dioxide laser was selected because of its familiarity to most practicing otolaryngologists, as well as its availability to otolaryngologists in the outpatient clinic and office settings. It is a very precise tool insofar as its ability to give very fine incisions, and its tissue interaction is favorable for this type of procedure. Although it is not the best coagulating laser available, it has adequate coagulation for the diameter of most vessels encountered with this procedure. The carbon dioxide laser is used at a power setting of between 15 and 20 watts, depending upon the thickness of tissue that is to be incised, and in a continuous mode. The beam is used in a focus mode for cutting, and it is used in a defocused mode for ablation and vaporization. A handpiece with a backstop to protect the posterior pharyngeal wall from stray laser energy should be used.

The surgeon prepares himself by wearing protective goggles, mask, and gloves, as well as protective clothing. All personnel in the room should wear adequate eye

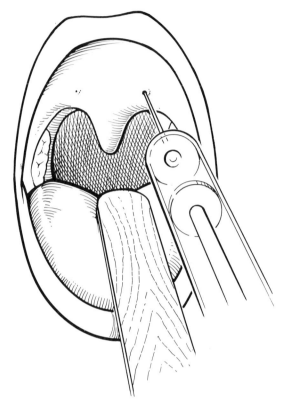

FIG. 2. Diagram showing the location of the injection points for the local anesthetic.

protection for the carbon dioxide laser. The standard safety precautions for use of the carbon dioxide laser should be followed at all times during the procedure.

Once the adequate level of anesthesia has been achieved in the soft palate, the carbon dioxide laser is then used to make bilateral vertical incisions through and through the palate at the base of the uvula (Fig. 3). These incisions are approximately 5° off the vertical and oriented from medial-inferior to lateral-superior, and the length of the incision is approximately 1 cm. The author uses the length of the backstop on the laser handpiece as the gauge for incision length. Taking the incisions much higher will usually result in increased postoperative pain for the patient, as well as some tendency to bleed at the apex of the incision. Once the palatal incisions have been made, then the uvula is shortened and reshaped. The uvula is reduced by approximately 50% of its length and is reshaped in a curved fashion, as a normal uvula would be shaped (Fig. 4). One can retract the tip of the uvula anteriorly and vaporize the central portion of the uvula muscle while leaving the mucosa intact. This may result in less postoperative pain. Once this has been accomplished, the procedure is finished. The patient is allowed to rinse the mouth with cool water

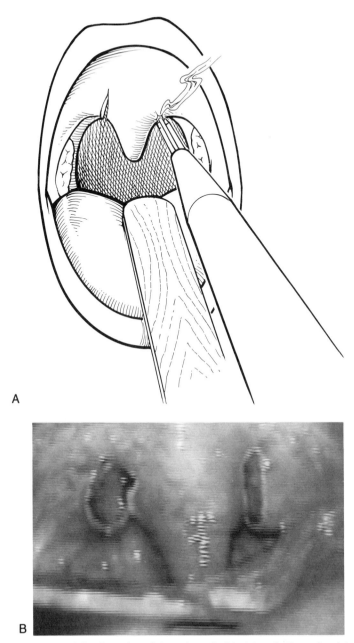

FIG. 3. A: Diagram of the through and through vertical incisions in the soft palate. **B:** Clinical photograph of the vertical palate incisions having been completed.

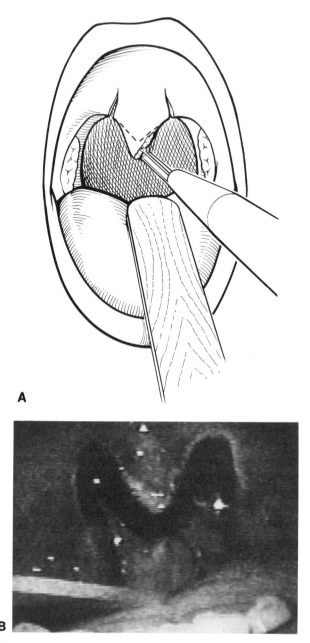

FIG. 4. A: Diagram showing the extent of laser ablation of the uvula. **B:** Clinical photograph of the uvula after the first stage of ablation.

(taking the heat out of the tissues) and can then leave the clinic and return either to home or to work.

Vaporization may also be accomplished by an instrument called a "Swiftlase" (Sharplan Lasers, Inc., 1 Pearl Ct., Allendale, NJ). This is used in a focused mode and the same power setting. This instrument rapidly rotates the beam in a 3-mm arch thus producing less char while ablating the tissue more rapidly.

POSTOPERATIVE PERIOD

After the procedure, the patient is given a prescription for pain medicine and antibiotic for approximately 5–7 days. The patient is instructed to gargle with a solution of 1 tablespoon of peroxide in a cup of water in the morning and evening to reduce the eschar on the tissue as rapidly as possible. The patient is also instructed to take acetaminophen in the morning and evening to take the edge off of the pain and to reduce the need for narcotic-type pain medication.

There are no absolute dietary restrictions; however, it is suggested that the patient stick to a soft diet the first day or two, and many patients find that extremes of temperature and carbonated fluids cause increased discomfort. It is also found that foods high in acid content, such as citrus drinks and foods containing tomatoes, will also give a burning sensation in the palate after this procedure has been performed. A topical anesthetic throat lozenge is often found to be beneficial in controlling discomfort around mealtime.

SUBSEQUENT PROCEDURES

The palate is allowed to heal over the next 3–4 weeks (Fig. 5). One may perform the next procedure sooner than that in the initial stages; however, as one reaches the final stages of the procedure, it is suggested that the healing phase of at least 4 weeks be allowed to occur so that one has an idea of how much retraction the palate will undergo before resecting any more.

The subsequent procedures are basically the same as the initial procedure, in that the palatal incisions are again created along with shortening and reshaping of the uvula. As one nears the completion of the treatment course, one must examine the palate and determine if attention is needed in other areas. Specifically, in some instances one will start to notice some increase in vibratory tissue laterally as the incisions extend towards the junction of the hard and soft palates. If this begins to occur, then the vaporization can be taken lateral to the palatal incisions to reduce this amount of tissue. Also as the retraction occurs, the palate will come anteriorly and superiorly, and this may tether the posterior tonsillar pillars, causing them to medialize. Should this occur and the pillars themselves begin to obstruct the airway, they can be released with a horizontal incision at the superior aspect of the pillar, through and through the pillar, thus releasing it (Fig. 6). At the same time, if the tonsils are still present, they may begin to rotate into the airway as well, and by the

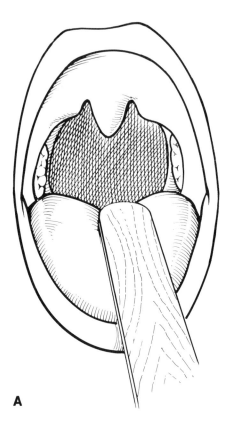

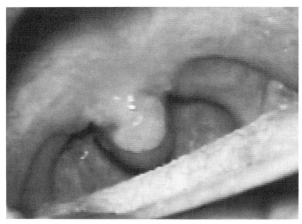

FIG. 5. A: Diagram of the soft palate and uvula after healing. Note the location of possible "dog ear" formation lateral to the incisions. These may need to be vaporized on subsequent sessions. **B:** Clinical photograph of the soft palate and uvula 4 weeks after the first stage of resection.

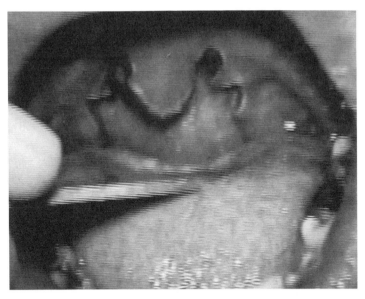

FIG. 6. The posterior tonsil pillars have been incised to release them. Note how the tissue tends to spread open without the need for vaporization.

third or fourth procedure if this is occurring, then they can be superficially vaporized after first anesthetizing this surface.

DETERMINATION OF ENDPOINT

The endpoint for this procedure is determined by any one or combination of the following factors:

1. If the patient is happy. When the patient's snoring is decreased and the patient and the spouse are now happy and do not wish to proceed with any further procedures, this is a legitimate point at which to stop.
2. If the snoring is gone. Again, this is the major goal of this procedure, and once the snoring has stopped, this indicates that the vibratory tissue is now gone and any further resection would run the risk of creating a situation of velopharyngeal incompetence.
3. If the patient is unable to make any snorting sound. If the patient still has noisy breathing but is unable to make a snorting sound, this should alert the surgeon that the patient is having noisy breathing from other tissue vibrating, such as in the region of the base of the tongue, and not necessarily at the soft palate. Any further resection of the soft palate after the patient is no longer able to snort will run the risk of excising too much tissue and creating velopharyngeal incompetence.

COMPLICATIONS

The complication rate for this procedure has been extremely low. There has been some postoperative bleeding which has occurred in the immediate post-op period, and this has responded to silver nitrate cauterization. The point of bleeding is usually at the apex of the incision and is generally due to overly aggressive incision.

Permanent voice changes, velopharyngeal insufficiency, temporary or permanent nasal reflux, and dehydration from the inability to take food or liquid orally have not been seen with this procedure.

The only infections that has been seen by the author has been two iatrogenic Candida infections of the oral cavity from the use of postoperative oral antibiotics. These have responded nicely to oral antifungal agents.

Pain associated with the procedure has not been incapacitating, and all patients have been able to attend classes or work in their normal routine. Most patients have reported some degree of weight loss, maximum being between 10 and 15 pounds over the course of the treatment. This has been a desirable side effect.

There has been an increased amount of pain associated with this procedure if the excision is more aggressive and more tissue is damaged. In our series of patients, approximately 20% have required only acetaminophen for pain management throughout the course of procedures, while 10% or 15% at the opposite end of the spectrum have required narcotic pain relief for upwards to 3 weeks after each procedure. On the average, there is little or no pain perceived for the first day or two, after which there is the acute onset of discomfort, which lasts from 7 to 10 days. During this time, narcotic-type pain reliever, such as acetaminophen with codeine, is required.

PROGRESSION OF RELIEF

The number of procedures required to achieve relief of symptoms has ranged between one procedure and seven procedures. With someone who has snoring without any evidence of apnea, the range is usually two to five procedures, and if apnea is present, there are usually five to seven procedures.

When there is less tissue to deal with, fewer procedures are needed—for example, in women who may have very long, thin palates and uvulas that are quite membranous and respond well to one or two treatments.

A decrease is seen in the subjective symptoms before a change in the objective symptoms. Usually after the first or second procedures the patients begin to feel that they are sleeping better and that they are better rested when they awaken in the morning, and the spouse will very often notice an improvement in mood. On the subsequent procedures one will start to see a decrease in the amount of snoring sounds, to the point that by the third or fourth procedure the snoring has been almost eliminated. The couples who have been sleeping apart are usually back in the same bedroom by the end of the third procedure.

CONCLUSION

This procedure opens the airway at the level of the palate and reduces vibratory tissue in the palate and uvula. It is a serial procedure assisted with a laser in an ambulatory office setting under local anesthetic. This is a cost-effective, simple, safe, and reliable procedure, and the author would suggest that surgeons consider adding this to their armamentarium of treatments for patients with sleep associated breathing disorders.

REFERENCES

1. Kamami Y-V. *Laser CO_2 for snoring: preliminary results. Acta Otorhinolaryngol Belg* 1990;44:451–456.
2. Sher A. *Obstructive sleep apnea and the otolaryngologist. Bull Am Acad Otolaryngol Head Neck Surg* 1991;10(9):12–13.
3. Crocker BD, Olson LG, Saunders NA, et al. *Estimation of the probability of disturbed breathing during sleep before a sleep study. Am Rev Respir Dis* 1990;142:14–18.
4. Young T, Palta M, Dempsey J, Skatrud J, Weber S, Badr S. The occurrence of sleep disordered breathing among adults. *N Engl J Med* 1993;328:1230–1235.

EDITOR'S NOTE

As of September 1993 the American Academy of Otolaryngology—Head and Neck Surgery had neither endorsed nor disputed the claims of effectiveness of laser-assisted uvulopalatoplasty for the treatment of snoring. Members of the Committee on Sleep Disorders of the Academy have expressed caution that there are no data as yet to support a claim of its being effective in treatment of obstructive sleep apnea. It is unfortunate, even embarrassing to our profession, that mass media publicity campaigns were launched well in advance of the scientific validation of this procedure's efficacy. (It is a marketing strategy reminiscent of the acupuncture movement of the 1970s and of other ill-fated medical "cures." See Fairbanks DNF. Unproven remedies for deafness. *Ear Nose Throat J* 1981;60:530–542. Also see *Miracle cures for deafness.* Triological Society thesis, 1975.)

Snoring and Obstructive Sleep Apnea, Second Edition,
edited by D.N.F. Fairbanks and S. Fujita.
Raven Press, Ltd., New York © 1994.

8

Limitations, Pitfalls, and Risk Management in Uvulopalatopharyngoplasty

George P. Katsantonis

Department of Otolaryngology, Saint Louis University Hospital, St. Louis, Missouri 63139

Uvulopalatopharyngoplasty (UPPP), which was introduced in 1979, continues to be the most commonly performed surgical procedure for obstructive sleep apnea (OSA) and socially disruptive snoring. The operation has been proven extremely successful for habitual snoring and effective in managing OSA in the majority (70%) of carefully selected patients. Because of satisfactory results and relatively low morbidity rate, UPPP is now performed widely. Nevertheless, the surgical procedure is associated with risks and complications of varying severity. Although the majority of the postoperative sequelae are mild, causing only an inconvenience to the individual, occasionally it can be associated with significant disability and may even have catastrophic consequences. Knowledge of the entire spectrum of complications is therefore important not only for their prevention and effective management once they have occurred but also for the correct preoperative counseling of the surgical candidates.

Complications of UPPP can be classified into three groups: (i) perioperative, (ii) early postoperative, and (iii) late postoperative. Perioperative complications are listed in Table 1. Regardless of the surgical procedure performed, patients with OSA are predisposed to specific complications because of anatomical abnormalities of the airway and the existence of the underlying OSA. Perioperative airway obstruction, or even narrowing of the pharyngeal lumen due to edema or hemorrhage which will accentuate the underlying OSA, is a potentially disastrous occurrence and is associated with high mortality rates. Almost all of the 16 deaths and 17 near-fatalities anecdotally reported by various surgeons following UPPP were caused by perioperative loss of the airway (1). Complications related to the airway represent approximately 75% of all perioperative complications of UPPP (2). Causes of perioperative airway loss are (a) airway flaccidity and collapse due to preoperative or intraoperative administration of narcotics, (b) unsuccessful intubation during induction of anesthesia, (c) postoperative pharyngeal edema, and (d) postoperative hemorrhage (Table 2).

Preoperative sedation should be avoided in patients with moderate or severe OSA

TABLE 1. *UPPP perioperative complications*

Airway obstruction
Cardiopulmonary sequelae
Loss of respiratory drive due to O_2 administration
Emergence of previously undiagnosed central apnea

because the additive effects of muscle relaxation, drowsiness, and ventilatory suppression will precipitously exacerbate OSA. It has been suggested that only muscle relaxants and anesthetics capable of rapid reversal should be used in patients with OSA (3). Depression of respiration due to narcotics [particularly the phenylpyridine derivatives (meperidine, fentanyl)] is dose-dependent, and their effect may persist for hours. In addition to respiratory depression by direct action on the brainstem respiratory centers, narcotics interfere with higher respiratory centers, resulting in increase of respiratory pauses, delayed expiration, and/or periodic breathing (4). The use of intraoperative narcotics (fentanyl or sufentanil), particularly in high doses (9.5 μg/min or 2.9 μg/kg), was found to be the most critical risk factor for airway loss in OSA patients, after extubation, by Esclamado et al. (2).

Unsuccessful intubation during induction of anesthesia may be a result of the anatomical abnormalities causing or contributing to the patient's OSA or individual variations of the upper airway anatomy. The anesthesiologist should carefully evaluate, in advance, the position of the hyoid bone, the relative placement of the larynx within the airway, the position and size of the base of the tongue, the thickness of the neck, adipose tissue deposits in the posterior cervical area, cervical spine limitations, and mandibular abnormalities. Induction of anesthesia and airway control in many OSA patients is a critical point, and fatalities have been reported due to airway loss at this stage (2). Preparedness is the best way to avoid a catastrophe. The anesthesiologist should be familiar with alternate intubation techniques (nasal blind intubation, awake intubation, fiberoptic intubation) and the surgeon and operating room personnel should be prepared for upper airway control by conventional tracheostomy or cricothyrotomy.

Postoperative pharyngeal and/or base of tongue edema will have a compounded effect on an already unstable airway and contribute to airway obstruction following extubation. The incidence of significant pharyngeal edema following an uncomplicated UPPP should be very low. According to Sanders et al. (5), there was no significant deterioration in OSA in the early postoperative period in patients undergoing UPPP. On the contrary, Powell et al. (6) have reported that base of tongue edema is a common occurrence following UPPP and may result in acute airway obstruction or

TABLE 2. *Causes of perioperative airway loss (in order of frequency)*

Use of narcotics
Unsuccessful intubation upon induction of anesthesia
Postoperative airway edema
Postoperative hemorrhage

exacerbation of OSA. If airway compromise is evident following extubation, then insertion of a nasopharyngeal airway will usually alleviate this problem. However, if airway compromise persists when the patient is fully awake, then a tracheostomy should be performed. If, on the other hand, airway instability is present only during sleep, then nasal continuous positive airway pressure (CPAP) application is recommended. In the author's series, patients with severe OSA were successfully fitted with nasal CPAP in the immediate post-UPPP period. Overnight endotracheal reintubation is another option.

Patients with moderate-to-severe OSA (those suffering a hundred or more apneic events per night with prolonged episodes and significant oxygen desaturations) are at highest risk for postoperative airway compromise (from the combined effects of surgical-site swelling, sedative/analgesics, and the disease itself). They are most safely managed with careful monitoring of respiration and oxygenation (oximetry) the first postoperative night. In many institutions the intensive care unit is the ideal place for such monitoring. Elsewhere in the hospital would be satisfactory if the nurses and attendants have been educated about the special risks and needs of these patients.

Airway loss may also occur because of postoperative hemorrhage. Hematoma formation in the submucosal compartments of the posterior and lateral pharyngeal walls, tonsillar fossa, and possibly tongue base may result in upper airway compromise. Active bleeding will also have an adverse effect on the upper airway either directly or because of iatrogenic manipulations. Therefore, tracheostomy may be necessary in such cases for securing the airway before surgical manipulations or induction of anesthesia for hemorrhage control.

The effect of O_2 administration in OSA patients, particularly in the postoperative period, remains a controversial issue. Decrease of respiratory drive because of loss of the hypoxemic stimulus in hypercapnic patients is a well-established phenomenon. However, in patients with OSA, several authors have demonstrated that O_2 administration prolongs apnea events, whereas others have observed no change or even reduction in apnea following O_2 administration (7–9). Patients with severe OSA may be susceptible to medical complications such as hypertension, cardiac arrhythmias, cor pulmonale, and congestive heart failure, conditions commonly associated with their underlying disease. Detailed analysis of these complications is beyond the scope of this chapter.

Early post-UPPP complications in order of frequency are: transient velopharyngeal incompetence (VPI), wound dehiscence, hemorrhage, and wound infection (Table 3). The incidence of early VPI ranges from 20% to 100% according to

TABLE 3. *Early post-UPPP complications (in order of frequency)*

Transient velopharyngeal incompetence
Wound dehiscence
Hemorrhage
Wound infection

various reports and is usually manifested with mild nasal regurgitation and less commonly with hypernasal speech (1). In the vast majority of patients, symptoms are mild and subside within 2–3 weeks. A small number of patients, however, continue to display mild regurgitation for prolonged periods of time or indefinitely. Self-training usually controls this problem and it rarely requires correction. Although hypernasal speech is less commonly noted, careful observation may show that fricative and plosive speech sounds are weaker in many patients.

Dehiscence of the lateral pharyngeal mucosal wounds is a common postoperative occurrence, but it is not clear whether this should be considered as a complication. According to Moran (10), the lateral pharyngeal wall wounds are left unsutured to heal by secondary intention. Many reports advocate the use of semipermanent sutures (polyglycolic acid or polyglactin) in order to minimize the chance of dehiscence (11,12). This author contends that nasopharyngeal dehiscence is caused by continuous pharygneal mobility during swallowing and tension of the pharyngeal mucosa and that the type of suture plays only a minimal role in this complication. Meticulous suturing without excessive tension and with substantial tissue "bites," as well as suturing in layers, will decrease the incidence of dehiscence postoperatively.

In the author's series there is approximately 4% incidence in delayed and 2% incidence in immediate post-UPPP bleeding. Nevertheless, no life-threatening hemorrhage early or delayed has been seen in this series. There are anecdotal reports of severe early postoperative bleeding occasionally associated with fatalities possibly due to iatrogenic injury of the carotid artery or other major arterial vessel. In one case a fatal delayed postoperative bleeding was thought to have been caused by a wound infection eroding into a major artery. Avoidance of transection of the pharyngeal constrictor muscle fibers is thought to be a major factor in avoiding severe postoperative bleeding.

There are no data concerning pharyngeal wound infection and/or the use of antibiotics after UPPP. Potentially all oropharyngeal wounds are infected due to contamination by the oropharyngeal flora. Nevertheless, infection subsides as the healing progresses and rarely constitutes an adverse factor in the postoperative course. Data collected from reports on antibiotic use after tonsillectomies suggest that the incidence of postoperative morbidity is lessened by antibiotic therapy, a fact which should apply to the UPPP operation (13).

Late post-UPPP complications are listed in Table 4. Approximately 20% of the patients complain of prolonged vague complaints related to their pharynx. This is usually expressed as "throat tightness," "dryness," "increased pharyngeal secretions," "food caught in throat," inability to initiate swallowing, disturbances of taste, and numbness of tongue. Some patients will also complain of persistent sore throat. The majority of these complaints are thought to be related to wound healing and contracture. These symptoms usually diminish with time. Nevertheless, a small number of patients may have these symptoms indefinitely. According to Finkelstein et al. (14), the absence of the uvula may be related to most of these symptoms. The uvula, according to this author, represents an active organ uniquely structured in humans. There is abundance of seromucinous salivary glands intermixed in a net-

TABLE 4. *Late post-UPPP complications (in order of frequency)*

Pharyngeal discomfort, dryness, tightness
Postnasal secretions
Food catching in throat
Inability to initiate swallowing
Prolonged sore throat
Taste disturbance
Speech disturbance
Tongue numbness
Permanent velopharyngeal incompetence
Nasopharyngeal stenosis

work of muscle fibers and large, voluminous excretory ducts. These histologic findings support the notion that the uvula is a lubricating organ particularly useful during speech, and possibly it is a phylogenetic development of an accessory speech organ. The likelihood of persistent throat dryness or other related minor, albeit bothersome, complaints should be mentioned during the preoperative counseling of patients undergoing UPPP.

It has also been reported that the loss of uvula following UPPP is responsible for the loss of vocal trill, which is a sound used in certain languages (Dutch, French, German, Arabic, Hebrew, Greek, Russian, Spanish, Persian, Turkish). The uvula is the primary structure implicated in the production of vocal trill. The loss of this sound may be extremely bothersome to individuals speaking these languages and could result in litigation (15).

The sensation of "food caught in the throat" is possibly a manifestation of mild velopharyngeal incompetence, caused by small food particles deposited on the dorsal surface of the shortened palate.

Occasionally patients complain of distortion of taste and or numbness of the tongue. The possible explanation is the prolonged pressure of the tongue base by the blade of the Crowe–Davis mouth gag. The bulkiness of the tongue encountered in many OSA patients may be a significant factor in this complication (16). Shifting the tongue blade from one side to the other or intermittently releasing the tension particularly during prolonged operations may lessen the incidence of this complication.

The incidence of permanent significant VPI severe enough to warrant surgical intervention is extremely low (0.5% according to the author's series). This complication usually manifests itself with nasal regurgitation. Permanent noticeable speech defect is extremely uncommon following UPPP (17).

Several techniques have been reported regarding the appropriate amount of palate removal in order to avoid VPI (18,19). Obviously, a maximal amount of palate must be removed while preserving the function of the velopharyngeal sphincter. It is reasonable to assume that the amount of palate to be removed will be directly proportional to the length of the palate and inversely proportional to the depth of the pharynx. Previously a fixed point, the caudal end of the levator palatini muscle, has

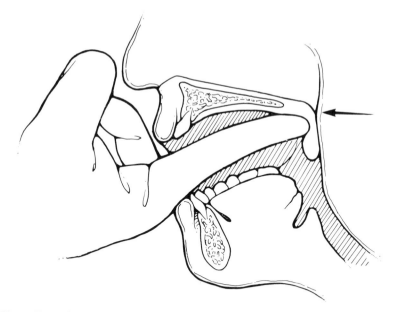

FIG. 1. The soft palate is displaced posteriorly to the point of contact with the posterior pharyngeal wall in order to determine the amount of palate to be resected.

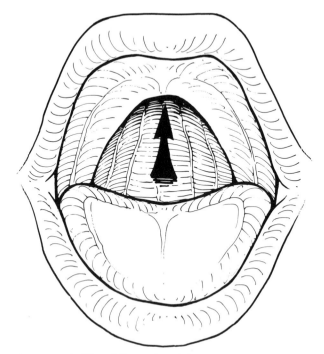

FIG. 2. Aggressive removal of the midline region of the soft palate will result in velopharyngeal incompetence.

been proposed as a landmark of the limit of resection. However, this point may overlap, or fall away from, the posterior pharyngeal wall, depending on the depth of the pharynx and the length of the palate. The amount of palate to be resected proposed by this author is as follows: After induction of anesthesia the midsection of the palate is displaced rostrally until the palate meets the posterior pharyngeal wall (Fig. 1). This point is marked on the ventral surface of the palate. The incision is then carried from this point laterally in a horizontal fashion, extending to the anterior tonsillar pillars and then curved down on the lateral aspect of the anterior pillars to the level of the inferior tonsillar pole. The central region of the palate is functionally the most important, and therefore aggressive resection in this area will result in insufficiency (Fig. 2). The configuration of the palatal incision ensures a conservative midline excision, where the velopharyngeal sphincter function is mostly needed; it also provides maximal resection laterally, resulting in enlargement of the oropharyngeal lumen (Fig. 3) (20).

If surgical correction for VPI is contemplated, the severity of the OSA should always be considered because the OSA will usually be exacerbated following correction of this complication. The author advocates against palate push-back procedures and nasopharyngeal flaps because they will invariably accentuate OSA. Teflon paste injection in the submucosal layer of the posterior pharyngeal wall has been reported as an effective method for treating VPI (21). Furthermore, the effects can easily be reversed by removing the injected substance if OSA recurs. The procedure of Teflon paste injection is simple and well-tolerated and can be performed

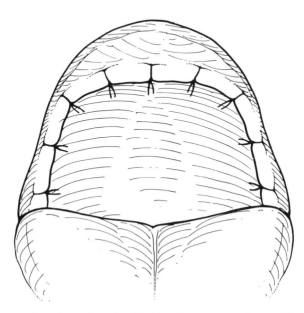

FIG. 3. Correct configuration of the palatal incision ensures competence of the velopharyngeal sphincter while providing maximal enlargement of the oropharyngeal lumen.

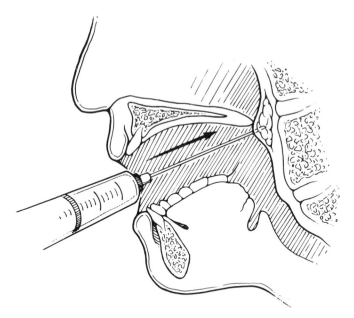

FIG. 4. Teflon injection into the posterior pharyngeal wall for treatment of post-UPPP velopharyngeal incompetence.

in an office setting (Fig. 4). This method has been used by the author to successfully alleviate nasal regurgitation in three patients with permanent VPI following UPPP.

Nasopharyngeal stenosis is a dreadful post-UPPP complication because it causes significant disability and is extremely difficult to correct. Prevention of this complication cannot be overemphasized. The surgeon should be aware of surgical pitfalls and predisposing factors to nasopharyngeal stenosis. Although this complication is usually attributed to problems with the operative technique, cases of spontaneous nasopharyngeal stenosis possibly caused by growth hormone overproduction in acromegalic patients have been reported (1). Surgical pitfalls and risk factors for nasopharyngeal stenosis are listed in Table 5. When excessive posterior tonsillar pillar resection has occurred, reapproximation of the mucosal edges superiorly at the area of the palatopharyngeal junction tends to produce retrodisplacement of the palate, thus bringing it close to the posterior pharyngeal wall (Fig. 5). This increases the

TABLE 5. *Risk factors in post-UPPP*
nasopharyngeal stenosis

Aggressive posterior pillar resection
Undermining of posterior pharyngeal wall mucosa
Excessive mucosa destruction
Infection
Necrosis
Excessive electrocautery
Acromegaly

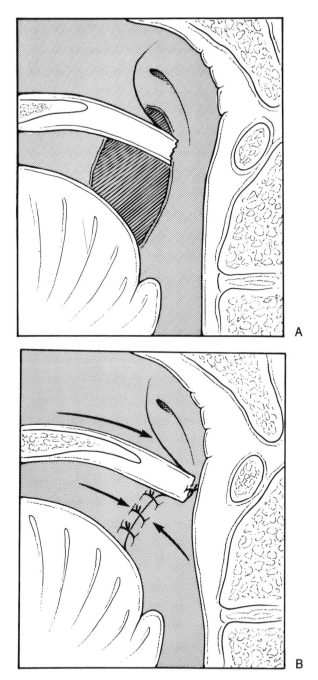

FIG. 5. A and **B:** In the case of excessive posterior tonsillar pillar resection, reapproximation of the wound edges brings the free edge of the palate in close proximity to the posterior pharyngeal wall.

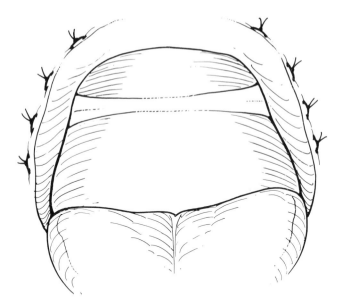

FIG. 6. "Tenting" of the posterior pharyngeal wall mucosa following suturing of the wound edges when excessive posterior pillar resection has taken place.

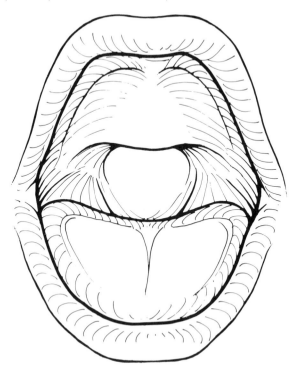

FIG. 7. Mild form of nasopharyngeal stenosis following UPPP.

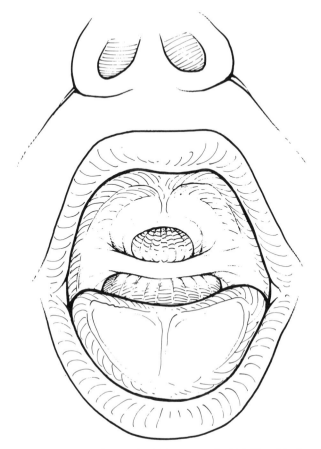

FIG. 8. Moderate nasopharyngeal stenosis. Note heavy cicatricial band in the posterior pharyngeal wall.

risk of nasopharyngeal stenosis. In addition, attempts to reapproximate the mucosa edges laterally in cases of excessive pillar resection produce a tenting effect of the posterior pharyngeal wall that will contribute to reduction of nasopharyngeal cross section (Fig. 6). Inattentive suturing of the mucosal edges of the palatopharyngeal junction may produce fusion of the palate to the posterior pharyngeal wall. Excessive undermining of the pharyngeal wall mucosa may compromise the blood supply to this area and predispose to necrosis and eventual scarring and contracture. It is obvious that aggressive resection of the posterior pillar mucosa is a major factor in the development of nasopharynx stenosis and that more conservative posterior pillar removal may prevent this complication. The use of electrocautery on the palatal incision and palatopharyngeal junction may produce retrograde necrosis of the mucosa and further increase the risk of excessive scarring. The role of simultaneous adenoidectomy may not be as significant as previously thought in the development of this complication. Many surgeons believe that adenoidectomy can be performed in association with UPPP (1).

Nasopharyngeal stenosis develops within 4–6 weeks after UPPP and can present with various grades of severity. The author prefers to classify nasopharyngeal stenosis into a mild, moderate, and severe form. The mild form is adherence of the lateral aspects of the palate to the posterior pharyngeal wall (Fig. 7). This type of deformity is not uncommon following UPPP but does not progress and is essentially asymptomatic. In moderate nasopharyngeal stenosis, only a small central section of the nasopharyngeal lumen remains open. This deformity is characterized by a heavy cicatricial band in the posterior pharyngeal wall (Fig. 8). It produces symptoms of partial nasal airway obstruction and not uncommonly velopharyngeal insufficiency. The latter is possibly the result of scar rigidity. In the severe form of nasopharyngeal stenosis, the palate is totally fused to the posterior pharyngeal wall (Fig. 9). However, the thickness of the scar formation, fibrosis, and length of obliteration of the nasopharynx usually vary.

Correction of nasopharyngeal stenosis is a formidable surgical task as indicated by the numerous techniques reported (22). Modern techniques include pharyngeal, palatal, and combination flaps, Z-plasty, skin grafting, and stenting. The author has experienced satisfactory results with a modified Mackenty technique (23,24). This

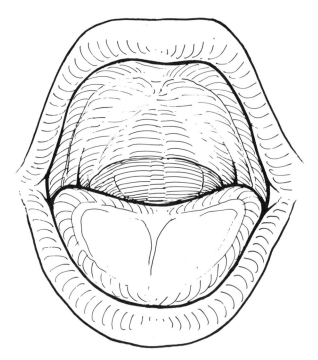

FIG. 9. Severe nasopharyngeal stenosis. Note complete fusion of the palate to the posterior pharyngeal wall.

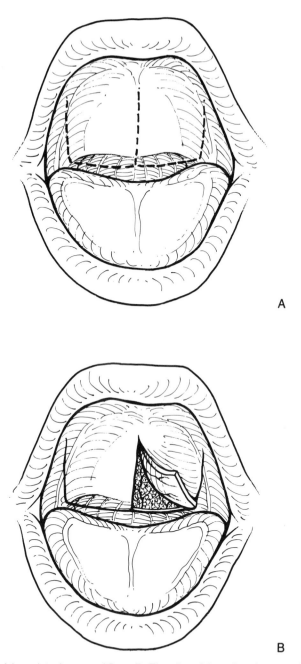

A

B

FIG. 10. A: Outline of the palatopharyngeal flaps. **B:** Elevation of the palatopharyngeal flaps. **C:** Rotation and suturing of the palatopharyngeal flaps to the dorsal surface of the palate.

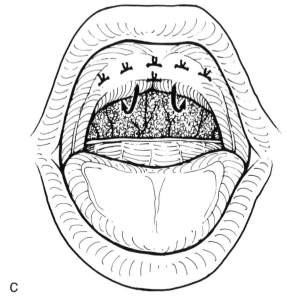

C

FIG. 10 *Continued*

approach is characterized by superiorly based palatopharyngeal flaps that are rotated to the dorsal surface of the palate (Fig. 10). The nasopharynx is stented post-operatively with a custom-made stent which is anchored on a maxillary dental plate and is worn intermittently for a period of 5–6 months (Fig. 11).

SUMMARY

Uvulopalatopharyngoplasty is a safe operation if performed according to standard techniques, and it appears to be well-tolerated by the vast majority of OSA patients and heavy snorers. Nevertheless, it may occasionally be associated with life-threatening complications such as airway loss, exacerbation of OSA, hemorrhage, and medical sequelae (hypertension, congestive heart failure, arrhythmias). Preparedness and coordinated team efforts by the surgeon, anesthesiologist, internist, and operating room personnel are extremely important in preventing or managing these complications. Intensive care monitoring and administration of nasal CPAP are necessary in the immediate postoperative period of patients with severe OSA.

The most common early post-UPPP complication is VPI. In the vast majority of patients, however, the symptoms are very mild and subside within 2–3 weeks after surgery. The most serious late post-UPPP complication is nasopharyngeal stenosis, but it is extremely rare.

In the overwhelming majority of cases, UPPP has produced successful and gratifying results with regard to elimination of snoring and reduction of OSA. When

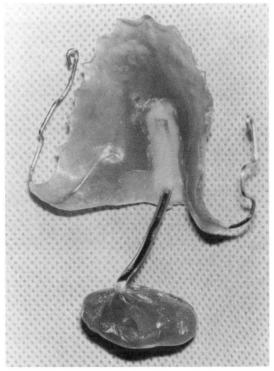

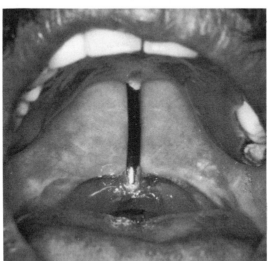

FIG. 11. A: Custom-made nasopharyngeal stent anchored on a dental plate. **B:** Nasopharyngeal stent in place.

appropriate precautions are taken, the benefits of UPPP largely outweigh the operative risks.

REFERENCES

1. Fairbanks DN. UPPP complications and avoidance strategies. *Otolaryngol Head Neck Surg* 1990; 102:239–245.
2. Esclamado RM, Glenn MG, McCulloch TM, Cummings CW. Perioperative complications and risk factors in the surgical treatment of obstructive sleep apnea syndrome. *Laryngoscope* 1989;99:1125–1129.
3. Koopman CF Jr, Moran WB Jr. Surgical management of obstructive sleep apnea. *Otolaryngol Clin North Am* 1990;23(4):787–808.
4. Bailey PL, Stanley TH. Pharmacology of intravenous narcotic anesthetics. In: Miller RD, ed. *Anesthesia.* New York: Churchill Livingstone, 1986;745–797.
5. Sanders MH, Johnson GT, Keller JEF, et al. The acute effects of uvulopalatopharyngoplasty on breathing during sleep and sleep apnea patients. *Sleep* 1988;11:75–89.
6. Powell NB, Riley RW, Guilleminault C, et al. Obstructive sleep apnea, continuous positive airway pressure and surgery. *Otolaryngol Head Neck Surg* 1988;99:362–369.
7. Gold AR, Schwartz AR, Bleckrer XY, et al. The effects of chronic nocturnal oxygen administration upon sleep apnea. *Am Rev Respir Dis* 1986;134:925–929.
8. Motta J, Guilleminault C. Effects of oxygen administration in sleep induced apneas. In: Dulimino C, Dement WC, eds. *Sleep apnea syndromes.* New York: Allan R Liss, 1978;137–144.
9. Martin RJ, Sanders MH, Gray BA, Pennock BE. Acute and longterm effects of hyperoxia on the adult sleep apnea syndrome. *Am Rev Respir Dis* 1982;125:175–180.
10. Moran WB. Uvulopalatopharyngoplasty: variations. In: Fairbanks DN, ed. *Snoring and obstructive sleep apnea.* New York: Raven Press, 1987;156–160.
11. Fairbanks DN. Uvulopalatopharyngoplasty: variations. In: Fairbanks DN, ed. *Snoring and obstructive sleep apnea.* New York: Raven Press, 1987;160–167.
12. Katsantonis GP. Uvulopalatopharyngoplasty for obstructive sleep apnea and snoring. *Oper Tech Otolaryngol Head Neck Surg* 1991;2(2):100–103.
13. Telian S, Fleisher G, Marsh R, et al. Effects of antibiotic use on recovery after tonsillectomy in children: a controlled study. *Otolaryngol Head Neck Surg [Suppl]*;1984:32.
14. Finkelstein MD, Meshorer A, Talmi WP, et al. *Otolaryngol Head Neck Surg* 1992;107(3):444–450.
15. Samelson CF. Sequela and complications of palatopharyngoplasty: impact on vocal trill. *Sleep* 1990;7:93–94.
16. Coleman MF. Limitations, pitfalls, and risk management in palatopharyngoplasty. In: Fairbanks DN, et al., eds. *Snoring and obstructive sleep apnea.* New York: Raven Press, 1987;171–184.
17. Sly DE, Coleman RF. Pre- and postoperative voice analysis of uvulopalatopharyngoplasty patients. *Arch Otolaryngol* December 1991;117(12):1345–1349.
18. Lusk RT, Accurate measurement of soft palate resection during uvulopalatopharyngoplasty. *Laryngoscope* 1986;96:697–699.
19. Kimmelman CP, Levine SB, Shore ET, et al. Uvulopalatopharyngoplasty, a comparison of two techniques. *Laryngoscope* 1985;95:1488–1490.
20. Katsantonis GP. Complications of surgical treatment for obstructive sleep apnea. *Oper Tech Otolaryngol Head Neck Surg* 1991;2(2):143–147.
21. Furlow LT Jr, Williams WN, Iescnbach CR II, et al. A longterm study on treating velopharyngeal insufficiency by teflon injection. *Cleft Palate J* 1982;19:47–56.
22. Stevenson DW. Cicatricial stenosis of the nasopharynx: a comprehensive review. *Laryngoscope* 1969;79:2035–2067.
23. Mackenty JE. Nasopharyngeal atresia. *Arch Otolaryngol* 1927;6:1–27.
24. Katsantonis GP, Friedman WH, Krebs FJ, et al. Nasopharyngeal complications following uvulopalatopharyngoplasty. *Laryngoscope* 1987;97:309–314.

Snoring and Obstructive Sleep Apnea, Second Edition,
edited by D.N.F. Fairbanks and S. Fujita.
Raven Press, Ltd., New York © 1994.

9

Laser Midline Glossectomy and Lingualplasty for Obstructive Sleep Apnea

*B. Tucker Woodson and †Shiro Fujita (1929–1993)

*Department of Otolaryngology and Human Communication, Medical College of
Wisconsin, Milwaukee, Wisconsin 53226; and †Department of Otolaryngology—Head and
Neck Surgery, Henry Ford Hospital, Detroit, Michigan 48202

Surgical treatment of obstructive sleep apnea (OSA) bypasses the site of obstruction (i.e., tracheotomy) or modifies the sites of obstruction or collapse. Infrequently, in the adult, specific pathology can be addressed which successfully cures OSA. Uvulopalatopharyngoplasty (UPPP), which removes redundant mucosa, tonsils, uvula, and soft palate, modifies the oropharynx and in many patients reduces snoring and other symptoms of the disease. Unfortunately, objective evaluation of UPPP reduces respiratory disturbance index (RDI) to clinically acceptable levels in only up to 50% of patients (1). The etiology of failure continues to be speculative, but airway obstruction at the tongue base and hypopharynx is suggested. Studies modifying the tongue base and hypopharyngeal airway with either skeletal advancement, soft tissue surgery, or dental appliances have reduced OSA (2,3). Objective manometric measures during sleep have observed complete tongue base obstruction in up to 50% of patients (4). UPPP failure is often associated with significant tongue base collapse with or without complete tongue base obstruction (5). Treatment modifying the upper airway needs to address not only the upper oropharynx and palate but also the lower oropharynx and tongue base.

Craniofacial surgery enlarges the airway by advancing the soft tissue attachments of the airway, particularly the tongue. These techniques have demonstrated excellent results. Alternatively, we have used primary soft tissue techniques to modify the shape and size of the obstructive tongue base, hypopharynx, and supraglottic tissues. Our initial experience with laser midline glossectomy (MLG) reduced RDI by 50% in 42% of patients. Although response was inadequate for a clinical cure, this group of severe apneics (mean RDI of 66 events/hr) required tracheotomy, and a reversal of the tracheotomy was possible in many patients following MLG (6). Subsequently, the procedure was modified to include lingualplasty. Results using this procedure with more stringent criteria to define surgical success has demonstrated an initial 67% clinical success rate in reducing RDI to less than 20 events/hr (7).

INDICATIONS

Indications for surgical treatment for OSA are determined by severity and the underlying anatomic structure. The goal of surgery is to cure the patient and not to reduce severity or symptoms. The definition of "cure" is controversial. Ideally, surgery would eliminate all sleep-related airflow limitation; however, this is not always achievable. Instead, the definition of acceptable surgical treatment must be to reduce the severity of disease to the level that no further medial or surgical treatment is indicated. The current "best" treatment is nasal CPAP; surgery should produce results that are equivalent.

Surgical treatment is performed in a staged fashion beginning with procedures with lower morbidity and progressing to procedures of higher morbidity. All segments of the upper airway that contribute to disease should be addressed. An aggressive approach to maximize the potential for cure should be considered with each stage of surgical treatment. Aggressiveness is tempered by the morbidity of the procedure, tolerance of the patient, underlying anatomic features, and airway safety. Because of its morbidity and the need for concurrent perioperative tracheotomy, in most patients, lingualplasty is indicated as a second-stage procedure for severe OSA. In selected cases with marked disproportionate anatomy of the tongue base, more aggressive treatment with lingualplasty may be indicated at an earlier stage. No rigid criteria exist to define patients, but should include symptomatic hypersomnolence and significant risk of morbidity due to respiratory disturbance. Relative indications include: (a) failure of prior UPPP, (b) obstructive tongue base anatomy (type IIb or type III airway on Fujita classification) on physical exam with hypertrophic lingual tonsils, and/or macroglossia causing near-complete collapse of the tongue base on supine endoscopy, and (c) redundant supraglottic tissues with floppy epiglottis, aryepiglottic folds, and arytenoids.

Contraindications for lingualplasty include patients with a prior history of significant swallowing difficulties, patients with poor pulmonary reserve (who would be at severe risk if swallowing difficulties developed), and patients with superior laryngeal or hypoglossal nerve abnormalities.

In addition to routine work-up, evaluation of all patients must include a complete nocturnal polysomnogram and postoperative sleep study, cephalometric x-rays or other equivalent objective airway measures, evaluation of swallowing function (if clinically indicated) with either functional endoscopic assessment or with video pharyngoesophagram, and assessment for significant gastroesophageal reflux.

SURGICAL PROCEDURE

The procedure is performed under general anesthesia, which is delivered via a permanent or temporary tracheotomy. The CO_2 laser requires attachment to the operating microscope, which makes exposure difficult and operating time longer. The CO_2 laser may produce less thermal injury. The KTP laser operates at higher temperatures, but ease of use and better exposure is beneficial. Studies of long-term healing results indicate no differences using different lasers.

The principle of the operation is to remove tongue soft tissue which is disproportionate for the available anatomic space, remove redundant hypopharyngeal tissues, and create a midline furrow in the tongue base. No objective measures allow the surgeon to determine what is enough or too little excision to create desired results. Preserving function is vital, and conservative resection combined with other modalities such as limited mandibular osteotomies and genioglossus advancement may be reasonable.

The patient is placed in the Rose position, and the teeth and tongue are protected with dental wax. Prophylactic antibiotics consisting of both a broad-spectrum cephalosproin (cephalexin) and anaerobic coverage (metronidazole) are administered perioperatively. Perioperative dexamethasone, 5–10 mg, is administered for three doses postoperatively. If gastroesophageal reflux is present or considered a risk, aggressive treatment with H_2 blockers and antacid is given. A Crow–Davis or similar mouth gag with tongue blade one size smaller than adult is set. For most patients a no. 3 "C-ring" tongue blade (Pilling Instrument Co., Philadelphia, PA) works well. This allows exposure of the tongue dorsum.

Midline glossectomy is performed first (Fig. 1). In this procedure the midline portion of the tongue beginning posterior to the circumvallate papillae is identified and marked with methylene blue. Care must be taken to stay in the midline. If any doubt exists during any portion of the procedure, direct laryngoscopy to confirm the position is done. The mucosal incisions for this glossectomy should be 2.0–2.5 cm. Sometimes the tongue folds on itself, and care must be taken to not mark and excise too much mucosal width. The laser is then used to excise a 4- to 5-cm-long midline portion of tongue. Excision is carried as deeply as possible and is assisted by vigorous countertraction on the excised segment using an Allis or similar clamp. Initial incisions should be deep to provide a firm purchase for the clamp because the strong countertraction needed cannot be performed with mucosa and requires that a solid portion of tongue muscle be grasped. Upon reaching the area of the valleculae, a hyoid branch of the lingual artery is often encountered and bleeding often requires suction electrocautery. After removal of the midline segment with the mouth gag in place, prolapse of tongue tissues may prevent further excision of redundant midline tissues including tongue, lingual tonsils, floppy epiglottis, and supraglottic tissues. Removing the mouth gag and using a laser laryngoscope, the surgeon can vaporize additional tissues as necessary. Conservative trimming of the epiglottis is often performed. This includes removal of all redundant tissue of the free portion, along with a "cookie bite" excision of epiglottic cartilage. Redundant arytenoid mucosa can be vaporized on the lateral and posterior margins to remove prolapsing tissue.

Lingualplasty may then be performed after replacement of the mouth gag and the no. 3 tongue blade. Beginning at the anterior corner of excision, an additional 1-cm-long wedge of lateral tongue is excised. This creates a defect. Laterally, this wedge excision should be superficial to ensure protection to the more deeply situated neurovascular structures. A 2-0 vicryl is then used to pull the posterior segment ante-

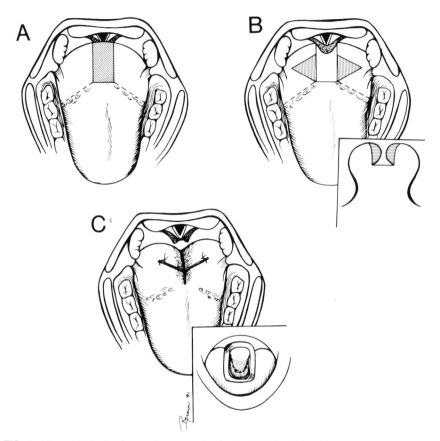

FIG. 1. Lingualplasty is shown diagrammatically. **A:** MLG (midline glossectomy) is performed first. Beginning posteriorly, a rectangular 2- to 2.5-cm mucosal width is marked and deeply excised. **B:** Redundant epiglottis is vaporized (*striped area*) using an appropriate laryngoscope (**insert**). Lingualplasty is performed by excision of a lateral wedge. The tongue is prolapsed into the defect, and we keep excision superficial laterally. **C:** Posterior tongue may be pulled anterior and laterally to demonstrate results. (From ref. 7, with permission.)

riorly and laterally. Bending the needle in a horseshoe shape may facilitate placement. This advances and modifies the shape of the tongue base, and enlargement of the posterior airway space can be appreciated. However, one must be aware that overly aggressive tongue excision or suture advancement may impair tongue mobility, thereby creating postoperative dysphagia and pain. Recent studies of healing indicate that scar contracture of the tongue following laser surgery produces complete closure of the wound with secondary healing. Therefore, suture placement may not be needed and may only increase dysphagia and pain by decreasing tongue mobility.

Patients can be started on a clear liquid diet on postoperative day 1, and this can be advanced as tolerated. Adequate fluid intake is often obtained by day 3; how-

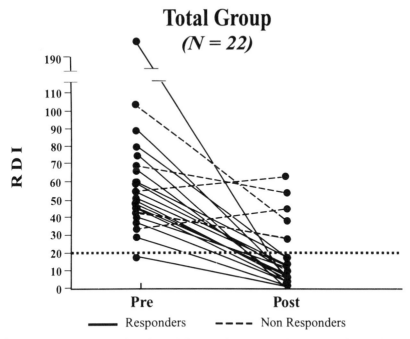

FIG. 2. Initial experience with 22 lingualplasty patients, most of whom had failed prior UPPP. Mean body mass index was 32.3 kg/m², and initial RDI was 58.6 events/hr. (From ref. 7, with permission.)

ever, some patients require vigorous swallow therapy to maximize and speed recovery. Aspiration may be a difficulty in the early postoperative period, and techniques similar to those used for supraglottic laryngectomy may be helpful in addressing swallowing dysfunction. Tracheotomy is capped during wakefulness at the discretion of the surgeon. A patent airway is common on day 1, but subcutaneous emphysema may occur with too early capping and associated vigorous coughing in patients with thick necks. When the tracheotomy is stable, capping is performed in the daytime. This is often performed prior to the discharge on day 3 or 4.

Initial results in 22 patients with severe apnea, most of whom had failed prior UPPP, demonstrated a successful response in 77%. In responders, RDI (respiratory disturbance index = apnea + hyponea/hours of sleep) decreased from 58.8 ± 39.5 to 8.1 ± 6.2 events/hr. Respiratory results in the total group are shown in Fig. 2. Complications from lingualplasty occurred in five patients and included bleeding, tongue edema, and prolonged dysphagia. All resolved with treatment, and no long-term complications have occurred. Many patients complained of transient changes in taste, but in most cases this did not persist as a complaint. All patients should be informed of this potential complication.

The advantage of lingualplasty is that this is able to address a specific pathology, such as lingual tonsillar hypertrophy, redundant supraglottic tissues, or disproportionate tongue base anatomy, if such is present. It has also been shown to be effective in many patients with severe OSA who have failed prior palatopharyngoplasty. Disadvantages include a relatively high complication rate, the need for tracheotomy (which creates its own morbidity and requires a longer hospitalization), and technical difficulty in exposing the tongue base in patients with small oral cavities. Lingualplasty improves results over palatopharyngoplasty alone, but results may be less successful than aggressive craniofacial techniques. However, in carefully selected patients, lingualplasty may be an alternative surgical treatment for OSA.

REFERENCES

1. Maisel RH, Antonelli PJ, Iber C, Mohowald M, Wilson KS, et al. Uvulopalatopharyngoplasty for obstructive sleep apnea: a community experience. *Laryngoscope* 1992;120:604–607.
2. Riley RW, Powell NB, Guilleminault C. Obstructive sleep apnea syndrome: a review of 306 consecutively treated surgical patients. *Otolaryngol Head Neck Surg* 1993;108:117–125.
3. Schmidt-Nowara WW, Meade TE, Hays MB. Dental appliances in sleep apnea. *Chest* 1991;99: 1378–1385.
4. Shepard JW, Thawley SE. Localization of upper airway collapse during sleep in patients with obstructive sleep apnea. *Am Rev Respir Dis* 1990;141:1350–1355.
5. Woodson BT, Wooten MR. Manometric and endoscopic localization of airway obstruction following uvulopalatopharyngoplasty. *Otol Head Neck Surg* 1994;in press.
6. Fujita S, Woodson BT, Clark JL, Wittig R. Laser midline glossectomy as a treatment for obstructive sleep apnea. *Laryngoscope* 1991;101:805–809.
7. Woodson BT, Fujita S. Clinical experience with lingualplasty as part of the treatment of severe obstructive sleep apnea. *Otolaryngol Head Neck Surg* 1992;107:40–48.

Snoring and Obstructive Sleep Apnea, Second Edition,
edited by D.N.F. Fairbanks and S. Fujita.
Raven Press, Ltd., New York © 1994.

10

Tracheostomy for Obstructive Sleep Apnea*

Indications and Techniques

David N. F. Fairbanks

Department of Otolaryngology, George Washington University School of Medicine,
Washington, D.C. 20037; and Ear, Nose, and Throat Medical Group,
Washington, D.C. 20037

Tracheostomy was utilized as an effective treatment for obstructive sleep apnea long before the disease was fully recognized as an entity or even named (1). While newer methods (discussed elsewhere in this book) have displaced tracheostomy as the *primary* treatment for the disease, tracheostomy is not yet obsolete.

The lifelong care of a tracheostomy is a nuisance to most patients, and to some patients (or spouses) it can be highly objectionable (2). But others adapt well to the new airway and find such a remarkable improvement in their quality of life that the annoyances of the tracheostomy become tolerable.

INDICATIONS

In theory, all patients who have obstructive apnea with debilitating daytime symptoms which threaten their jobs and all patients whose polysomnograms show many oxygen desaturations below 80% or cyclic bradycardias below 40–45/min with arrhythmias are candidates for tracheostomy. However, continuous positive airway pressure (CPAP) can be an effective palliative measure against obstructive sleep apnea, and uvulopalatopharyngoplasty (UPPP) can cure or considerably improve some cases (3,4). The problem lies in predicting, on the basis of a physical examination, who is a good candidate for a UPPP—and thus has a good chance of escaping the need for tracheostomy—because no completely clear guidelines exist. It seems only moderately clear that three types of patients are not good candidates: morbidly obese patients, patients with small mandibles, and patients whose endo-

---

*This chapter has been largely derived from the work of F. Blair Simmons, and it is modified from his chapter of the same title in the first edition of this volume.

TABLE 1. *Indications for tracheostomy for obstructive sleep apnea*

Morbid obesity
Hypo/retrognathia
Excessive hypopharyngeal tissue obstructing mirror exam of larynx
Oxygen desaturations below 50% on polysomnography
Significant cardiac arrhythmias during apneas

larynges cannot be seen by mirror examination because of excessive hypopharyngeal tissue.

Current policy is to recommend tracheostomy for the above three types of patients when they have failed to improve with (or tolerate) CPAP, particularly for patients whose oxygen desaturations are frequently below 50% or who have cyclic bradycardias below 40–45/min, especially when associated with significant arrhythmias (Table 1). It should also be noted that most patients with morbid obesity and associated moderate pulmonary hypoventilation syndrome also continue to have some problems after tracheostomy.

When tracheostomy is required, patients are offered concurrent UPPP under the same general anesthetic. Some patients will have a favorable UPPP outcome and can later have the tracheostomies closed. All patients are restudied at about 6 months after their tracheostomies have been plugged nightly for a week preceding the studies. They are then decannulated if oxygen saturation remains about 80% and there are no severe arrhythmias. However, it is not sufficient to plug the tracheostomy only for the sleep studies because it can take several days for the syndrome to recur.

PREOPERATIVE EVALUATION

Part of the treatment is to convince the patient that therapy is required. The typical patient is a 50-year-old man whose wife started the diagnostic process months earlier. He is usually still unconvinced. Abnormal polysomnogram results dictate the need for tracheostomy or a lifetime of treatment with CPAP. Weight reduction is not a choice here. Surgery has the usual risks plus some unusual ones because these persons' responses to a general anesthetic can be unpredictable and frightening.

The patient and his spouse are explicitly told that managing the short-term results of a tracheostomy can be both alarming and occasionally repugnant. They are told that after 2–3 months, tracheostomies are usually not a problem except for hygiene, and that expectorations will be by mouth when the tube is occluded. All patients should be able to live relatively normal lives, except that they should not go swimming.

At least half of these patients are hypertensive. Hypertension should be under adequate management before surgery.

There are occasional patients with truly severe and "unmanageable" hypertension for whom a general anesthetic is a major risk. Tracheostomy under a local anesthetic is advised but may not be possible if the patient is severely obese. In these circumstances, a temporary cricothyrotomy can be performed, followed by a tracheostomy 2–3 weeks later when the hypertension will have substantially resolved. An alternative is a course of CPAP treatment.

No apnea patient should ever be allowed to receive preoperative sedation. If an anesthesiologist insists, the assistance of another anesthesiologist should be sought. Sedatives can precipitate an acute airway emergency in these patients and can make unsafe the margin for rapid reversal of a general anesthetic should it become necessary to do so if intubation fails. Severe sleep apnea patients can be the most challenging of cases for an anesthesiologist.

Fortunately, most inductions and intubations are uneventful. However, two or three unsuccessful passages of the endotracheal tube with subsequent bleeding or edema can precipitate an airway crisis. Preferably, induction should not include muscle relaxants or anesthetic agents not capable of rapid reversal. If the anesthesiologist is having intubation trouble, it is far safer to wake the patient, do a temporary cricothyrotomy as a means of intubation, and then proceed with an orderly tracheostomy through the same incision.

OPERATIVE MANAGEMENT

Once the airway has been intubated, placement of the tracheostomy is fairly routine, although there are exceptions: (a) An "extra" 2 inches of operating exposure can be created in the excessively fat neck by using a 2-inch elastoplast as a snood or "Barton bandage" under the chin to pull the chin and neck fat upward and out of the way; (b) the incisions must fit the curve of the tracheostomy tube in the normal position of the neck and not the hyperextended position on the operating table. Failure to realize that these two positions are quite different has resulted in the insertion of poorly fitting tracheostomy tubes. Thus, the skin incision must be opposite the cricoid cartilage, and the trachea opening must be at the third or fourth ring.

In large necks, a self-retaining thryoid retractor is a very useful extra instrument. Right-angle clamps also help if the thyroid gland must be divided (as it usually must). Electrocautery is not recommended for hemostatis deep in the platysma muscle because coughing by the patient in the recovery ward can open even innocuous-looking veins and precipitate a trip back to the operating room.

The trachea is opened only after intraluminal injection of a few cubic centimeters of local anesthetic with the endotracheal tube cuff temporarily deflated. This prevents nearly all coughing at surgery. A 5- × 5-mm segment of the third tracheal ring is removed, and then the fourth ring is cut in the midline.

The size of the tracheal lumen is sometimes smaller than one would expect for the body size of the patient. When so, the tracheostomy tube can be fenestrated so it does not overly occlude the tracheal lumen.

The most satisfactory tracheostomy tube is the #6 Moore uncuffed silicone rubber tube manufactured by Dow Corning. It has an inner cannula and is considerably longer than other tubes available. Sometimes this length is needed, and anything extra can be cut off. Available separately is the "anesthesia flange" inner cannula with a metal extension which will prevent neck fat from overlapping the outer opening in very obese patients. A cuffed endotracheal tube is used rather than a cuffed tracheostomy tube (which may be typically too short) as a temporary measure in very obese patients with moderate pulmonary hypoventilation syndrome. The chances are about 50:50 that some ventilatory assistance will be needed for a day or two. These types of patients also do much better sitting up than lying down.

A number of writers have advocated various procedures for "permanent" flap-type tracheostomies to either speed up healing and the postoperative hospital stay or to produce a more manageable end result (5,6).

The following is Fee and Ward's (5) description of the permanent tracheostomy: The skin incisions for the average adult are 2–3 cm horizontally and 1–1.5 cm vertically and will result in an eventual permanent stoma 8–10 mm in diameter as shown in Fig. 1. One should allow for approximately 30–40% ultimate narrowing of the initial stoma created. The incisions should be placed as inferiorly as possible, allowing finger occlusion for convenient speaking. The exact incision location should be determined with the head and neck in the neutral position. The greater the amount of subcutaneous adipose tissue present, the more difficult it is to execute this procedure. Thus, in the obese, one sacrifices a large pad of subcutaneous fat underneath the skin flaps.

Two cervical skin flaps with attached subcutaneous tissue are raised in a plane above the platysma muscle fascia and retracted with either fine suture material or delicate skin hooks. Undermining of the surrounding skin is then performed to facilitate advancement of all flaps. The superficial and middle layers of the deep cervical fascia are divided vertically, and the thyroid isthmus is incised and over-sewn. The pretracheal fascia is incised, and the soft tissues between tracheal rings are injected with lidocaine and epinephrine to prevent cough and achieve hemostasis.

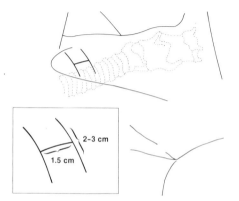

FIG. 1. Skin incisions with average dimensions. (From ref. 5.)

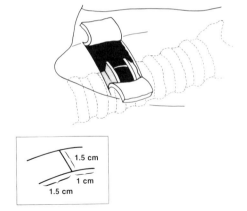

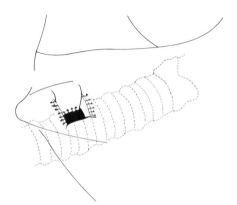

FIG. 2. Tracheal incisions with average dimensions. (From ref. 5.)

Figure 2 shows the tracheal incisions. The length of the tracheal incision averages 1.5 cm inferiorly and 1 cm superiorly. The superior and inferior lengths of the tracheal flaps to be created depend upon the distance from the trachea to the skin. Care must be exercised in the lateral-most placement of the incisions to avoid possible recurrent nerve damage. The tracheal flaps are raised and retracted superiorly and inferiorly and are sewn to the skin with 3-0 polyglycolic acid (Dexon "S") sutures. The cervical skin flaps are then sewn to the trachea as shown in Fig. 3.

A tracheostomy tube is used because frequent suctioning is anticipated immediately postoperatively and because positive pressure ventilation and oxygen inhalation may be desired.

POSTOPERATIVE MANAGEMENT

Immediate postoperative care has been reported (Table 2) (7,8). Self-care of the tracheostomy begins on the second day, and the patient is discharged by the fifth day. With a flap-type tracheostomy, the stoma is well enough healed that the patient

FIG. 3. Skin and tracheal flaps rotated into place, thereby creating the final stoma. (From ref. 5.)

TABLE 2. *Protocol for postoperative care of the sleep apnea patient after tracheostomy*[a]

1. First 2 hr postoperative:	Tracheostomy suctioning every 15 min
Next 4 hr:	Tracheostomy suctioning every 30 min
First 24 hr:	Continuous mist to tracheostomy; apply antibiotic to tracheostomy stoma
2. Second 24 hr:	During waking hours, 20 min off mist, 10 min on mist; apply antibiotic ointment (polymyxin B-bacitracin) to tracheostomy stoma
3. Third 24 hr:	During waking hours, 40 min off mist, 20 min on mist, 5 ml normal saline solution down tracheostomy in middle of off-mist period; apply antibiotic ointment
4. Fourth 24 hr:	During waking hours, off mist continually, 5 ml normal saline solution down tracheostomy every 2 hr; apply antibiotic ointment
5. Fifth 24 hr:	Home mist may be supplied at home by several commercial agencies for nighttime use

6. Train patient to clean own tracheostomy tube and to suction himself or herself; train how to use both suction and mist machines
7. Suggest criteria for ability of patient to return home:
   a. Ability to care for tracheostomy, including cleaning the inner cannula, self-suctioning, wound care
   b. Patient must feel at ease with tracheostomy
   c. No evidence of respiratory rate increase from that of admission
   d. Patient ambulating vigorously about ward
   e. Amount and character of secretions from tracheostomy not suggestive of pulmonary infection
   f. Have patient's sleeping habits improved since surgery?
8. Have Social Service arrange for suction and mist machines for patient to take home or have available when he or she returns home

[a]Three factors influence hospital discharge: (a) ability of patient (and spouse or friend) to care for tracheostomy; (b) ability to do without mist while still keeping secretions moist; (c) infection. Orders are written with the following instructions in mind: Antibiotic ointment must be applied to the tracheostomy stoma t.i.d.; decrease mist use as rapidly as possible (this varies from patient to patient) by substituting saline drops; insist that patient and family participate in daily care by the fourth day. On anticipated discharge from the hospital, some decisions must be made about individual patients, specifically with regard to mist use. If there is no one at home besides the patient, he or she will need home mist for nighttime sleeping for approximately 3 weeks. If there is someone at home who can put 3 ml saline solution into the tracheostomy tube every 2–4 hr for the first week or so, a mist machine will not be needed. A suction machine is needed, and we recommend purchase, not rental, since there will be an intermittent need for suction indefinitely. Purchase is less expensive than renting. (From ref. 8.)

can change his or her entire tracheal tube (including outer tube) by the second or third day. A speaking tube is then inserted (i.e., #8 fenestrated cuffless Shiley tube). We advise purchase of a suction apparatus and the temporary use of a collar-type mist machine for the first 3 weeks of home care. In our experience, the most common reason for a prolonged hospital stay has been delay in obtaining the home suction.

Intermediate management of the tracheostomy involves two common problems: normal wound healing and the proper fit of the tube. About half of patients will have problems with granulation tissue formation. This begins at 1 month and continues for several months and is usually manifested by minor bleeding episodes. We remove the granulations by knife or punch (such as adenoid punch), and then we cauterize the base. Continued recurrence of granulation tissue indicates that the patient is not especially concerned about the problem; that is, he or she is not diligently applying an antibiotic ointment to the stoma at least four times a day, nor is he or she changing the gauze pad when wet. We are firm about this requirement because otherwise we are forced to snip and cauterize granulations *ad infinitum*.

About half of patients will have one of two problems with the fit of the tracheostomy tube. Head or neck position may cause an inordinate amount of coughing, or patients cannot breathe completely with the tube plugged during the daytime. Coughing with neck movement usually means that a better tube fitting is needed. This should be evaluated with lateral tomograms of the neck with the patient in a normal and comfortable position to see what needs to be done. The tube length or curvature is then adjusted accordingly. The patient with daytime plugged-tube breathing problems is either the recipient of a poor intratracheal fit or has a small trachea. Adjusting the fit or fenestrating the tube should solve the problem.

With a flap-type tracheostomy, it is not entirely predictable how much narrowing will occur in the weeks and months postoperatively. Many of these patients need to wear no tracheal appliance at night, and they simply wear a stomal plug in the daytime. Others need the tube to prevent a progressive narrowing, and some need one simply to keep fatty, flabby neck skin from falling onto the opening. This type of stoma will not close by itself on decannulation, and a deliberate surgical closure is required when the need for the tracheostomy is gone.

LONG-TERM MANAGEMENT

The patient should be experiencing no difficulties and show no granulation tissue by 4 months after the tracheostomy. At about this time, follow-up polysomnograms should be done. It is important to do this because even though the patient may be feeling much better and tracheostomy is purported to be 100% curative, very obese patients may still be having subclinical problems or the tube may become occluded during the night. If no problems are found at this time, the patient is discharged from routine follow-up care to return on an "as needed" basis, although we do recommend periodic regular evaluations by the patient's personal physician.

SUMMARY

Obstructive sleep apnea can be diagnosed by nighttime sleep monitoring alone. Tracheostomy is the only 100% successful treatment, but it should be reserved for severe obstructive sleep apnea patients who are unsuitable for (or have failed with) surgery or CPAP. Preoperative counseling can save the physician and patient considerable problems later. Selection of the anesthesiologist is important. Very obese patients may need postoperative ventilatory support.

APPENDIX: SPECIAL PROBLEMS PATIENTS HAVE
WITH A TRACHEOSTOMY

Editor's note. The following informative communication is reprinted from *JAMA* 1983;249(6):702, with permission.

A year ago, I fell asleep at midday while driving and demolished my car. It was eventually determined that I was one of an estimated 50 million people with sleep apnea. A permanent tracheostomy was performed so that I could breathe through the tube at night (the tube is plugged during the day). It sounds simple enough, but the problems involved were such that it took a year to find solutions that would allow me to return to near-normal function.

The two major problems are air leakage, which makes it difficult to talk, and hygiene. The tracheostomy was meant to be a temporary expedient for bed patients, not for someone who is up and around. For example, there is no plug designed for the tube; Comfit ear plugs work perfectly. The only place to get the little brush necessary to clean the inside of the tube is in the hospital tracheostomy kits complete with rubber gloves, sterile drape, plastic tongs, scissors, and woven ribbon, which ties around the neck, most of which is not needed. The Kellog Brush Manufacturing Co. (Easthampton, MA 01027) makes a small tube brush for coffee percolators that can be cut off and curved for cleaning inside the tube; a toothbrush works well for the outside. Small elastic cord tied to hooks from hook-and-eye sets are much better for daily use than the ribbon ties. Ivory Snow is a soap free of any perfume or chemicals that could be irritating. Plastic containers for false teeth are good for washing and storing the tube.

Covering the tube and stoma is difficult. In addition to making it hard to talk, the air leakage is uncomfortably hot, especially when covered. One can't button the collar of a shirt or blouse because it would press on the tube and cause the wearer to gag. The stoma is too high to be concealed by an ascot or scarf, but a tailor can make a dickey with a tubular band to go around the neck, through which elastic can be threaded and secured at the back by Velcro buttons. Because the "apneic" does not need the tube to breath during the day, the happiest discovery I made was Stomahesive, a material made by Squibb for attaching colostomy bags. Stomahesive can be bought from medical supply stores in 4-in. squares without the colostomy fitting. This can be cut into 3.5- × 5-cm patches that will effectively cover the stoma, eliminating most of the problems. If you don't use anything oily, such as preshave or aftershave around the neck, the patch will usually stay airtight all day. Painting the area around the stoma with benzoin before placing the patch makes it stick better and also makes it easier to remove without irritating the skin. It's a good idea to carry a spare patch in case of a blowout.

This information can greatly reduce the physical and emotional impact on those who must have a permanent tracheostomy.

John P. Dye
Newport Beach, California

REFERENCES

1. Simmons FB, Guilleminault C, Dement WC, Tilkian AG, Hill M. Surgical management of airway obstructions during sleep. *Laryngoscope* 1977;87:326–338.
2. Conway WA, Victor Lyle D, Magilligan DJ, Fujita F, Zorick FJ, Roth T. Adverse effects of tracheostomy for sleep apnea. *JAMA* 1981;246:347–350.
3. Fujita S, Conway W, Zorick F, et al. Surgical corrections of anatomic abnormalities in obstructive sleep-apnea syndrome: uvulopalatopharyngoplasty. *Otolaryngol Head Neck Surg* 1981;89:923–934.
4. Simmons FB, Guilleminault C, Silvestri R. Snoring and some obstructive sleep apnea can be cured by oropharyngeal surgery: palatopharyngoplasty (PPP). *Arch Otolaryngol* 1983;109:503–507.
5. Fee WE, Ward PH. Permanent tracheostomy. *Ann Otolaryngol* 1977;86:635–637.
6. deBerry-Borowiecki B, Sassin JF. Surgical treatment of sleep apnea. *Arch Otolaryngol* 1983;109: 508–512.
7. Hill MW, Simmons FB, Guilleminault C. Tracheostomy and sleep apnea. In: Guilleminault WC, Dement WC, eds. *Sleep apnea syndromes*. New York: Alan R Liss, 1978;347–352.
8. Simmons FB. Tracheostomy in the sleep apnea syndrome. *Ear Nose Throat J* 1984;63:222–226.

Snoring and Obstructive Sleep Apnea, Second Edition,
edited by D.N.F. Fairbanks and S. Fujita.
Raven Press, Ltd., New York © 1994.

11

The Nose and Its Impact on Snoring and Obstructive Sleep Apnea

Michael J. Papsidero

Mount Sinai Nasal/Sinus Center, Cleveland, Ohio 44106; and Cleveland Ear, Nose, Throat & Facial Surgery Group, Inc., Garfield Heights, Ohio 44125

While observations consistent with obstructive sleep apnea syndrome (OSAS) have appeared in the literature since 1877, characterization of this syndrome has evolved slowly (1). In the 1960s, reports appeared describing patients with nasopharyngeal obstruction, hypersomnolence, cor pulmonale, right heart failure, and alveolar hypoventilation (2–7). In 1973, sleep apnea as a syndrome was first described by Guilleminault et al. (8); shortly thereafter, Simmons and Hill (9) reported the otolaryngologic manifestations of OSAS. These reports, as well as most subsequent reports, have focused on the role of the nasopharyngeal inlet, oropharynx, tongue, and mandible as the primary pathogenic structures in the development of OSAS (10–14). There is, however, an increasing body of evidence which suggests that nasal obstruction plays an important role in the development of mild-to-moderate obstructive sleep apnea (OSA). Additionally, nasal obstruction appears to play a pathogenic role in the development of snoring, sleep fragmentation, and excessive daytime somnolence in some patients.

HISTORICAL BACKGROUND

Many anecdotal reports exist in the literature extending back into the 1800s which describe conditions consistent with OSAS and which establish an association with nasal obstruction and snoring. In 1892, Carpenter (15) noted the association between disrupted sleep and impairment of daytime intellectual performance and memory. He attributed this impairment to nasal obstruction. In 1898, Wells (16) described 10 patients who had nasal obstruction. Eight of the 10 patients also experienced associated severe daytime somnolence. This condition was alleviated when the nasal obstruction was corrected. The pioneering electroencephalographic work of Aserinsky and Jouvet, decades later, established an association between sleep stages and the postural relaxation observed in patients with sleep apnea and snoring (17,18). In the 1960s, case reports describing children with nasal obstruction on the

179

basis of tonsillar and adenoid hyperplasia, and consequent cor pulmonale, were introduced into the literature (5–7). In 1978, Cottle (19) described the nasal-nocturnal syndrome, which associated restless sleep with snoring, gasping respirations, and nasal obstruction. In the 1980s, Lavie et al. (20) and others (21–26) better defined the relationship between nasal obstruction and sleep disorders.

That there is a close relationship between nasal obstruction, snoring, and OSAS has been well established by these researchers as well as others. Moreover, it is a common clinical observation that nasal obstruction and associated intranasal structural abnormalities are present in snorers. It has also been clearly established that the severity of snoring directly correlates with the severity of OSA. Therefore, an understanding of the relationship between nasal obstruction and snoring is important to understanding the pathogenesis of OSAS.

NASAL OBSTRUCTION AND SNORING

Snoring is a noise produced by vibrations of the soft palate and pharynx, occurring as a result of partial upper airway obstruction, and consequent turbulent airflow. Snoring occurs during sleep and may present as a mild condition, unassociated with oxygen desaturation or arousal. However, it may also occur in association with obstructive sleep apnea and its attendant severe pathophysiologic consequences. Snoring may be continuous, occurring with virtually every inspiration. Most commonly, this type of snoring is not associated with severe OSA. Snoring may also be cyclical, characterized by intermittent quiet intervals subsequently interrupted with snorts. This type of snoring is often associated with OSAS.

Recognition of the importance of snoring has evolved slowly in the rhinologic literature. In Proetz's landmark book entitled *Essays on the Applied Physiology of the Nose* (27), published in 1941, hardly any mention is made of snoring. Snoring at that time, and until relatively recently, was considered a mere nuisance to the sleeper and to the bed partner and was thought to be of little physiologic importance. The development of comprehensive sleep disorders laboratories has resulted in a much better characterization of snoring as an essential component in the evolution of OSAS. Virtually all patients with OSA are snorers, and most have been heavy snorers for years prior to the diagnosis. This observation suggests a pathogenic relationship between snoring and OSAS.

Further confirmation of the pathogenic association of snoring and OSAS is to be found in the work of Lugaresi et al. (28–30), who have shown that, during sleep, alveolar ventilation can decrease in heavy snorers, with an associated elevation in pulmonary artery pressure. They also noted an association between snoring and elevation of systemic blood pressure. It has been postulated that the paradoxical thoracoabdominal motion which occurs during snoring may indeed interrupt normal cardiorespiratory mechanics (31). Furthermore, a number of epidemiologic studies have indicated a correlation between snoring, arterial hypertension, cardiac disease, and brain ischemia (32–38). Based on current evidence, there can be little doubt that snoring, in addition to being a social nuisance, represents a potentially significant medical condition.

Loud snoring is generally associated with nasal obstruction, and it occurs almost exclusively with mouth breathing. While the relationship between nasal obstruction, snoring, and mouth breathing is somewhat ill-defined, it has been recently clarified by several authors (39–44). Fairbanks (45) elaborated on this association in the study of 113 patients undergoing nasal septoplasty/submucous resection of turbinates for nasal airway impairment, 47 of whom were snorers preoperatively. Snoring was significantly improved following nasal surgery alone in 77% of them. This study certainly implicates nasal obstruction as a major contributor to the development of snoring.

PATHOPHYSIOLOGIC ASPECTS OF NASAL OBSTRUCTION IN SNORING

The noxious noise which we define as snoring is produced by partial obstruction of the upper airway. For our purposes, the upper airway may be divided into two segments, namely, the nose and the oropharynx. Snoring and obstructive apnea result from the partial occlusion of the oropharynx as a byproduct of the negative endothoracic pressure which occurs during inspiration. The degree of negative endothoracic pressure is partly a function of (a) the amount of upstream nasal resistance which is present and (b) the compliance of oropharyngeal tissues (Fig. 1). On this basis, individuals with significant nasal obstruction are at more risk for the development of snoring and OSA. In addition, the turbulent flow which occurs in the face of nasal obstruction also contributes to oropharyngeal collapse, by creating pockets of subatmospheric pressure. A variety of structural and mucosal nasal abnormalities may contribute to a nasal obstruction and snoring (Table 1).

It is of note that heavy snorers, while awake, may also have abnormally increased negative endothoracic pressure during inspiration. This indicates that increased re-

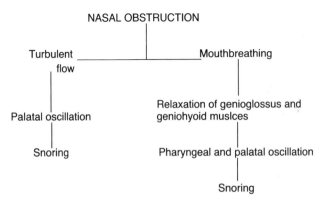

FIG. 1. Schematic representing the relationship between nasal obstruction and snoring.

TABLE 1. *Conditions of nose and nasopharynx associated with OSAS and snoring*

Nose
Deviated septum
Polyps, papillomas
Turbinate enlargement
Choanal atresia
Rhinitis: allergic, nonallergic
Nasopharynx
Adenoid hyperplasia
Nasopharyngeal stenosis
Nasopharyngeal tumors
Pharyngeal flap
Posterior nasal packing
Nasopharyngitis

sistance to airflow in the upper airways may continue during wakefulness (30,39). This observation may be explained on the basis of persistent nasal obstruction, oropharyngeal collapse, and/or increased peripheral pulmonary resistance in these patients.

The actual snoring sound is largely produced by oscillation of the soft palate. This appears to depend, at least in part, upon the tension provided by the tensor veli palatini muscle. It has been noted that snoring increases through sleep stage IV, but then diminishes during rapid eye movement (REM) sleep. This is the time when obstructive sleep apnea is at its worst. Presumably, the relaxation of the tensor veli palatini muscle during REM sleep results in a reduction in snoring while airway obstruction increases. In addition to nasal obstruction, nasopharyngeal obstruction has also been shown to be correlated with both snoring and OSAS (46–50). It is a common clinical observation that snoring will abate following adenoidectomy, or following tonsillectomy with adenoidectomy, in children with hyperplasia of these structures. Adenoid hyperplasia alone has been shown to contribute not only to snoring but also to OSAS (5–7,46–48). Adenoidectomy has been curative in these patients.

While snoring is clearly correlated with nasal and nasopharyngeal obstruction, it is also correlated with mouth breathing. Snoring occurs almost exclusively when mouth breathing. It is unclear as to whether or not this association is due to a higher incidence of nasal obstruction in mouth breathers, or rather is a byproduct of the combination of partial nasal obstruction and oral respiration, resulting in enhanced vibration of the soft palate.

RELATIONSHIP BETWEEN NASAL OBSTRUCTION AND OSAS

Nasal obstruction, snoring, and OSA can be described as existing on a parallel continuum. Mild snoring and nasal obstruction are generally associated with mini-

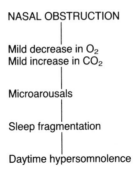

NASAL OBSTRUCTION
|
Mild decrease in O_2
Mild increase in CO_2
|
Microarousals
|
Sleep fragmentation
|
Daytime hypersomnolence

FIG. 2. Schematic representing the relationship between nasal obstruction and daytime hypersomnolence.

mal or no obstructive sleep apnea, whereas heavy snoring, frequently associated with significant nasal obstruction, is virtually always present when significant OSA occurs. This association, however, is not inviolate. Certainly, some patients with severe OSA have no significant nasal obstruction. The association with snoring per se is probably more direct, with severe OSA almost always accompanied by significant snoring. Mild snoring may be accompanied by minimal or no desaturations and by microarousals, whereas very often severe snoring is associated with significant desaturations and full arousals. This, of course, results in sleep fragmentation and daytime hypersomnolence in many of these patients (Fig. 2, Table 2).

The relationship between snoring and OSAS, and its parallel association with nasal obstruction, cannot be ignored in assessing the patient with sleep apnea. Treatment programs should be designed to address the issue of nasal obstruction, as well as oropharyngeal obstruction. Many patients may benefit by the addition of nasal surgery to a treatment program typically involving nasal continuous positive airway pressure (CPAP) or uvulopalatopharyngoplasty.

CLINICAL EVIDENCE FOR THE ROLE OF NASAL AND NASOPHARYNGEAL OBSTRUCTION IN OSAS

In the late 1970s, Cottle (19) defined the nasal-nocturnal syndrome in children. This study linked sleep fragmentation and respiratory embarrassment to nasal obstruction.

McNicholas et al. (51) demonstrated that nasal obstruction due to allergic rhinitis is associated with both sleep fragmentation and OSAS. This condition appeared to be reversible with treatment of the allergic rhinitis. Lavie et al. (52) made similar observations of disordered breathing in association with allergic rhinitis.

Abnormalities such as septal deviation and nasal valve obstruction have also been reported to result in sleep disturbance and OSAS. Dayal and Phillipson (26) demonstrated that relief of nasal valve obstruction is directly correlated with alleviation of OSAS. Lavie et al. (53) demonstrated similar findings and suggested that nasal

TABLE 2. *Causes of sleep fragmentation and hypersomnolence*

Psychological and behavioral
Nasal/nasopharyngeal obstruction
Obstructive sleep apnea
Narcolepsy
Primary alveolar hypoventilation

surgery may result in a demonstrable improvement in sleep parameters and/or subjective reduction in sleepiness.

These studies, however, did not control for other associated factors known to cause disorders of excessive somnolence.

In an effort to clarify the role of nasal obstruction alone in the development of sleep fragmentation and excessive daytime somnolence, a group of seven patients was identified from 150 consecutive patients undergoing one or two night polysomnograms in our sleep laboratory. In order to eliminate factors (other than nasal obstruction) known to cause daytime somnolence, the seven patients were selected to meet each of the following criteria: (a) excessive daytime somnolence as measured by multiple sleep latency testing, (b) normal apnea/hypopnea indices, (c) positive subjective and rhinomanometric evidence for nasal obstruction, (d) normal spirometry, (e) absence of nocturnal myoclonus, (f) normal psychometric battery, and (g) anatomic intranasal abnormalities resulting in nasal obstruction (Table 1).

Table 3 summarizes the pretreatment patient data, and Table 4 summarizes the pre- and postoperative results.

All patients underwent septoplasty and turbinate cautery and outfracture. All patients experienced significant improvements in subjective and objective measures of nasal breathing. Six of seven demonstrated a significant improvement in snoring. All had a marked reduction in hypersomnolence as measured by improvement in postoperative multiple sleep latency test (MSLT) scores.

These findings further corroborate the impression that nasal obstruction alone, in the absence of other factors known to cause sleep fragmentation, may result in

TABLE 3. *Summary of pretreatment patient data*

Age	Sex	Subjective breathing impairment preoperatively	Snoring	Spirometry	Nocturnal myoclonus	Psychometric battery[a]
58	M	Moderate	Yes	NL[b]	NL	Negative
34	M	Severe	Yes	NL	NL	Negative
43	M	Mild	No	NL	NL	Negative
62	M	Moderate	Yes	NL	NL	Negative
38	M	Severe	Yes	NL	NL	Negative
66	M	Mild	Yes	NL	NL	Negative
48	F	Moderate	Yes	NL	NL	Negative

[a]Cornell Medical Index, Stanford Sleep Inventory, and MMPI.
[b]NL, no evidence for airways disease.

TABLE 4. *Preoperative and postoperative results*

Pre MSLT[a] (min)	Prerhinomanometry, % change	Apnea/ hypopnea index	Subjective improvement	Post rhinometry, % change	Post MSLT (min)	Snoring
3.2	36	10.1	Yes	44	9.2	Minimal
4.2	35	2.4	Yes	40	8.9	Minimal
4.9	39	11.0	Yes	42	9.8	Minimal
4.7	34	15.5	Yes	39	9.0	Minimal
3.0	36	2.2	Yes	44	8.5	Minimal
4.9	37	19.0	Yes	46	9.3	Minimal
4.6	35	11.8	Yes	45	8.5	Minimal

[a]MSLT, multiple sleep latency test.

significant hypersomnolence. The elimination of nasal obstruction through surgical repair, likewise, may result in (a) a reduction in sleep fragmentation and (b) improvement in the disabling symptoms of daytime hypersomnolence in some patients.

PATHOGENIC RATIONALE FOR THE ROLE OF NASAL OBSTRUCTION IN OSAS

While the role of the nasopharyngeal inlet, pharynx, and tongue in OSAS appears intuitively evident, the role of nasal obstruction per se is not (Fig. 3). The pharynx represents a distensible tube weakly supported by surrounding structures and dilator musculature. With inspiration, the pressure differential created by the diaphragm results in flow, but it also creates a negative (i.e., subatmospheric) intrapharyngeal pressure. This negative intraluminal pressure results in collapse of the compliant soft tissues of the pharynx. The degree of collapse is dependent upon a variety of factors, including the effect of dilator and abductor musculature, the diameter of the nasopharynx and oropharynx, central factors, and the degree of subatmospheric intraluminal pressure created. The degree of reduction in the intraluminal pressure has been shown to be directly correlated with the amount of resistance upstream to the oropharynx. This resistance is largely produced by the nose.

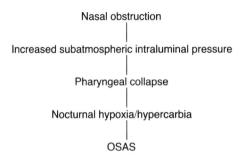

FIG. 3. Schematic representation of the role of nasal obstruction in OSAS.

Under normal circumstances, the nose is responsible for approximately 50% of upper respiratory resistance to airflow. Nasal resistance is dynamic and is a product of a variety of factors including the structure of the bony nasal pyramid, the nasal septum, the nasal valve and, of course, the mucosally covered erectile tissue of the turbinates. It is also a function of position, exercise, and environmental conditions. Daily variations in nasal resistance occur largely on the basis of (a) the so-called nasal cycle and (b) other vasomotor influences on the erectile tissue of the turbinates.

The nasal cycle involves an alternate engorgement of the turbinates of one side of the nose, with constriction of the turbinates on the other side. This cycle appears to occur in approximately 90-min intervals. It results in an increased nasal resistance on one side, with a decreased nasal resistance on the other. However, total nasal resistance remains unchanged.

There may be several additional nasal reflexes which play a role in human respiration (54–56). For decades it has been known that strong stimulation of the nose and nasopharynx may result in a vagally mediated apneic response. This is clearly demonstrated in the diving reflex of infants.

Cole and Haight (57) demonstrated that lateral recumbency decreases the patency of the ipsilateral side of the nose and increases the patency of the contralateral side. Thus, unilateral obstruction of the nose may be manifested as a disease state when in certain positions of recumbency.

The so-called nasal–pulmonary reflex has been implicated by a number of authors in the development of alveolar hypoventilation and OSA (Fig. 4). While this reflex is poorly understood, in many patients with nasal obstruction there appears to be an associated increase in peripheral pulmonary resistance. The nasal obstruction may be unilateral or bilateral, and it has been seen in patients with partial as well as total nasal obstruction.

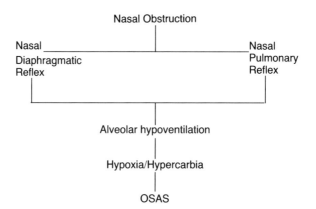

FIG. 4. Schematic representation of the relationship between nasal obstruction, nasal reflexes, and OSAS.

Corroborative clinical evidence occurs in the form of studies performed on patients with posterior nasal packing (58,59). These studies have shown alveolar hypoventilation and an increased peripheral pulmonary resistance in these patients. However, it remains unclear as to whether or not this is a true reflex action.

Further supportive evidence comes from studies of patients who have undergone pharyngoplasty flaps for correction of velopharyngeal insufficiency (60–62). Kravath et al. (60) described a group of three children in whom severe OSA developed following a pharyngoplasty flap. Despite the ability to mouth breathe, these children all developed significant OSA, and one died in her sleep after surgical intervention. Guilleminault et al. (63) described a group of five children who were defined as near-miss sudden infant death syndrome (SIDS) patients. OSA later developed in these children. Three children were treated with adenoidectomy, and one underwent adenoidectomy and uvulectomy. Adenoidectomy was successful in correcting OSA in the four patients. Both Olsen et al. (62) and Zwillich et al. (21,64) have demonstrated that artificial obstruction of the nose, both unilateral and bilateral, results in sleep fragmentation and OSA. One of the proposed explanations for this phenomenon is the nasal–pulmonary reflex. Lavie et al. (65) similarly showed that unilateral or bilateral nasal obstruction in normal subjects can result in apnea. However, large individual variations in response to nasal obstruction were noted. In many cases, significantly disordered sleep occurred.

There is some evidence to suggest that a nasal–diaphragmatic reflex relationship occurs (Fig. 4). The presumption is that nasal airflow alone may be stimulatory to breathing, and that such airflow results in stimulation of nasal mucous membrane receptors which increase diaphragmatic activity. The interruption of nasal airflow then results in a reduction in diaphragmatic activity and an associated reduction in ventilation. This relationship was first alluded to by Rochester and Braun (66) in studying the relationship between the diaphragm and dyspnea in patients on respirators. Further supportive evidence is given by Mathew et al. (67) and White et al. (68), who showed that diaphragmatic response to negative pharyngeal pressure was abolished when nasopharyngeal topical anesthesia was administered.

Therefore, nasal reflexes may, during sleep, influence the normal respiratory process. When nasal pathology is present, this effect may be significant and may result in a predisposition to OSA.

In summary, there appear to be two general mechanisms by which nasal obstruction may contribute to OSAS. Nasal obstruction results in increased upstream resistance to the oropharynx, leading to increased diaphragmatic effort and an associated reduction in intrapharyngeal pressure. This process results in pharyngeal collapse, hypoxia and hypercarbia, and OSAS. The second mechanism is through proposed nasal reflexes. Nasal obstruction may result in a reflex increase in peripheral pulmonary resistance and associated reduction in alveolar ventilation. This results in hypoxia, hypercarbia, and a worsening of underlying OSA. The second nasal reflex mechanism could be termed the nasal–diaphragmatic reflex, in which reduction in nasal airflow results in a reduction in stimulation of nasal receptors responsible for enhanced diaphragmatic activity. With a reduction in diaphragmatic activity, an associated reduction in ventilation occurs, resulting in hypoxia, hypercarbia, and a further enhancement of underlying OSA.

MOUTH BREATHING

While infants may be obligatory nasal breathers, maturation appears to diminish this requirement. Therefore, why would a patient with severe nasal obstruction not simply opt for mouth breathing? Presumably, this would result in reduced airway resistance and a decreased tendency for pharyngeal collapse. The assumption is that opting for mouth breathing would effectively reduce airway resistance and the work of breathing.

Under normal circumstances, humans show a strong predilection for nasal breathing. The reasons for this are numerous, but primarily relate to the physiologic function of the nose. Specifically, the lungs benefit from nasal function which includes filtration, warming, and humidification. Furthermore, expiratory resistance enhances alveolar filling and gaseous exchange.

Mouth breathing may, in fact, not be the pathway of least resistance in the sleeping and recumbent individual.

Olsen et al. (62), in an intriguing study, demonstrated (from measurements of respiratory effort in the same position and stage of sleep) that oral airway resistance is actually greater than nasal airway resistance while sleeping. This study suggests that oral breathing appears to be a higher net resistance pathway during sleep than nasal breathing in some individuals. While this may be explained in some instances by invoking the nasal reflexes previously referenced, there are other explanations.

The open mouth posture unfavorably alters the pharyngeal airway by creating a relatively unstable lumen. The opening of the mouth releases the anterior portion of the tongue, producing a posterior–superior movement to the genioglossus muscle. In addition, by effectively shortening the muscle belly, less anterior force is exerted on the tongue. This results in a reduction in the anterior–posterior diameter of the oropharyngeal lumen at this level by 1 cm or more. Consequently, airway obstruction may be worsened by mouth breathing during sleep (Fig. 5).

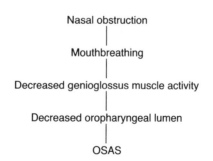

Nasal obstruction
|
Mouthbreathing
|
Decreased genioglossus muscle activity
|
Decreased oropharyngeal lumen
|
OSAS

FIG. 5. Schematic of role of mouth breathing in OSAS.

SUMMARY

There is strong clinical and experimental evidence, as well as historical support, for the role of nasal obstruction in the development of sleep fragmentation, snoring, and OSAS.

Nasal obstruction may result in sleep fragmentation by causing small variations in oxygen and carbon dioxide levels which, in sensitive individuals, result in micro-arousals and sleep fragmentation.

Nasal obstruction contributes to the development of OSA through complex mechanisms, which include (a) direct reduction in intrapharyngeal pressure with associated pharyngeal collapse and (b) stimulation of nasal reflexes. Either pathway will result in alveolar hypoventilation, hypoxia and hypercarbia, and OSA.

In patients who are snorers or who have symptoms consistent with OSAS, a careful history eliciting evidence for possible nasal obstruction, as well as a thorough nasal examination, is necessary. If nasal obstruction is present, intervention should be considered as part of a comprehensive treatment program for the patient with snoring, sleep fragmentation, or OSAS.

EDITOR'S ADDENDUM

To assess the nasal component of the airway problem in snoring or OSA, the following simple diagnostic exercise can be useful. The patient is given a small sample bottle of oxymetazoline (Afrin) decongestant nasal spray with an instruction sheet that states the following:

Nose Spray Test

Three sprays in each nostril
one-half hour before bedtime
every *other* night this week.

Compare snoring on spray nights
versus snoring on non-spray nights.

(This is a test only; the spray
is not intended for use as a
remedy for snoring or stuffy nose.)

When the patient returns or telephones with the test result, the physician can judge the advisability (or nonadvisability) of nasal treatments for snoring (or apnea). For example: If snoring completely disappeared on the nose-spray nights, the nose constitutes a major factor in the disorder and nasal treatment can likely relieve snoring. But if snoring was improved only somewhat by the spray, then it would be improved only somewhat by nasal treatment (surgical, etc.). And if snoring was not improved at all by the nose spray—even though nasal breathing was much improved—then nasal treatments would likely be disappointing as a snoring (or apnea) cure.

Generally it is the ordinary (or mild apneic) snorer with associated nasal complaints/abnormalities who will be cured of snoring by nasal therapy alone (69). But many snorers and mild to moderately severe apneics who have not been fully cured by UPPP can gain additional relief with subsequent nasal surgery as adjunctive therapy. Severe obstructive sleep apneics almost always suffer from other causes that overshadow the nasal factor, and nasal surgery requiring packing (which aggravates obstructive sleep apnea) could be a hazardous undertaking (70).

REFERENCES

1. Broadbent WH. Cheyne–Stokes respiration in cerebral hemorrhage. *Lancet* 1877;1:307–309.
2. Luke MJ, Mehrizi A, Folger GM, Rowe RD. Chronic nasal pharyngeal obstruction as a cause of cardiomegaly, cor pulmonale, and pulmonary edema. *Pediatrics* 1966;37:762.
3. Menashe VD, Farrehi C, Millier M, et al. Hypoventilation and cor pulmonale due to chronic airway obstruction. *J Pediatr* 1965;67:198–263.
4. Noonan J. *Reversible cor pulmonale due to hypertrophied tonsils and adenoids: studies in two cases* [Abstract]. American Pediatric Society, May 6–8, 1965, p. 48.
5. Luke MJ, Mehrizi A, Folger GM Jr, Rowe RD. Chronic nasopharyngeal obstruction as a cause of cardiomegaly, cor pulmonale, and pulmonary edema. *Pediatrics* 1966;37:762–768.
6. Lubart J. Nasal obstruction and the cardiorespiratory mechanism. *Eye Ear Nose Throat Monthly* 1968;47:49–54.
7. Levy AM, Tabakin BS, Hanson JS, Narkewicz RM. Hypertrophied adenoids causing pulmonary hypertension and severe congestive heart failure. *N Engl J Med* 1967;277:506–511.
8. Guilleminault C, Eldrige FL, Dement WC. Insomnia with sleep apnea: a new syndrome. *Science* 1973;181:856–858.
9. Simmons FB, Hill MW. Hypersomnia caused by upper airway obstructions: a new syndrome in otolaryngology. *Ann Otol Rhinol Laryngol* 1974;83:670–673.
10. Mata J, Guilleminault C, Schroeder JS, Dement WC. Tracheostomy and hemodynamic changes in sleep induced apnea. *Ann Intern Med* 1978;89:454–458.
11. Hill MW, Guillemet HC, Simmons FB. Fiberoptic and EMG studies in hypersomnia–sleep apnea syndrome. *Sleep apnea syndromes*. New York: Alan R Liss, 1978.
12. Fujita S, Conway W, Zorick F, Ruth T. Surgical correction of anatomic abnormalities in obstructive sleep apnea syndrome: uvulopalatopharyngoplasty. *Otolaryngol Head Neck Surg* 1981;89:923–934.
13. Guilleminault C, Korobkin R, Winkle R. A review of 50 children with obstructive sleep apnea syndrome. *Lung* 1981;159:275–287.
14. Olsen KD, Suh K, Staats BA. Surgically correctable causes of sleep apnea syndrome. *Otolaryngol Head Neck Surg* 1981;89:726–731.
15. Carpenter JG. Mental aberation and attending hypertrophic rhinitis with subacute otitis media. *JAMA* 1892;19:539–542.
16. Wells WA. Some nervous and mental manifestations occurring in connection with nasal disease. *Am J Med Sci* 1898;116:677–692.
17. Aserinsky E, Kleitman N. Regular occurring periods of eye motility and concomitant phenomena during sleep. *Science* 1953;118:273.
18. Jouvet M, Michel M, Courjon J. Sur une étude d'activité électrique cérébrale rapide au cours du sommeil physiologique. *Ec R Soc Biol (Paris)* 1959;1953:1024.
19. Cottle M. Nasal nocturnal syndrome. Presented at the meeting on Current Medical, Surgical and Physiologic Aspects of Rhinology, Rochester, Minnesota, June 1–3, 1978.
20. Lavie P, Fischel N, Zomer J, Eliaschar I. The effects of partial and complete mechanical occlusion of the nasal passages on sleep structure and breathing in sleep. *Acta Otolaryngol* 1983;95:161–166.

21. Zwillich CW, Zimmerman J, Weil JV. Effects of nasal obstruction on sleep in normal man [Abstract]. *Clin Res* 1979;27:405A.
22. Zwillich CW, Pickett C, Hanson FN, Weil JV. Disturbed sleep and prolonged apnea during nasal obstruction in normal man. *Am Rev Respir Dis* 1981;124:158–160.
23. Irvine BW, Dayal VS, Phillipson EA. Sleep apnea due to nasal valve obstruction. *J Otolaryngol* 1984;13:37–38.
24. Himer D, Scharf SM, Lieberman A, Lavie P. Sleep apnea syndrome treated by repair of deviated nasal septum. *Chest* 1983;84:184–185.
25. Rubin AH, Eliaschar I, Joachim Z, Alroy G, Lavie P. Effects of nasal surgery and tonsillectomy on sleep apnea. *Bull Eur Physiopathol Respir* 1983;19:612–615.
26. Dayal VS, Phillipson EA. Nasal surgery in the management of sleep apnea. *Ann Otol Rhinol Laryngol* 1985;94:550–554.
27. Proetz A. *Essays on the applied physiology of the nose.* St. Louis: Annals Publishing Company, 1941.
28. Lugaresi E, Cirignotta F, Coccagna G, Montagna P. Clinical significance of snoring. In: Saunders N, Sullivan CE, eds. *Sleep and breathing.* New York: Marcel Dekker, 1984.
29. Lugaresi E, Cirignotta F, Mondini S. Snoring. *Bull Eur Physiopathol Respir* (in press).
30. Lugaresi E, Coggagna G, Cirignotta F, et al. Breathing during sleep in man in normal and pathological conditions. In: Fitzgerald RS, Gautier H, Lahiri S, eds. *The regulation of respiration during sleep and anesthesia.* New York: Plenum, 1984.
31. Lugaresi E, Cirignotta F, Coccagna G, Piana C. Some epidemiological data on snoring and cardiocirculatory disturbances. *Sleep* 1980;3:221–224.
32. Mondini S, Zucconi M, Cirignotta F, et al. Snoring as a risk factor for cardiac and circulatory problems: an epidemological study. In: Guilleminault C, Lugaresi E, eds. *Sleep/wake disorders: natural history, epidimiology and long term evolution.* New York: Raven Press, 1983.
33. Partinen M. Palomaki H. Snoring and cerebral infarction. *Lancet* 1985;2:1325–1327.
34. Gislason T, Alberg H, Taube A. Snoring and systemic hypertension—an epidemiological study. *Acta Med Scand* 1987;222:415–421.
35. Koskenvuo M, Kaprio J, Telakivi T, et al. Snoring as a risk factor for ischaemic heart disease and stroke in men. *Br Med J* 1987;294:16–19.
36. Norton PG, Dunn EV. Snoring as a risk factor for disease: an epidemiological survey. *Br Med J* 1985;231:630–632.
37. Koskenvuo M, Kaprio J, Partinen M, et al. Snoring as a risk factor for hypertension and angina pectoris. *Lancet* 1985;1:893–896.
38. Williams AJ, Houston D, Finberg S, et al. Sleep apnea syndrome and essential hypertension. *Am J Cardiol* 1985;55:1019–1022.
39. Lugaresi E, Coccagna G, Farneti P, et al. Snoring. *Electroencephalogr Clin Neurophysiol* 1975; 39:59–64.
40. Lugaresi E, Mondini S, Zucconi M, et al. Staging of heavy snorers disease: a proposal. *Bull Eur Physiopathol Respir* 1983;19:590–594.
41. Issa FG, Sullivan CE. Alcohol, snoring and sleep apnea. *J Neurol Neurosurg Psychiatry* 1982; 45:353–359.
42. Bradley TD, Brown IG, Grossman RF, et al. Pharyngeal size in snorers, nonsnorers and patients with obstructive sleep apnea. *N Engl J Med* 1986;315:1327–1331.
43. Brown IG, Bradley TD, Phillipson EA, et al. Pharyngeal compliance in snoring subjects with and without obstructive sleep apnea. *Am Rev Respir Dis* 1985;132:211–215.
44. Cirignotta F, Lugaresi E. Some cineradiographic aspects of snoring and obstructive apneas. *Sleep* 1980;3:225–226.
45. Fairbanks DNF. Snoring: surgical vs nonsurgical management. *Laryngoscope* 1984;94:1188–1192.
46. Grundfast KM, Wittich DJ Jr. Adenotonsillar hypertrophy and upper airway obstruction in evolutionary perspective. *Laryngoscope* 1982;92:650–656.
47. Freeman WJ. Adenoid hypertrophy, cyanosis and cor pulmonale in children with congenital heart disease. *Laryngoscope* 1973;83:238–249.
48. Jaffee IS. Adenotonsillectomy as the treatment of serious medical conditions: five case reports. *Laryngoscope* 1974;84:1135–1141.
49. Konno A, Togawa K, Hoshino T. The effect of nasal obstruction in infancy and early childhood upon ventilation. *Laryngoscope* 1980;90:699–707.
50. Morris HD, Doyle PJ, Riding KH, Morton JW. The effects of posterior packing on pulmonary function in posterior epistaxis. *Trans Am Acad Ophthalmol Otolaryngol* 1976;82:504–508.

51. McNicholas WT, Tarlo S, Cole P, et al. Obstructive apneas during sleep in patients with seasonal allergic rhinitis. *Am Rev Respir Dis* 1982;126:625–628.
52. Lavie P, Gertner R, Zomer J, Podoshin L. Breathing disorders in sleep associated with "microarousals" in patients with allergic rhinitis. *Acta Otolaryngol (Stockh)* 1981;92:529–533.
53. Lavie P, Fischel N, Zomer J, et al. The effects of partial and complete mechanical obstruction of the nasal passages on sleep structure and breathing in sleep. *Acta Otolaryngol (Stockh)*1983;95:161–166.
54. Ramos J. On the integration of respiratory movements. 111. The fifth nerve afferents. *Acta Physiol Lat Am* 1960;10:104–113.
55. Arbour P, Kern EB. Paradoxical nasal obstruction. *Can J Otolaryngol* 1975;4:333–338.
56. Angell James JE, Daly M de B. Nasal reflexes. *Proc R Soc Med* 1969;62:1287–1293.
57. Cole P, Haight JSJ. Posture and nasal patency. *Am Rev Respir Dis* 1984;129:351–354.
58. Cassisi NJ, Biller HF, Ogura JH. Changes in arterial oxygen tension and pulmonary mechanics with the use of posterior packing in epistaxis: a preliminary report. *Laryngoscope* 1971;81:1261–1266.
59. Morris HD, Doyle PJ, Riding KH, Morton JW. The effects of posterior packing on pulmonary function in posterior epistaxis. *Trans Am Acad Ophthalmol Otolaryngol* 1976;82:504–508.
60. Kravath RE, Pollack CP, Borowiecki B, Weitzman ED. Obstructive sleep apnea and death associated with surgical correction of velopharyngeal incompetence. *J Pediatr* 1980;96:645–648.
61. Crysdale WS. Otorhinolaryngologic problems in patients with craniofacial anomalies. *Otolaryngol Clin North Am* 1981;14:145–155.
62. Olsen KD, Kern EB, Westbrook PR. Sleep and breathing disturbance secondary to nasal obstruction. *Otolaryngol Head Neck Surg* 1981;89:804–810.
63. Guilleminault C, Souquet M, Ariagno RL, Korobkin R, Simmons FB. Five cases of near-miss sudden infant death syndrome and development of obstructive sleep apnea syndrome. *Pediatrics* 1984;73:71–78.
64. Zwillich CW, Picket C, Hanson FN, Weil JV. Disturbed sleep and prolonged apnea during nasal obstruction in normal men. *Am Rev Respir Dis* 1981;124:158–160.
65. Lavie P, Fischel N, Zomer J, Eliaschar I. The effects of partial and complete mechanical occlusion of the nasal passages on sleep structure and breathing in sleep. *Acta Otolaryngol* 1983;95:161–166.
66. Rochester DF, Braun NMT. The diaphragm and dyspnea: evidence from inhibiting diaphragmatic activity with respirators. *Am Rev Respir Dis* 1979;119(Suppl):77–80.
67. Mathew OP, Abu-Osba YK, Thach BT. Influence of upper airway pressure changes on genioglossus muscle respiratory activity. *J Appl Physiol* 1982;52:438–444.
68. White DP, Cadieux RJ, Lombard RM, et al. The effects of nasal anesthesia on breathing during sleep. *Am Rev Respir Dis* 1985;132:972–975.
69. Fairbanks DNF. Effect of nasal surgery on snoring. *South Med J* 1985;78:268–270.
70. Fairbanks DNF. Uvulopalatopharyngoplasty complications and avoidance strategies. *Otholaryngol Head Neck Surg* 1990;102:239–245.

Snoring and Obstructive Sleep Apnea, Second Edition,
edited by D.N.F. Fairbanks and S. Fujita.
Raven Press, Ltd., New York © 1994.

12

The Hypopharynx

Upper Airway Reconstruction in Obstructive Sleep Apnea Syndrome

*†Nelson B. Powell, *†Robert W. Riley,
and †Christian Guilleminault

*750 Welch Road, Suite 317, Palo Alto, California 94304; and
†Stanford Sleep Disorders Clinic, Stanford, California 94305

It is now well established that there are multiple sites of obstruction in obstructive sleep apnea syndrome (OSAS) (1–4). In the past, these regional sites have often been treated independently, and unfortunately the overall control rates have reflected this approach (5). An understanding of these problems would suggest that a concept of comprehensive upper airway reconstruction (UAR) should now include all anatomic regions that may contribute to nocturnal airway obstruction. This reconstructive approach should improve clinical outcomes from surgical intervention. The regions of the nose, nasopharynx, and pharynx are generally managed with soft tissue surgery. Surgery to these individual regions has been very successful when the obstructive anatomy was isolated to one of these specific sites, and the outcome is reflected by acceptable control rates at those levels (6–8). The remaining region, the hypopharynx, includes the genioglossus–hyoid complex, epiglottis, and ary-epiglottic folds (supraglottic larynx). A combination of soft tissue and skeletal reconstruction of the hypopharynx can lead to control rates that are comparable to those achieved at the upper levels and that are statistically competitive with current medical management (CPAP) (9). A review of the soft tissue and maxillofacial surgical techniques are to be described using a protocol formulated by our surgical group at the Stanford Sleep Disorders Center.

SURGICAL INDICATIONS (GENERAL)

All patients with documented OSAS [by history (subjective) and polysomnogram (objective)] and with sufficient symptoms and clinical findings to treat medically are candidates for surgical intervention. This assumes they are medically healthy and psychologically stable and that their respective age does not create undesirable risks. Specifically, surgical indications must include two parameters of OSAS. These are excessive daytime somnolence (EDS) (behavioral derangement) and cardiorespiratory derangements. EDS currently is an important indicator for treatment on an equal basis with hypoxemia and arrhythmia (cardiorespiratory derangements). Parameters from the polysomnogram are used to include the respiratory disturbance index (RDI), sleep architecture, and oxygen desaturation. An RDI≥20 is used as a general criterion for treatment of OSAS. This level of sleep derangement is usually associated with EDS and thus chosen as a baseline for treatment. There are, as would be expected, exceptions where EDS is noted below an RDI of 20. There is even a smaller subgroup with low RDIs whose daytime somnolence is secondary to upper airway resistance syndrome (10). These must be carefully examined individually and assessed because many could also benefit from surgical intervention. Furthermore, oxygen desaturation is limited to only a few drops in oxygen saturation below 90%, with any major hypoxemia $SaO_2 \leq 85$ being a more positive indicator for treatment (Table 1).

METHODS OF EVALUATION: HYPOPHARYNGEAL

The discussion of surgical intervention in the patient with OSAS must be linked to discovery of "disproportionate anatomy" in the upper airway (2). Each region of the airway is carefully examined clinically, fiberoptically, and radiographically to determine the most likely sites of obstruction. From a compilation of the patient's symptoms, health, polysomnographic data, and results of therapeutic and diagnostic trials of CPAP, along with our clinical evaluation (as previously described), we can logically direct surgical management. Because this discussion is limited to the hypopharynx, it will be assumed that these same methods discussed above should have been applied and utilized when evaluating the remaining upper airway in OSAS. This is absolutely essential because anywhere along the upper airway "tube" a blockage not recognized and corrected above or below will ensure failure to the level treated. Hence, the concept of complete upper airway evaluation and reconstruction must be vigorously adopted and pursued.

The most consistent pathologic finding in our examination of the hypopharynx in OSAS is a narrow posterior airway space (PAS) and low hyoid bone position (MP-H) (11). Both depict a posterior placed base of tongue (BOT). Often the clinical finding of a mandibular deficiency is noted. As usual, there are many associated factors such as weight, age, body habitus, skeletal deficiencies, and current health

TABLE 1. *General indications for treatment*

Altered daytime performance [excessive daytime somnolence (EDS)]
RDI ≥ 20
Oxygen desaturation < 90
Arrhythmias associated with obstructions

TABLE 2. *Two-phase surgical approach for OSAS treatment*

Phase I surgery[a]
Nasal reconstruction
Uvulopalatopharyngoplasty (UPPP)
Genioglossus advancement-hyoid myotomy (GAHM)
Phase II surgery[a]
Bimaxillary advancement (MMO)
Subapical mandibular osteotomy[b]
Base of tongue surgery

[a]Staged as indicated.
[b]For class I cases when sufficient overjet is not present.

that also impact management. These multifactorial associations combine to challenge our abilities in evaluation and treatment.

PRINCIPLES OF TREATMENT

Surgical treatment of the hypopharynx in OSAS is not straightforward; this is due to the varied multifactorial combinations which impact this region. Our ability to consistently predict a favorable outcome has therefore been difficult. This problem has seen significant improvement in recent years, although there is still more work to be done to perfect the process. Until then, for these precise reasons, we advocate a phased surgical intervention. At our center, there are two surgical phases with individual steps (stages) in each (Table 2). The first phase is the most conservative approach to the tongue base and relies on a limited tongue advancement/ hyoid suspension without movement of the jaw or teeth. The rationale for this procedure stems from the fact that the forward movement of the geniotubercle and genioglossus muscle places tension on the tongue, thereby decreasing the probability it will prolapse into the PAS during sleep. Those patients who have failed to respond sufficiently (i.e., surgical cure) may be considered for phase II intervention which is a bimaxillary advancement [maxillary mandibular osteotomy (MMO)]. This procedure is a routine maxillofacial technique adapted and modified specifically to treat and enlarge the posterior airway space (PAS) (12–18). The framework for bimaxillary surgery was developed to improve the results found with movement of the mandible alone in treating OSA (19–22). The advancement of the midface provides more room for the tongue and places additional tension on the tongue/ hyoid complex. We have defined our phases (I and II) and individual stages in each phase into a protocol to attain a number of objectives. This protocol and the principles of treatment can be used as a tool to evaluate, diagnose, and plan management as well as to gather objective and subjective data for clinical outcomes. It additionally has been used to limit unnecessary surgery and minimize risks to the patients. This protocol and the principles of treatment have been outlined in previous publications, and only the highlights are presented (23–25) (Table 3).

TABLE 3. *Principles of treatment protocol*

Treatment to cure
Logically direct management
Full patient disclosure of options and risks
Stage surgical management
Follow-up all treatment

INDIVIDUAL TREATMENT METHODS

At present, base of tongue obstruction is surgically managed by maxillofacial techniques and/or by direct surgical or laser excision of the tongue base and portions of the supraglottic larynx. Our phase II protocol does occasionally include tongue reduction; however, this technique is infrequently used by our center and has been limited to cases where the tongue is a major problem due to its size (i.e., acromegaly or idiopathic macroglossia). Additionally, tongue reduction has been used very selectively as a recovery technique in patients who have improved in phase I or II but could benefit by further enlargement at the PAS.

Fujita and Woodson (26,27) have devised two excellent methods for soft tissue management of the tongue base, specifically laser glossectomy and midline lingualplasty. They will present these procedures and usage in Chapter 9 (*this volume*). We have preferred to advance the tongue first by maxillofacial techniques before reverting to these methods but support and subscribe to their important role in the treatment of hypopharyngeal obstruction. The maxillofacial methods presently used are an anterior mandibular osteotomy with genioglossus and hyoid advancement (AMO-H) [this procedure will be referred to as a *genioglossus advancement–hyoid myotomy* (GAHM) in the remaining text] (phase I protocol) and bimaxillary advancement (MMO) (phase II protocol).

GENIOGLOSSUS ADVANCEMENT–HYOID MYOTOMY: HISTORY AND TECHNIQUE

This is a surgical method which, without moving the jaw or teeth, moves the genioglossus and its attachment at the inferior lingual aspect of the mandible (geniotubercle) forward approximately the full thickness of the respective mandible. This distance is usually 10–14 mm. No additional room is gained for the tongue; however, the tongue is placed on tension. In combination with this maxillofacial technique, the hyoid is suspended and fixed as an adjunct to the genioglossus forward tension (28,29). Because this portion is not considered a maxillofacial procedure, it will be described separately. The GAHM procedure improves PAS in most patients. However, it has been difficult and impractical to predetermine the amount of forward advancement necessary to effect a cure at this level. Despite the many hundreds of these we have performed over the years, we are always surprised

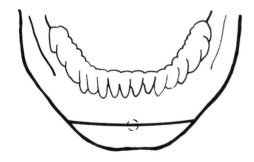

FIG. 1. A horizontal osteotomy cut across the anterior mandible which attempts to include a portion of the genioglossus attachment (*dotted circle* depicts geniotubercle). (Procedure abandoned because of fracture risk.)

at the extreme variations found in the elasticity of the genioglossus. Some advancements are difficult to move even 6–10 mm due to the extreme tension of the genioglossus, whereas others are so lax that the segment is "floppy" and we have had to resort to placing a graft behind the advanced section to gain additional tension and stability. Through the years, every attempt has been made to improve this technique and its outcome. The original method was nothing more than a high genioplasty which would include only a portion of the genioglossus muscle (Fig. 1). Results were absolutely discouraging, and with any reasonable advancement of the geniotubercle the chin was protrusive and could be unsightly. The mandible was often weakened enough that mandibular fracture was a concern. This technique was abandoned after only a few trials. The next generation was an inferior sagittal osteotomy with genioglossus advancement (ISO) which was a very satisfactory procedure in our hands (Fig. 2). Unfortunately it was technically very difficult and it too could weaken the inferior border sufficiently to set up a fracture site. This concern and reports of fractures from a few who had attempted the surgery convinced us that if the rationale and technique for this procedure was to survive and become popular it would be important to redesign the technique so that it would be safer and more easily performed by most surgeons. The next generation was an anterior mandibular osteotomy (AMO) where a segment of bone was cut through and through to include the geniotubercle and genioglossus (Fig. 3). This segment was rectangular, and when pulled forward the lingual surface (inner) of the mandible with the tubercle attached was now at the outer surface of the labial cortex

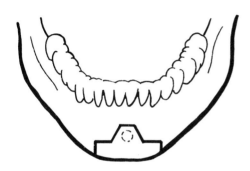

FIG. 2. An inferior sagittal osteotomy cut at the inferior border extending up and including the geniotubercle (*dotted circle* depicts geniotubercle). The cuts are sagittal to allow an advancement with locking of the wings of the cut on the outer surface. (Fracture risk exists.)

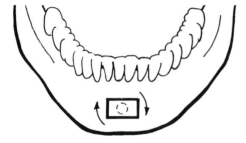

FIG. 3. The anterior mandibular osteotomy is made in a rectangular form with 2.2-cm horizontal and 0.8-cm vertical limbs and parallel walls. This cut includes the entire geniotubercle (*dotted circle* depicts geniotubercle). The segment is advanced and turned 90° to lock the inner (lingual) surface of the mandible and geniotubercle at the outer (labial) surface. The inferior border is maintained intact. (Preferred procedure.)

(outer). The rectangular segment was then turned 90° like a key and locked from pulling lingually. The outer surface was smoothed, and one small titanium screw was used for rigid fixation. This procedure was very simple, and there were minimal changes in the external contour of the chin after removal of the outer cortex. The disadvantages were that hemostasis of the bony cuts was more difficult and that the geniohyoids, which attached lower, were not advanced as well as they had been in prior techniques which advanced the entire inferior border (ISO). The major advantage was its simplicity and stability from any fractures due to the fact that the inferior border was solidly intact.

In our continued attempt to improve outcomes, we decided to again redesign the technique to be a composite of the ISO and the AMO where the genioglossus was separately isolated and the inferior border was sectioned (Fig. 4). This seemed reasonable because the geniohyoids would be subjected to some additional tension from advancement of the inferior segment. Hence, a two-piece mandibular procedure similar to the ISO was developed, but it differed in that the inferior border was reestablished and fixed, thereby creating improved stability. This new step did provide more access for improved hemostasis, and it theoretically gained some additional tension on the geniohyoids not achieved in the AMO technique.

After clinical use and assessment of this modification, we did not see a clinically significant improvement in our outcomes which would justify continuing use. In addition, this procedure was very similar to the ISO; and although it was easier to technically accomplish, it still had approximately the same risks of fracture. We have presently settled for the AMO (Figs. 5 and 6) and have done so because (a) sufficient tension is possible, (b) it is easy to do surgically, and (c) the inferior border is protected. This procedure has fewer potential risks and is more likely to be used by surgeons in our field.

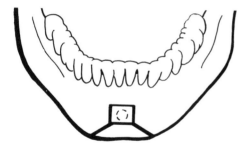

FIG. 4. The anterior mandibular osteotomy cut combines the methods shown in Figs. 2 and 3 and is done in two separate pieces. Advancement of the geniotubercle is then made, and the inferior segment of the mandibular border is reestablished (*dotted circle* depicts geniotubercle). (Fracture risk exists.)

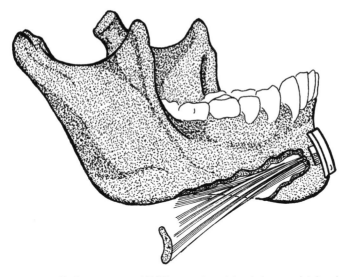

FIG. 5. Anterior mandibular osteotomy (AMO) procedure, lateral view: geniotubercle advancement showing anterior repositioning of genioglossus and geniohyoids.

The exact surgical procedures which include the hyoid myotomy and suspension have been described in detail in the literature (24,30) and, like the bimaxillary advancement, will not be reviewed in any specific detail.

HYOID MYOTOMY AND SUSPENSION

The hyoid is an integral determinant to base of tongue position. We have used this concept to combine advancement procedures with hyoid surgery to improve the

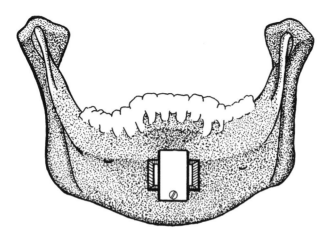

FIG. 6. Anterior mandibular osteotomy (AMO) procedure, frontal view: geniotubercle advancement.

TABLE 4. *Indications for surgical intervention genioglossus advancement–Hyoid myotomy*

An RDI of 20 or greater and/or documented excessive daytime somnolence with an RDI of less than 20[a].
Oxygen saturation below an Sao$_2$ of 90%[a].
Both of the above with a base of tongue obstruction as seen by clinical examination, lateral cephalometric head film, and fiberoptic endoscopy.
A BMI of less than 33.
No significant skeletal facial deformity (SNB ≥ 75).
Patients with severe obstructive apnea who are being prepared for bimaxillary surgery in a step sequence in our phased protocol. This includes the patients with a BMI greater than 33 or SNB less than 75.

[a]General indications for treatment of OSAS.

overall outcomes. Previously and up to December 1991, we had used a technique that suspended the hyoid upward and forward with fascia lata. Over the years, this procedure has also undergone attempted refinements as directed by other reports and our own hands-on experience (31,32). The suspension was done to the inferior anterior mandible utilizing variations of stainless steel wire, temporalis fascia, pericranium, permanent sutures, and finally fascial lata. The most predictable and reliable was suspension with fascia lata, and the vast majority were done with fascia. A few cases were also done by sectioning the hyoid as described by Patton and Thawley (32). Titanium miniplates were used for expansion, or the expansion was done using a sliding osteotomy of the hyoid body if the hyoid was sufficiently calcified. These were found, in most, to be unstable and not predictable enough to continue usage. In January 1992 a modified technique was adopted which suspends the hyoid to the larynx for improved clinical outcomes. At present we are evaluating this simpler method which does not require a fascial graft. The numbers thus far are too small to report on although very promising, and hence we will defer presentation until it is appropriate. Suffice to say that the original method has been a reliable adjunct to the geniotubercle advancement (GA) and should not be ignored as a method to improve the PAS.

SPECIFIC INDICATIONS FOR TREATMENT WITH GENIOGLOSSUS ADVANCEMENT–HYOID MYOTOMY (GAHM)

The indications and rationale for this surgical technique must include those cited as general indications for treatment of OSAS (Table 4). This group must then additionally have the findings of type II or III obstruction as classified by Fujita (33) (Table 5). This is simply the finding of base of tongue obstruction (hypopharyngeal

TABLE 5. *Classification of obstructive region by Fujita*

Type I:	Palate (normal base of tongue)
Type II:	Palate and base of tongue
Type III:	Base of tongue (normal palate)

obstruction). It is a misconception that patients who have a very-small-PAS micrognathism (SNB<75°) may not be candidates for this procedure. This finding simply decreases the odds for success. A small number of these patients simply depict a subclass that will require phase II surgery as well. When this group is identified, the patients should pass through phase I in preparation for phase II. We know from our data that there is a modest possibility that patients in this subgroup may improve sufficiently and be controlled without utilization of phase II. Hence, all patients are studied after the first step (phase I). Patients who failed phase I surgery and are selected for phase II will conceptually be more adequately prepared and will be a safer group to manage immediately postsurgically. This is because by protocol the nose and pharyngeal region either would be nonobstructed or would have been optimally cleared surgically during phase I. Important also is that the tongue, in those with hypopharyngeal obstruction, would be on maximum tension from a GAHM prior to a bimaxillary advancement. This fact has, we believe, improved our outcomes and creates in most situations excess tension to the tongue which may well protect the patient from relapse (i.e., protective overcorrection).

CLINICAL OUTCOMES

Criteria for the evaluation of success have been selected and consistently applied in all of our previous papers and recently have been upgraded to comply with continuing knowledge of this syndrome. This upgrading was in step with new data on morbidity and mortality as well as medical success with the use of nasal CPAP or BiPAP. All patients in our reports underwent a complete clinical examination combined with fiberoptic nasopharyngolaryngoscopy, cephalometric analysis, and polysomnography pre- and postoperatively. Surgical procedures were logically directed by these findings, and patients were placed in a phased protocol as previously described. Many in each phase were on CPAP prior to surgery and maintained on CPAP after surgery until a follow-up polysomnogram was performed. Patients were restudied with polysomnography 4–6 months following each phase, and weights [body mass index (BMI), expressed in kg/m^2)] were documented. Polysomnography was done almost exclusively at the Stanford Sleep Disorders Center. Recorded were the RDI, number of Sao_2 falls below 90%, and the nadir Sao_2. In more recent reports, sleep architecture and esophageal pressures (PES) are included. Subjective data on snoring and daytime performance were attained in all. Several of our papers have compared the results of surgery to the results of CPAP prior to surgery (9,34). These studies have modified our definition of a favorable clinical outcome. Recent papers have used this comparison to assess cure or control rates for the individual procedures. Prior to this we used the following criteria to define control: a postoperative RDI of 20 or less and/or at least a reduction of the RDI of 50% (i.e., a patient with an RDI of 28 would need to have a postoperative RDI of 14 to be a responder). In addition, postoperative Sao_2 must be normal or only have a few minimal falls below 90%. After 1990, sleep architecture and CPAP comparison were included.

GAHM CLINICAL OUTCOMES

In 1989, 55 patients had undergone genioglossus advancement and hyoid suspension and were reported on using the original criteria for success (28). Polysomnographically, 37 patients (67%) had been positive responders and 18 patients (33%) were not. This was a reasonably large series, and prior reports of ours and others confirmed similar improvements and control (35–37). Experience from these series suggested additional criteria to use to further select patients who may have favorably responded to phase I protocol. Included were normal pulmonary function, normal mandibular development, and the absence of morbid obesity. Those who were in the nonresponder group were then candidates for phase II surgical protocol or continued on CPAP. Recently we have reported on 306 consecutively treated patients from a group of 415 patients (34). A two-phase surgical protocol was adhered to when the patient had not initiated surgical treatment elsewhere. Otherwise they were accepted "as is" regardless of previous management. Phase I surgery consisted of a uvulopalatopharyngoplasty (UPPP) for palatal obstruction (type I Fujita) and a genioglossus advancement with hyoid (GAHM) for type II and or type III (Fujita). Follow-up polysomnograms were done a minimum of 6 months after surgery. The postoperative polysomnogram was compared to the preoperative study. In those cases where patients were also concomitantly treated with nasal CPAP (121 patients), their second-night nasal CPAP polysomnogram was also compared. Polysomnographic parameters were RDI, lowest O_2 saturation (LSAT), number of falls <90%, and sleep architecture. Outcomes were considered favorable (i.e., cure) if surgery was equivalent to nasal CPAP (second-night study) or if the postoperative RDI was less than 20 with normal oxygen saturation (no or minimal Sao_2<90%).

In phase I, 239 patients were treated and restudied: 233 had both a UPPP and a GAHM, 6 had only a GAHM, and 10 underwent UPPP as an isolated procedure. The respective success rates for these groups were 61% (145 of 239) overall, 57% (133 of 233), 66% (4 of 6), and 80% (8 of 10) (Table 6). The mean age of the group (35 women and 271 men) as a whole (306 patients) was 47.2 years (SD 11.2). The mean BMI was 30.5 kg/m^2 (SD 5.8) (normal <27.8 kg/m^2). Thus, most were moderately obese. Mandibular deficiency was seen with a mean SNB of 76.5% (SD 5.3). This group had moderate-to-severe OSAS with a mean RDI preoperatively of 55.8 (SD 26.7) and LSAT mean of 70% (SD 15.8) (Table 7). Preoperative CPAP and postoperative data are seen in Table 8. There were sufficient numbers of pa-

TABLE 6. *Phase I surgical protocol results*

Surgery groups	Number of successful patients/total	Success rate (%)
GAHM + UPPP	133/233	57
GAHM	4/6	67
UPPP	8/10	80
Total	145/239	61

TABLE 7. *Baseline data 306 patients with OSAS*

Age:	47.2 years (SD 11.2)
Sex:	35 F /271 M
Weight (BMI):	30.5 (SD 5.8)
RDI:	55.8 (SD 26.7)
LSAT:	70.5 (SD 15.8)

tients in this series to correlate severity against outcomes using the RDI and LSAT (Table 9). There was no statistically significant change in weight (BMI) in pre- and post-treatment measurements. Forty-four patients had 1–4 years follow-up. All patients in this study were loud snorers and experienced EDS. After treatment, snoring and EDS as a group were significantly improved. Those who did not attain a positive clinical outcome were offered phase II surgery or continued CPAP.

INDICATIONS FOR BIMAXILLARY ADVANCEMENT (MMO) (PHASE II)

This procedure (phase II) is offered to patients with severe OSAS who have failed all other methods of surgical or medical management. This group is usually obese and unable to lose weight. Previous reports of mandibular advancements alone have demonstrated successful improvements. However, those of bimaxillary advancement have even been more predictable and successful. The specific criteria for our phase II protocol are listed in Table 10.

MMO HISTORY AND TECHNIQUE

Originally, the major impetus for developing bimaxillary surgery for OSAS was to offer an alternative to tracheotomy and decannulate patients who had tracheostomies and who were not doing well due to hygiene, chronic bronchitis, and psychologic reasons. A bimaxillary procedure was selected instead of a single advancement of the mandible because movement of only one jaw limited sufficient

TABLE 8. *Surgical results phase I (GAHM)*

Parameter	Preoperative CPAP	CPAP	Postoperative CPAP
RDI	48.3 (SD 25.8)	7.2 (SD 4.9)	9.5 (SD 9.5)
LSAT	75.0 (SD 12.6)	86.4 (SD 11.0)	86.6 (SD 4.5)
TST	360 (SD 72)	363 (SD 67)	379 (SD 63)
% Stage 3–4	4.4 (SD 5.6)	11.1 (SD 10.8)	8.5 (SD 7.7)
% REM	11.9 (SD 5.8)	18.3 (SD 7.0)	17.7 (SD 5.6)
SNB	77.5 (SD 5.2)		
PAS	5.5 (SD 1.6)		8.5 (SD 2.1)
BMI	29.2 (SD 5.2)		28.8 (SD 4.9)

TABLE 9. *Surgical results for phase I*

OSAS severity	Number of successful patients/total	Success rate (%)
RDI<20[a] LSAT>85	20/26	77
RDI 20–40[b] LSAT>80	45/58	78
RDI 40–60[c] LSAT>70	36/51	71
RDI>60[d] LSAT<70	44/104	42

[a]Mild.
[b]Moderate.
[c]Moderate-severe.
[d]Severe.

improvement to the PAS. This surgical procedure is used much more infrequently than phase I because success rates in phase I have been reasonable. From our experience we must caution others that it does not make good medical or surgical sense to proceed with this procedure (phase II) unless the more conservative measures have been exhausted first. Patients in this last group are generally morbidly obese with a BMI greater than 33 kg/m^2, an RDI greater than 60, and a mean SNB less than 75° (reflecting mandibular deficiency). Because of the severity of the patient's OSAS and the extent of surgery required, our protocol includes a more rigorous set of contraindications. Patients who have severe chronic lung disease with an FEV 1 less than 70% and/or an RV/TLC greater than 40% have been excluded. We have also been reticent to accept patients for treatment who are aged and whose health may significantly alter recovery from this major surgical procedure. Those who are drug-dependent or psychiatrically unstable are also excluded. It is obvious that this procedure may not be appropriate to all patients in this group (phase II). Each patient must be fully counseled concerning the other possible options, as well as the risks and benefits, so that they may become educated enough to make an informed consent. To date, all surgical management of bimaxillary advancement has been done in conjunction with orthodontic treatment to help ensure a stable occlusion postoperatively.

It is the specific goal of the bimaxillary surgical procedure to move the maxilla and mandible as far forward as possible (see Fig. 7), keeping in mind three important factors. The first is stability of the segments, which minimizes any significant relapse. The second would be limiting aesthetic changes of the face from excessive forward movements, and the third would be the overall goal of clearing the PAS.

TABLE 10. *Bimaxillary advancement: indications for treatment*

Severe OSAS
Morbid obesity BMI>33
Satisfactory desire and health to undergo and recover from surgery
Failure of other forms of treatment

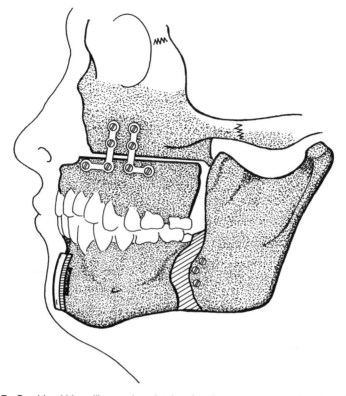

FIG. 7. Combined bimaxillary and geniotubercle advancement procedure, lateral view.

During the work-up of patients with severe OSAS, we have found that many of these patients have a class II malocclusion demonstrating a mandibular deficiency with overjet (the distance between the upper and lower teeth with mouth closed). The remaining patients are those who have a class I occlusion, which is a normal bite with the central incisors and bicuspid molars interdigitating so that the teeth meet evenly (less than 1- to 2-mm overjet). The patient with a mandibular deficiency (class II) can usually proceed with an advancement of the maxilla and the mandible into a class I dental occlusion. This stabilizes the arch as well as maximizes the amount of advancement to the maxilla and mandible and thus gains additional PAS. A more complicated problem is seen in patients who have a normal occlusion (class I). The decision then must be made whether to move the upper and lower jaw forward as one unit. This movement, in most patients, usually gains a maximum advancement of 8–10 mm. This is due, in part, to the fact that the maxillary wall is thin and that extreme advancements (greater than 10 mm) create instability and possible aesthetic disharmony. If, after an individual evaluation of the specific case, it is felt that the PAS was improved in phase I, then a bimaxillary advancement will probably open the airway sufficiently to justify a bimaxillary advancement as one unit. Hence, both jaws are brought forward and the class I occlusion is maintained. In the case where there is concern that the PAS is narrowed and very little improvement has been seen in phase I, an attempt to gain further room by an intermediate procedure is planned. This is a total subapical mandibular osteotomy with repositioning of the inferior alveolar nerves bilaterally. In this step the second molar teeth are removed from the mandible bilaterally to gain 8–10 mm of room. Then the inferior alveolar nerves are isolated from the bone and carefully moved laterally out of the way of the planned subapical osteotomy. A cut below all of the roots of the teeth extending back to the second molar extraction site is then finished. After this procedure has been performed, which it should be pointed out is quite challenging, a distalization of the alveolus and the teeth into the space made by removing the second molar teeth is completed. The body of the mandible maintains its original position. This creates approximately 8–10 mm of additional overjet (a change from a class I occlusion to a class II occlusion). A period of 6–8 weeks for healing is planned and then the bimaxillary procedure is scheduled. The advantage of this surgical procedure is that when the maxilla is moved forward 6–8 mm the mandible is able to move forward approximately twice the distance that the maxilla is moved. The additional room that is gained and the effort required is not always necessary, and the decision to proceed with this intermediate step must be made on an individual basis with each selected patient.

MMO CLINICAL OUTCOMES

Our current report reviewing 306 patients had 91 patients placed into phase II protocol. The group of patients who declined phase II treatment and opted for CPAP or no further treatment were older and had a mean age of 51.8 years (SD 9.8). The mean age of the remaining patients who were placed in the phase II protocol was lower: 43.5 years (SD 11.5). From this group of 91 patients, 24 patients had unsuccessfully passed through phase I and 60 patients had been referred after previous unsuccessful surgical management at other centers. Many of these had portions of phase I surgery already completed. Seven patients did not require UPPP; however, they underwent GAHM. All patients were restudied at 6 months using the protocol previously described with comparison to CPAP. The mean RDI preoperatively was 68.3 (SD 23.3) and the LSAT was 63.2 (SD 17.5). The mean postoperative RDI was 8.4 (SD 5.7) and the LSAT was 86.6 (SD 3.4). These were compared to those who were utilizing CPAP on the second night of nasal CPAP adjustments, with the finding that the mean nasal CPAP RDI was 7.6 (SD 5.9) and the LSAT was 87 (SD 3.9) (Table 11). In this group of patients the mean follow-up was approximately 9 months. Twenty-seven of the patients who entered into this protocol had follow-up studies ranging from 1 to 4 years. There were two failures in this group (2 of 91). Success rate and clinical outcomes utilizing CPAP as a parameter for cure showed that 97% were registered as successful (Table 12).

TABLE 11. *Surgical results for phase II (MMO)*

Parameter	Preoperative CPAP	CPAP	Postoperative CPAP
RDI	68.3 (SD 23.3)	7.6 (SD 5.9)	8.4 (SD 5.9)
LSAT	63.2 (SD 17.5)	87.0 (SD 3.9)	86.6 (SD 3.4)
TST	373 (SD 60)	354 (SD 72)	381 (SD 63)
% Stage 3–4	2.9 (SD 4.4)	12.0 (SD 13.6)	8.2 (SD 7.7)
% REM	8.9 (SD 4.0)	20.8 (SD 8.8)	19.1 (SD 6.0)
SNB	74.0 (SD 8.1)		76.7 (SD 6.2)
PAS	4.3 (SD 1.8)		9.4 (SD 2.2)
BMI	31.1 (SD 6.3)		30.5 (SD 5.9)

CLINICAL OUTCOMES: MORBIDITY, MORTALITY

In this series of 306 patients there was no mortality. The morbidity of the procedures is very low and can be credited to a very systematic medical and surgical work-up which utilizes (a) nasal CPAP with surgery (38) and (b) a staged method of management. The mean hospital stay for patients in phase I surgery is 2.1 days (SD 0.5). The phase II hospital stay is 2.4 days (SD 0.7). In the 233 patients who underwent a combined GAHM and UPPP, three patients required control in the operating room for postoperative bleeding. None of these patients required a blood transfusion. It should be further pointed out that none of the 306 patients in the complete series were given or required banked blood. The patients who have undergone UPPPs have experienced a minor amount of transient reflux, and this has resolved within approximately 3–6 weeks. No difficulties have been seen with speech or swallowing in any of the procedures. The patients requiring maxillofacial surgical procedures in phase II have experienced transient anesthesia in the cheek and chin region especially after a subapical osteotomy with repositioning of the inferior alveolar nerves. Eighty-seven percent of these anesthesias, paresthesias, or dysesthesias have resolved in 6–12 months. No patient has experienced any motor nerve involvement from the procedures, and none has required readmission for an infectious process.

TABLE 12. *Phase II (MMO) surgical protocol results*

Surgery groups	Number of successful patients/total	Success rate (%)
Failed phase I (GAHM + UPPP)	24/24	100
Skeletal deformity (without UPPP)	7/7	100
Failed UPPP[a]	58/60	97
Total	89/91	98

[a]Outside referral; severe OSAS did not enter protocol.

DISCUSSION

This series of 306 patients is, at present, one of the largest published surgical series of UAR for OSAS in the world. Not only the experience gained from intervention, but also the evaluation of the data, has substantiated surgical treatment for OSAS. The results of diligent surgical management are now comparable to those of CPAP. This is, at present, germane because new studies on nasal CPAP have objectively shown excellent initial efficacy; however, long-term compliance has been poor. These studies further suggest that as a result of this problem, quality sleep is rarely seen in those who are treated with CPAP (39–41). The surgical arm of treatment for OSAS will become more important in management because many of the failures from CPAP resurface for treatment. Surgical intervention will be important for those who wish a more permanent solution. It is apparent that with proper selection, preparation, and postoperative management, soft tissue and maxillofacial surgery combined with the use of CPAP will result in adequate control of most patients with OSAS.

REFERENCES

1. Borowiecki B, Pollak C, Weitzman E, Rakoff S, Imperato J. Fibro-optic study of pharyngeal airway during sleep in patients with hypersomnia obstructive sleep-apnea syndrome. *Laryngoscope* 1978; 88:1310–1313.
2. Rojewski T, Schuller D, Clark R, Schmidt H, Potts R. Videoendoscopic determination of the mechanism of obstruction in obstructive sleep apnea. *Otolaryngol Head Neck Surg* 1984;92:127–131.
3. Wilms D, Popovich J, Fujita S, Conway W, Zorick F. Anatomic abnormalities in obstructive sleep apnea. *Ann Otol Rhinol Laryngol* 1982;91:595–596.
4. Crumley R, Stein M, Golden J, Gamsu G, Dermon S. Determination of obstructive site in obstructive sleep apnea. *Laryngoscope* 1987;97:301–308.
5. Riley R, Guilleminault C, Powell N, Simmons B. Palatopharyngoplasty failure, cephalometric roentgenograms, and obstructive sleep apnea. *Otolaryngol Head Neck Surg* 1985;93:240–243.
6. Sher AE, Thorpy MJ, Shprintzen RJ, Spielman AJ, Burack B, McGregor PA. Predictive valve of Müller maneuver in selection of patients for uvulopalatopharyngoplasty. *Laryngoscope* 1985;95: 1483–1487.
7. Katsantonis GP, Walsh JK. Somnofluoroscopy: its role in the selection of candidates for uvulopalatopharyngoplasty. *Otolaryngol Head Neck Surg* 1986;94:56–60.
8. Katsantonis GP, Maas CS, Walsh JK. The predictive efficacy of the Müller maneuver in uvulopalatopharyngoplasty. *Laryngoscope* 1989;99:677–680.
9. Riley RW, Powell NB, Guilleminault C. Maxillofacial surgery and nasal CPAP. A comparison of treatment for obstructive sleep apnea syndrome. *Chest* 1990;98:1421–1425.
10. Guilleminault C, Stoohs R, Duncan S. Snoring. Daytime sleepiness in regular heavy snorers. *Chest* 1991;99:40–48.
11. Riley R, Guilleminault C, Herran J, Powell N. Cephalometric analyses and flow-volume loops in obstructive sleep apnea patients. *Sleep* 1983;6:303–311.
12. Riley RW, Powell NB, Guilleminault C. Maxillofacial surgery and obstructive sleep apnea: a review of 80 patients. *Otolaryngol Head Neck Surg* 1989;101:353–361.
13. Riley R, Powell N, Guilleminault C. Current surgical concepts for treating obstructive sleep apnea syndrome. *J Oral Maxillofac Surg* 1987;45:149–157.
14. Riley R, Powell N, Guilleminault C, Nino-Murcia G. Maxillary, mandibular, and hyoid advancement: an alternative to tracheostomy in obstructive sleep apnea syndrome. *Otolaryngol Head Neck Surg* 1986;94:584–588.
15. Cote E. Obstructive sleep apnea—an orthodontic concern. *Angle Orthod* 1988;293–307.

16. Guilleminault C, Quera-Salva MA, Powell NB, Riley RW. Maxillo-mandibular surgery for obstructive sleep apnoea. *Eur Respir J* 1989;2:604–612.
17. Hoffstein V, Wright S. Improvement in upper airway structure and function in a snoring patient following orthognathic surgery. *J Oral Maxillofac Surg* 1991;49:656–658.
18. Waite PD, Wooten V, Lachner J, et al. Maxillomandibular advancement surgery in 23 patients with obstructive sleep apnea syndrome. *J Oral Maxillofac Surg* 1989;47:1256–1261.
19. Bear SE, Priest JH. Sleep apnea syndrome: correction with surgical advancement of the mandible. *J Oral Surg* 1980;38:543–550.
20. Kuo PC, West RA, Bloomquist DS, McNeil RW. The effect of mandibular osteotomy in three patients with hypersomnia sleep apnea. *Oral Surg Oral Med Oral Pathol* 1979;48:385–392.
21. Powell N, Guilleminault C, Riley R, Smith L. Mandibular advancement and obstructive sleep apnea syndrome. *Bull Eur Physiopathol Respir* 1983;19:607–610.
22. Martin PR, Lefebvre AM. Surgical treatment of sleep-apnea-associated psychosis. *CMA J* 1981; 124:978–980.
23. Powell NB, Riley RW. Obstructive sleep apnea. Orthognathic surgery perspectives, past, present, and future. *Oral Maxillofac Surg Clin North Am* 1990;2:843–856.
24. Powell NB, Riley RW, Guilleminault C. Maxillofacial surgery for obstructive sleep apnea. In: Guilleminault C, Partinen M, eds. *Obstructive sleep apnea syndrome: clinical research and treatment.* New York: Raven Press, 1990;153–182.
25. Powell NB, Riley RW, Guilleminault C. Rationale and indications for surgical treatment in obstructive sleep apnea syndrome. *Oper Tech Otolaryngol Head Neck Surg* 1991;2:87–90.
26. Fujita S. Midline laser glossectomy with linguoplasty: a treatment of obstructive sleep apnea syndrome. *Oper Tech Otolaryngol Head Neck Surg* 1991;2:127–131.
27. Woodson BT, Fujita S. Clinical experience with lingualplasty as part of the treatment of severe obstructive sleep apnea. *Otolaryngol Head Neck Surg* 1992;107:40–48.
28. Riley RW, Powell NB, Guilleminault C. Inferior mandibular osteotomy and hyoid myotomy suspension for obstructive sleep apnea: a review of 55 patients. *J Oral Maxillofac Surg* 1989;47:159–164.
29. Riley R, Guilleminault C, Powell N, Derman S. Mandibular osteotomy and hyoid bone advancement for obstructive sleep apnea: a case report. *Sleep* 1984;7:79–82.
30. Powell NB, Riley RW, Guilleminault C. Maxillofacial surgical techniques for hypopharyngeal obstruction in obstructive sleep apnea. *Oper Tech Otolaryngol Head Neck Surg* 1991;2:112–119.
31. Kaya N. Sectioning the hyoid bone as a therapeutic approach for obstructive sleep apnea. *Sleep* 1984;7:77–78.
32. Patton T, Thawley S. Expansion hyoidplasty for sleep apnea. *Ear Nose Throat J* 1984;63:88–101.
33. Fujita S. Pharyngeal surgery for obstructive sleep apnea and snoring. In: Fairbanks DNF, Fujita S, Ikematsu T, Simmons FB, eds. *Snoring and obstructive sleep apnea.* New York: Raven Press, 1987;101–128.
34. Riley RW, Powell NB, Guilleminault C. Obstructive sleep apnea syndrome: a review of 306 consecutively treated surgical patients. *Otolaryngol Head Neck Surg* 1993;108:117–125.
35. Rintala A, Nordström R, Partinen M, Ranta R, Sjöblad A. Cephalometric analysis of the obstructive sleep apnea syndrome. *Proc Finn Dent Soc* 1991;87:177–182.
36. Metes A, Direnfeld V, Haight J, Hoffstein V. Resolution of obstructive sleep apnea following facial surgery. *J Otolaryngol* 1991;20:342–344.
37. Johnson NT, Chinn J. Uvulopalatopharyngoplasty and inferior sagittal mandibular osteotomy with genioglossus advancement for treatment of obstructive sleep apnea. *Chest* 1994;105:276–283.
38. Powell NB, Riley RW, Guilleminault C, Nino-Murcia G. Obstructive sleep apnea, continuous positive airway pressure, and surgery. *Otolaryngol Head Neck Surg* 1988;99:362–369.
39. Kribbs NB, Redline S, Smith PL, et al. Objective monitoring of nasal CPAP usage in OSAS patients. *Sleep Res* 1991;20:270–271.
40. Kribbs NB, Pack AI, Kline LR, et al. The effects of one night without nasal CPAP treatment on sleep and sleepiness in patients with obstructive sleep apnea. *Am Rev Respir Dis* 1993;147:1162–1168.
41. Kribbs NB, Pack AI, Kline LR, et al. Objective measurement of patterns of nasal CPAP use by patients with obstructive sleep apnea. *Am Rev Respir Dis* 1993;147:887–895.

Snoring and Obstructive Sleep Apnea, Second Edition,
edited by D.N.F. Fairbanks and S. Fujita.
Raven Press, Ltd., New York © 1994.

13

Anesthesia for Obstructive Sleep Apnea Patients

Risks, Precautions, and Management

*Mary K. Craddock and †David E. Lees

*Department of Anesthesia, Sibley Memorial Hospital, Washington, D.C. 20016; and
†Department of Anesthesia, Georgetown University Medical Center, Washington, D.C. 20007

Patients requiring surgical treatment of obstructive sleep apnea syndrome present significant challenges for safe and successful anesthetic management. The frequently robust appearance of these patients belies the presence of a pathologically fragile airway, the source of the sleep apnea syndrome.

The special anesthesia risks attending these patients include the following:

1. Muscular relaxation of sleep, sedation, or anesthetic induction allows the soft palate to collapse against the posterior pharynx, the tongue to fall back against the posterior oropharynx, and the fleshy lateral walls of the hypopharynx to collapse medially on inspiration (1,2). The excessive redundancy of these tissues in the apnea patient makes the lumen resemble the interior of an intestine, and the path of the airway easily becomes lost among the folds. Even the lightest sedation carries the potential to create an airway crisis.

2. Typical anatomical features of apnea patients include a receding chin; a short, stocky neck; a bulky tongue; and a short mandible that resists wide opening of the mouth. These are well-known impediments to easy peroral endotracheal intubation, and it sometimes requires considerable muscular effort to expose the larynx to direct view. Indeed, it is not unusual to encounter one of these patients in whom conventional intubation is completely impossible. Induction should not begin without a contingency plan to establish an airway by some other means.

3. Cor pulmonale, hypertension, and cardiac arrythmias often accompany these patients as part of the sleep apnea syndrome, adding risk to all facets of anesthesia (3).

A thoughtful anesthetic approach to the obstructive sleep apnea patient avoids sedative and narcotic premedication which might alter respiratory drive or influence the tone of the genioglossus and geniohyoid muscles. Premedication with atropine or glycopyrrolate is desirable for the antisialagogue properties in the event that repeated intubation maneuvers become necessary. A preoperative visit to establish rapport with the patient and give him or her confidence in the anesthesiologist is an excellent method of making the patient free of apprehension and fully cooperative on the day of surgery. During the preoperative visit, the anesthesiologist will be afforded the opportunity to assess the extent of the obstructive sleep apnea syndrome by the patient's history and from the sleep laboratory testing results. Examination of the oropharynx, assessment of temporomandibular joint motion, demonstration of neck mobility, and judgment of the relative position of the larynx to the mandible aid in predicting difficulty of airway management. The anesthesiologist may observe adipose deposits in pharyngeal tissue or hypertrophied tonsils, which may contribute to airway obstruction. Inability of the patient to place his or her lower incisors anterior to the upper incisors will reflect limitations of the temporomandibular joints (4). Distance, measured with the neck in full extension, between the inferior border of the mandible and the thyroid notch may be a useful predictor of intubation difficulty. If that distance is 6.0 cm or less in the adult, visualization by direct laryngoscopy is probably impossible; between 6.0 and 6.5 cm, visualization is possible but difficult; a distance of greater than 6.5 cm from the lower edge of the chin to the thyroid notch corresponds to an easy intubation (5). Also, the location of the larynx relative to the cervical spine influences the degree of difficulty. Normally the larynx extends from the third to the sixth cervical vertebra. When the larynx is relatively high on the cervical column in the "short, thick-necked" patient (a phrase not infrequently used to describe the sleep apnea patient), the angle between the oral cavity and the pharynx will be so acute that visualization beyond it by direct laryngoscopy is impossible (6). Additional factors such as prominent teeth and receding chin will also increase the difficulty of tracheal intubation. In predicting the degree of difficulty through his or her preoperative visit, the anesthesiologist has the opportunity to select techniques which he or she believes will give reasonable expectation of securing an airway. Emergency tracheostomy after failed attempts at establishment of an endotracheal airway is exceedingly rare, but the anesthesiologist should arrange for this option to be immediately available should the need arise during anesthetic induction.

Because a patient who is awake is able to maintain his or her own airway during anesthetic induction, awake intubation is the preferred technique in the suitably prepared, cooperative patient with a difficult airway. Topical anesthesia of the upper airway, when achieved with thoroughness and patience, produces a comfortable, relaxed patient and, therefore, easier working conditions for the anesthesiologist. Mild sedation, administered in small incremental intravenous doses in preparation for the intubation attempt, can facilitate patient relaxation and may be used as long as the patient is able to maintain his or her airway. Topical anesthesia of the mouth and oropharynx can be accomplished by a 2% viscous lidocaine gargle or a local anesthetic spray, such as 4% lidocaine or Cetacaine (benzocaine, butamben, and tetracaine combination) (7). Anesthesia produced by gargling is best accomplished when the patient sits with his or her head back in full extension and is encouraged to gargle vigorously until coughing occurs, indicating some aspiration and therefore a well-anesthetized glottis. Anesthesia of the nasopharynx includes the goal of vasoconstriction to reduce the incidence of epistaxis and enlarge the nasal passages. This can be accomplished with 4–6% cocaine as a spray or applied to the nasal mucosa on cotton pledgets or with 4% lidocaine plus 0.5% phenylephrine as a spray. Because cocaine is a controlled substance and the drugs have been proven to be equally efficacious, the lidocaine–phenylephrine combination may be preferred on the basis of easier handling and storing (8).

Two nerve blocks may be added to the topical anesthesia to ensure a completely anesthetic upper airway. A block of the superior laryngeal nerves may be desirable because the internal laryngeal branch of the superior laryngeal nerve supplies sensation to the mucous membranes of the pharynx and larynx just above the glottis. With the patient supine, the injection of several cubic centimeters of a local anesthetic between the thyroid cornu and the hyoid cartilage bilaterally will block both the internal laryngeal nerve and the external laryngeal nerve which supplies the cricothyroid muscle, the only extrinsic muscle of the larynx (9). Because the recurrent laryngeal nerve supplies sensation below the level of the vocal cords, a transtracheal (translaryngeal) block will be required to prevent coughing as the endotracheal tube passes into the trachea. A concentrated local anesthetic such as 3–4 ml of 4% lidocaine is injected midline through the cricothyroid ligament between the inferior border of the thyroid cartilage and the cricoid cartilage. Rapid removal of the needle upon injection is necessary, since the patient will involuntarily cough with the introduction of the local anesthetic to the trachea (10).

With the upper airway comfortably anesthetized, intubation of the trachea is possible while the patient continues to maintain his or her own airway in the awake state. Depending upon the degree of difficulty predicted for the tracheal intubation and the skills of the anesthesiologist, a variety of techniques are available for awake intubation.

BLIND NASAL INTUBATION

A well-lubricated endotracheal tube is gently inserted through a nostril and into the pharynx. Once breath sounds are heard coming from the endotracheal tube, the anesthesiologist positions the tube and the patient's head so that as the tube is advanced the breath sounds increase in volume until the tube passes through the glottis. Problems arise when repeated attempts become necessary, since repositioning the nasotracheal tube inevitably results in epistaxis with the attendant coughing or expectoration, suctioning, and possibly loss of patient rapport. Successfully performed, this technique has the advantage of requiring no special equipment and no instrumentation other than the endotracheal tube (11).

INTUBATION WITH DIRECT LARYNGOSCOPY

Suitable anatomy and a fully cooperative patient are the ingredients for success with this technique. It is important to position the patient to carefully align the axes of the mouth, pharynx, and trachea: the head is elevated with firm padding, the cervical spine is flexed, and the head is extended at the atlantooccipital joint. The patient then voluntarily opens his/her mouth and relaxes his/her tongue and neck while a laryngoscope is introduced with as little stimulation as possible. With steady upward pressure the laryngoscope is eased forward at the base of the tongue until the glottis is exposed for intubation.

TRANSILLUMINATION-GUIDED INTUBATION

Devices with a lighted tip such as a fiberoptic laryngoscope or a flexible light wand (Flexilum by Concept Inc. of Clearwater, Florida) have been used in conjunction with a darkened room as a valuable aid for the difficult intubation. The fiberoptic laryngoscope or the flexible light wand is positioned to just inside the tip of the endotracheal tube, and the tube is advanced toward the glottis, with or without a laryngoscope. When transillumination of the trachea is brightest, the endotracheal tube can be advanced into the trachea (12–15).

TRANSTRACHEAL RETROGRADE CATHETER GUIDE

Retrograde passage of a small catheter or guide wire via a needle puncture of the cricothyroid membrane through the glottis and exiting from the oral cavity supplies a guide for the endotracheal tube insertion (16,17). A 14- or 16-gauge needle is used to puncture the cricothyroid membrane, and, with the needle directed toward the larynx, the catheter or wire is threaded cephalad through the vocal cords and into the oropharynx. The catheter or guide wire should be of sufficient length to allow easy handling, such as the 36-in. epidural catheters or the 120-cm Swan-Ganz introducer wire (18). The catheter or wire exits the mouth either when the patient produces it with his/her tongue or when the anesthesiologist sweeps the patient's mouth with his/her finger. The endotracheal tube is then placed over the guide and threaded through the glottis into the trachea. The catheter or wire may then be removed from either end.

If the passage of the endotracheal tube is thwarted by soft tissue obstruction, a variation of this technique is invariably successful: After retrograde passage, the catheter or wire is securely tied through the Murphy eye of the endotracheal tube. A stylet with an appropriate curve is placed in the endotracheal tube, and under direct laryngoscopy the tube is advanced toward the glottis with an assistant pulling steadily on the guide catheter/wire. With the catheter/wire held in tension between the tip of the endotracheal tube and the cricothyroid, the epiglottis tents and elevates over the guide, while the trachea realigns its axis and the intubation can proceed under direct vision. The guide catheter/wire is removed with the endotracheal tube during extubation.

FIBEROPTIC LARYNGOSCOPY

Improvement of flexible fiberoptic laryngoscopes and the addition of adequate suctioning capabilities have done much to advance the popularity of this technique for managing difficult intubations (19–21). The technique still requires experience on the part of the operator and familiarity of the airway appearance through the fiberoptic device. The flexible laryngoscope (or bronchoscope) is passed through an orally positioned endotracheal tube. Under direct vision through the fiberoptic eyepiece, the laryngoscope is passed through the vocal cords; the endotracheal tube is then sheathed down the laryngoscope into the trachea to complete the intubation. When the oral route is chosen, a bite block or airway is recommended to protect the fiberoptics from damage by a patient who might inadvertently bite down during instrumentation; the airway will also help keep the tongue in a forward position, thereby enhancing access to the larynx. An alternative to the flexible fiberoptic laryngoscope in oral intubation is the fiberoptic stylet laryngoscope, in which the fiberoptic system is a malleable stylet for the endotracheal tube. The fiberoptic stylet is placed within 3–4 mm of the endotracheal tube tip, and the stylet and tube are inserted orally. The operator then uses the eyepiece to direct the stylet and tube toward the glottis, then slides the tube off the stylet into the trachea, timing it with patient inspiration.

In nasotracheal intubation, the endotracheal tube is inserted through a nostril to the posterior pharynx. The fiberoptic laryngoscope is then passed beyond the tube toward the glottis, and the laryngoscope tip is manipulated until the epiglottis and vocal cords are identified. The laryngoscope is passed through the glottis into the trachea, and the endotracheal tube is threaded over it. This technique is associated with a very high success rate in the hands of experienced operators: One series reports only four failures in 413 cases of fiberoptic laryngoscopy for anticipated difficult intubations (22). Control of bloody or mucous secretions appears to be a critical factor in achieving success; a preoperative antisialagogue, minimization of trauma, and adequate suction port on the fiberoptic equipment can substantially contribute to reducing problems with secretions.

INTUBATION WITH A FIBEROPTIC ENDOSCOPE

The Bullard laryngoscope is a rigid fiberoptic endoscope that is useful in cases of difficult intubation. It consists of a rigid, anatomically curved blade and a fiberoptic system with the eyepiece at the level of the laryngoscope handle (23). The image bundle runs under the blade and emerges under the distal tip, enabling indirect visualization of the larynx. The blade height is narrow (a maximum distance of 6 mm), requiring a small area of mouth to be opened (24). A dedicated stylet positions the endotracheal tube beneath the blade and guides the tube through the glottis, with minimal manipulation on the part of the operator (25). When used with well-applied topical oropharyngeal anesthesia, it is suitable for a comfortable awake oral intubation.

Because the Bullard laryngoscope mates fiberoptic capability with the traditional laryngoscopy technique, the learning curve associated with flexible fiberoptic intubation is avoided. This may, in part, account for its popularity with some anesthesiologists.

POSTOPERATIVE MANAGEMENT

Postoperative extubation is considered only after the patient regains consciousness, reflexes are restored, and postoperative edema is regarded as unlikely to compromise airway patency. Monitoring respiratory status in the intensive care setting for the first 24–48 hours is strongly recommended.

SUMMARY

Patients with obstructive sleep apnea should, by definition, be considered to have difficult airways for management. Steps to prepare for anesthetic airway management include a preoperative visit to assess airway appearance and to enable the patient to establish trust in the anesthesiologist. Atraumatic awake intubation in the topically anesthetized and cooperative patient is the ideal goal. Choice of suitable awake intubation techniques rests in the experience of the anesthesiologist and the physical limitations of the airway itself.

REFERENCES

1. Sanders MH, Martin RJ, Pennock BE, Rogers RM. The detection of sleep apnea in the awake patient. *JAMA* 1981;245:2414–2418.
2. Weinberg S, Kravath R, Phillips L, Mendez H, Wolf G. Episodic complete airway obstruction in children with undiagnosed obstructive sleep apnea. *Anesthesiology* 1984;60:356–358.
3. Hall JB: The cardiopulmonary failure of sleep-disordered breathing. *JAMA* 1986;255:930–933.
4. Rosenberg H, Rosenberg H: Airway obstruction and causes of difficult intubation. In: Orkin FK, Cooperman LH, eds. *Complications in anesthesiology.* Philadelphia: JB Lippincott, 1983;125–136.
5. Patil VU, Stehling LC, Zauder HL. Predicting the difficulty of intubation utilizing an intubation gauge. *Anesthesiol Rev* 1983;10 (8):32–33.
6. Vandam LD: Functional anatomy of the larynx. *Weekly Anesthesiol Update* 1977;1:Lesson 5.
7. Adriani J, Savoie A, Naraghi M. Scope and limitations of topical anesthetics in anesthesiology practice. *Anesthesiol Rev* 1983;10(7):10–15.
8. Sessler CN, Vitalitti JC, Cooper KR, Jones JR, Powell KD, Pesko LJ. Comparison of 4 percent lidocaine/0.5 percent phenylephrine with 5 percent cocaine: Which dilates the nasal passage better? *Anesthesiology* 1986;64:274–277.
9. Katz J. Superior laryngeal nerve block. *Atlas of regional anesthesia.* New York: Appleton–Century–Crofts, 1985;58.
10. Katz J. Larynx. *Atlas of regional anesthesia.* New York: Appleton–Century–Crofts, 1985;56.

11. Stoelting RK. Endotracheal intubation. In: Miller RD, Churchill L, eds. *Anesthesia*, vol 1, 2nd ed. 1986;536.
12. Stone DJ, Stirt JA, Kaplan MJ, McLean WC. A complication of light wand-guided nasotracheal intubation. *Anesthesiology* 1984;61:780–781.
13. Weis FR, Kaiser RE. Light wand-guided nasotracheal intubation is an effective technique. *Anesthesiology* 1985;62:839–840.
14. Watson CB, Claphem M. Transillumination for correct tube positions; use of a new fiberoptic endotracheal tube. *Anesthesiology* 1984;60:253.
15. Hammer M, Garry B. Transillumination of the trachea with Flexilum. *Anesth Analg* 1985;64:91–92.
16. Waters DJ. Guided blind intubation using a sheath stylet. *Anesthesiology* 1985;63:567.
17. King HK. Translaryngeal guided intubation using a sheath stylet. *Anesthesiology* 1985;63:567.
18. Roberts KW. New use for Swan–Ganz introducer wire. *Anesth Analg* 1981;60:67.
19. Watson, CB. Fiberoptic bronchoscopy for anesthesia. *Anesthesiol Rev* 1982;9(9):17–26.
20. Marshall, WK. Management of the difficult airway. *Anesthesiol Rev* 1984;11(4):18–22.
21. Kraft M: Stylet laryngoscopy for oral tracheal intubation. *Anesthesiol Rev* 1982;9(11/12):35–37.
22. Ovassapian A, Yelich SJ, Dykes MHM, Brunner EE. Blood pressure and heart rate changes during awake fiberoptic nasotracheal intubation. *Anesth Analg* 1983;62:951–954.
23. Saunder PR, Giesecke AH. Clinical assessment of the adult Bullard laryngoscope [Abstract]. *Can J Anaesth* 1989;36:5118–51119.
24. Gorback MS : Management of the challenging airway with the Bullard laryngoscope. *J Clin Anesth* 1991;3:473–477.
25. Borland LM, Casselbrandt M. The Bullard laryngoscope: a new indirect oral laryngoscope (pediatric version). *Anesth Analg* 1990;70:105–108.

Snoring and Obstructive Sleep Apnea, Second Edition,
edited by D.N.F. Fairbanks and S. Fujita.
Raven Press, Ltd., New York © 1994.

14

Snoring and Obstructive Sleep Apnea in Children

William P. Potsic and Roger R. Marsh

Department of Otolaryngology and Human Communication, The Children's Hospital of Philadelphia, Philadelphia, Pennsylvania 19104

Airway obstruction in children, and its manifestations, can be every bit as subtle or as dramatic as in adults. The etiology is varied and, as in adult cases, the treatment differs accordingly. Special considerations in both diagnosis and treatment apply to the management of children, such as the inability of a child to submit to invasive, uncomfortable, or unfamiliar tests. This makes the evaluation of a child with obstruction and sleep apnea a challenge.

The concerns of this chapter are chronic nocturnal upper airway obstruction, causing snoring that is louder in inspiration than exhalation, and interruption or cessation of airflow in the presence of inspiratory effort. Obstructive sleep apnea (OSA) is not a separate entity. It is just the extreme on a continuum of obstruction that ranges from very mild to severe. We are concerned here only with pharyngeal obstruction. Other causes of obstruction, like laryngotracheal anomalies, may produce stridor, a sound very different from snoring, and may cause severe airway obstruction, but they will not be considered here.

We use Guilleminault's definition of apnea as a cessation of airflow of at least 10-sec duration (1). However, we believe that frequent periods of cessation of airflow of less than 10 sec are also significant. We and others have also seen patients who exhibit depressed Po_2 or Sao_2 without apnea, a pattern that has been termed *obstructive sleep dyspnea* (2,3). The definitions of degrees of airway obstruction short of apnea are not well-standardized. We employ distinctions that can be made on the basis of observation of the patient and analysis of respiratory sounds. "Snoring" is imprecise; some children rattle the windows and others gasp almost inaudibly as if breathing through a straw. The loudness of snoring is not a proven correlate of severity of obstruction. The deviations from normal patterns are quantifiable, however. Along the continuum from normal, quiet respiration to apnea, we define the following degrees of obstruction: elevated inspiratory effort, irregular respiratory rate, pauses of less than 10 sec without airflow, and apnea greater than 10 sec. Snoring of some kind is invariably associated with airway obstruction of any of these degrees. Thus we shall use "obstruction" to mean "upper airway obstruction with or without apneic episodes," and we shall use "apnea" to mean OSA. OSA— frequent obstructive apneas during sleep—is distinguished from OSA syndrome, which comprises OSA and associated features such as cor pulmonale and daytime hypersomnolence.

CAUSES

By far the most common cause of snoring and apnea in childhood is hyperplasia of the tonsils and adenoids. It has been argued that the incidence of obstruction has actually increased in recent years as the number of tonsillectomies has declined (4). There are no definitive population studies of the incidence of airway obstruction due to lymphoid hyperplasia; but hyperplasia, rather than recurrent infection, is the indication for surgery in nearly 80% of the adenotonsillectomies in our department (5). In a prospective study of 100 children scheduled for surgery on the basis of hyperplasia causing airway obstruction, snoring was reported by parents in 98% of patients, as opposed to 36% in an age-matched group of children without obstruction who had not had tonsils or adenoids removed (6). Episodes of "breath holding" during sleep were reported by 70% of parents for the adenotonsillectomy group, as opposed to less than 3% for the controls. We infer that snoring is not rare at this age but that the degree of obstruction found in the patient group is not prevalent in the population in general. Few of these patients had OSA as conventionally defined; it is our belief that obstruction need not progress to that point to affect the child adversely.

Enlargement of the adenoids is normal in childhood, and it is uncertain why some children develop sufficient hyperplasia to cause obstruction while others do not. As summarized by Crepeau et al. (7), studies differ as to the time course of hyperplasia, but it is nearly universal from the fourth through the sixth year of life. In various series, the mean ages of patients undergoing adenotonsillectomy for obstruction are 4.8–5.8 years (6,8–10). OSA involving the tonsils or adenoids can appear much earlier; in a series of 14 patients under 18 months of age, symptoms were reported to have appeared at 2–6 months of age (11). Neither thickness of the adenoids nor size of the airway, determined radiographically, strongly predicts obstruction (7,8). Among patients with large tonsils, size of the tonsils (but not weight!) was weakly associated with obstruction (9). The same study did find a clear association between obstruction and short soft palates, but did not infer causality.

Numerous craniofacial syndromes have been associated with snoring and apnea. The list includes achondroplasia, facio-auriculo-vertebral sequence, and Pierre Robin, Treacher Collins, Klippel–Feil, Crouzon, and Apert syndromes (12–15). Mandibular hypoplasia is the anomaly most often implicated in OSA (Fig. 1), but there is variation in the mechanism of obstruction from syndrome to syndrome and even within a diagnosis (15). OSA in patients with craniofacial malformation may

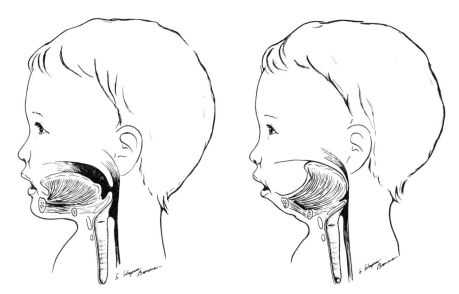

FIG. 1. Airway anatomy in mandibular hypoplasia. **Left:** Normal child. **Right:** Child with mandibular hypoplasia. Pharyngeal obstruction results from the posterior displacement of the tongue. (From ref. 41, with permission.)

develop at any time, up through adulthood. Even if the child is free of OSA at the initial examination, there is no assurance that the airway will not later become compromised. The tonsils and adenoids are often the primary cause of obstruction or play some role in these cases. A marginal airway is vulnerable to obstruction by relatively minor hyperplasia, and removal of a normal volume of adenoids can restore adequate function in some congenitally compromised airways. Even in syndromes not primarily involving craniofacial anomalies, the incidence of obstruction may be high. Nearly all Down's syndrome children snore, and apnea may develop (16–18). Hunter and Hurler cases frequently are complicated by upper airway obstruction (19). Although these children may initially respond to adenotonsillectomy, there is progressive deterioration of the airway, making management a frustrating experience (20).

Iatrogenic obstruction must be acknowledged. Snoring is to be expected when pharyngeal flaps are constructed in patients with cleft palate, and apnea, possibly with disastrous consequences, may ensue (21,22).

Although the Pickwickian syndrome is probably the most sensational presentation of OSA, obesity is not a common feature among children with OSA. To the contrary, reports abound of OSA patients who are much below normal for weight. Certainly OSA syndrome associated with obesity is encountered in the pediatric practice (4,23), but failure to thrive with weight well below the 25th percentile is the more common pattern in OSA (4,10,12,24,25).

Other causes of obstruction and OSA deserve mention. Masses of various sorts may be encountered, such as nasopharyngeal cysts, tumors, and encephaloceles.

Rarely, the lingual tonsils may enlarge enough to obstruct the airway (26). Deviated nasal septa have also been implicated (27). Airway obstruction and OSA also appear in children with neuromuscular disorders where a combination of poor pharyngeal muscular tone and hyperplasia of the tonsils and adenoids produce nighttime obstruction.

EFFECTS

OSA syndrome in children has many of the same features that it does in adults. Cor pulmonale and daytime hypersomnolence, reversible by restoration of the airway, are well-documented (1). There is, however, some feeling that findings are more variable among children; in particular, hypersomnolence may not be observed as consistently. Polysomnographic findings are similar to those in adults (1).

Certain problems are more likely in children. Body weight is often well below normal (4,10,12,24,25). Rapid catch-up weight gain after restoration of the airway is typical, demonstrating that the low weight is a consequence of obstruction. The precise relation between obstruction and low weight has not been defined, but dysphagia is often a feature of obstruction. These children are slow eaters and dislike food that requires chewing. Swallowing is difficult and uncomfortable, and food may lack appeal if the obstruction renders the child anosmic. It has been suggested, without confirmation, that impaired sleep in these children leads to growth hormone deficiency (10,28). There are suggestions in the literature of OSA causing developmental delay (10,24); but documentation is limited, and the delay, apparent or real, might be secondary to daytime hypersomnolence or sleep deprivation rather than hypoxia.

Airway obstruction need not progress to apnea to affect the child adversely (Table 1). Even without OSA, sleep disturbances are frequently reported by parents and

TABLE 1. *Manifestations of adenotonsillar hyperplasia with airway obstruction*

Manifestation	Percent of patients[a]
Sleep-related	
Snoring	98
Breath holding	70
Fatigue during day	31
Night cough	25
Daytime	
Mouth breathing	75
Slow eating	60
Dry mouth	42
Trouble swallowing	37

[a]Based on parental responses to questionnaire for 100 patients scheduled for adenotonsillectomy for airway obstruction (6).

have been documented by polysomnography (27). These children are restless sleepers, moving around in the bed all night and waking frequently. Nocturnal enuresis may persist or reappear in the obstructed child (1,29). Daytime tiredness and morning crankiness are appreciably more common in children with obstruction than among unobstructed controls, and they are also more troublesome in the obstructed children before corrective surgery than afterwards, according to parental reports (6). Other daytime manifestations—trouble swallowing, anosmia, and mouth breathing—serve as reminders that these children are always obstructed. Chronic mouth breathing also has been associated with orthodontic malformations and changes in craniofacial development (30,31), although causality, and even the existence of the association, have been questioned (32).

DIAGNOSIS

If unequivocal OSA syndrome were the sole ground for concern, then polysomnography might be the only diagnostic tool. However, we consider lesser degrees of obstruction important. History and physical examination typically provide an adequate basis for the diagnosis of airway obstruction due to adenotonsillar hyperplasia (6,33). If confirmation of OSA is required, the analysis of nocturnal breathing sounds is nearly as definitive as polysomnography and far less expensive (3). In such cases radiographic studies may aid in the diagnosis, but they are not conclusive.

In taking a history, it is perhaps obvious that parents should be questioned about the child's breathing at night and sleep habits, yet physicians may hesitate to accept parental reports as clear evidence of obstruction. Two independent studies have shown that parental responses to questions about difficulty in breathing, apnea, and snoring clearly differentiate obstructed from unobstructed children (6,34). Although the two groups differ in many other respects—appetite, behavior, daytime mouth breathing, and the like—it is the respiratory patterns during sleep that are both sensitive and specific for obstruction.

On physical examination, mouth breathing and large tonsils are characteristic. If tonsils and adenoids are enlarged in the child experiencing airway obstruction at night, a strong presumption exists that they are the culprits. In most cases of OSA in children with hypertrophic tonsils and adenoids and in nearly all the cases of lesser obstruction, the patients have responded unequivocally to adenotonsillectomy (6, 10,16,27).

The lateral neck film aids in the evaluation of the airway in cases of lymphoid hyperplasia, but is not definitive as to degree of obstruction (7,8,35). The airway responds to so many factors—posture, muscle tone, airflow, and pressure—that a static radiograph cannot adequately represent the dynamic effects of hypertrophy during sleep. Radiography also has a place when obstruction has been diagnosed but the etiology is obscure, in that radiographic examination might well demonstrate an unexpected anomaly of the upper airway.

In those cases where there is any question as to the severity of airway obstruction, definitive answers can be had by arranging for parents to tape record the child's breathing sounds during sleep. Whereas central apnea might be difficult to differentiate acoustically from very quiet breathing sounds, snoring is the hallmark of upper airway obstruction; and the practiced ear can readily recognize apneic and hypopneic episodes, as well as the ragged patterns associated with moderate degrees of obstruction. We use a more refined method of recording and analyzing breathing sounds, which we term *sleep sonography* (6,36); but we still prefer to listen to the breathing sounds to appreciate fully the parents' concern.

For sleep sonography, we lend the parents a stethoscope–microphone assembly and a tape recorder whose automatic gain control has been suitably modified. The parents attach the small stethoscope with microphone at the suprasternal notch and record two 1-hr samples. The instrument is then returned to the laboratory in a prestamped mailer, which we also provide. In the laboratory, the tape is subjected to analog and digital processing to generate displays of the sort illustrated in Fig. 2. We have demonstrated very good reliability in the interpretation of these displays, both as to agreement between observers and between recordings obtained on successive nights (37). It is our experience also that sleep sonography and polysomnography correlate well in identification of apneas and hypopneas (3).

There are certain cases where sleep sonography is particularly valuable. On occasion, one wonders whether reports of disordered nocturnal respiration are distorted by parental concern. It would certainly be understandable if apneic spells were misjudged as to duration. We have found that most often the parents have not been exaggerating, and they may welcome the opportunity to demonstrate the severity of the child's problem. In some such instances, sleep sonography has a clear advantage over polysomnography. If the obstruction varies in severity from night to night, a polysomnographic study (at considerable expense and inconvenience to all involved) may prove negative if done on the wrong night. In such cases it is more productive to lend the parents the recording apparatus with instructions to wait (for weeks if needed) until the child does have the breathing problems they are concerned about.

Polysomnography is of undeniable value in those cases where apnea is suspected but history and the physical findings are ambiguous. Examples are (a) children with neuromuscular disorders where lack of muscle tone is the primary problem and (b) patients in whom central or mixed apnea is suspected.

When polysomnography is performed for evaluation of OSA, the most important measures are those that address respiratory physiology rather than electroencephalography. Separate channels should be available for oral and nasal airflow, although it can be difficult to maintain the position of the sensors during the sleep disturbances that apnea can elicit. It is also useful to record respiratory sounds on tape, along with a graphic representation of the sound on the polygraph. Thoracic movement need not be quantified, but must be recorded at least qualitatively to permit differentiation of obstructive from central apnea. This can often be done most conveniently by recording the output of a cardiorespiratory monitor. Pulse

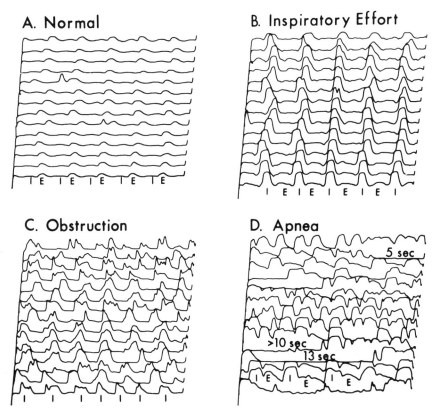

A. Normal

I E I E I E I E I E

B. Inspiratory Effort

I E I E I E I E I

C. Obstruction

D. Apnea

5 sec

>10 sec

13 sec

I E I E I E

FIG. 2. Sleep sonography. Breathing sounds are recorded under controlled conditions, then subjected to digital and analog processing. The computer-generated displays can reliably differentiate degrees of obstruction. Each line represents a 20-sec sample, with selected inspirations (I) and exhalations (E) labeled. **A:** Child free of significant tonsillar hypertrophy. **B:** Respiration is remarkably loud, but rate is stable. **C:** Inspiratory phase is prolonged and respiratory rate shows variations from one trace to the next. **D:** Patterns reflect severe obstruction; two apneas and a shorter pause are labeled. (From ref. 6, with permission.)

oximetry has largely replaced ear oximetry and transcutaneous Po_2 measurement, being convenient and accurate, but movement artifact during strenuous inspiratory effort may interfere with measurement. Recording the pulse signal from the pulse oximeter, along with the electrocardiogram from the cardiorespiratory monitor, will aid in detecting artifact. Finally, electro-oculography and electromyography permit identifying rapid eye movement (REM) sleep and the arousals that typically terminate apneic episodes.

TREATMENT

In the great majority of cases in children, lymphoid hyperplasia causes the obstruction, and adenotonsillectomy is the definitive treatment. If only the most obvious culprit, either tonsils or adenoids, is removed, obstruction often recurs, requiring a second procedure (10). It is therefore advisable to remove tonsils and adenoids together. Close observation, and even aggressive airway management, may be necessary postoperatively in patients who had severe OSA preoperatively (38,39), in part because these children may have reduced ventilatory drive, having developed tolerance to chronic hypercarbia. Patients with sickle cell disease also require special management as with any major surgery (40).

Children with craniofacial anomalies and obstructive sleep breathing also respond to adenotonsillectomy, even when the absolute mass of lymphoid tissue appears relatively small. On some occasions, improvement is considerable but adenotonsillectomy does not relieve all of the obstruction. This is particularly true in anomalies such as Crouzon's syndrome, where the cranial base severely restricts the anterior–posterior dimension of the nasopharynx. Airway management in these patients can present special challenges to the surgeon and anesthesiologist (41).

The uvulopalatopharyngoplasty (UPPP) has a place in pediatric otolaryngology. It appears to be successful in certain children with neuromuscular disorders affecting muscle tone and tissue composition (42,43). Although the basic etiology may be physiological rather than anatomical, the operation may provide an airway that is competent in spite of the underlying neuromuscular pathology. A modified procedure has been reported to benefit children with Down's syndrome as well (17).

The nasopharyngeal (NP) tube must not be forgotten (24). In cases where surgery must be deferred—acute obstruction with infection or cardiopulmonary involvement—the NP tube provides immediate relief by stenting open the obstructing NP tissues. Rarely, an endotracheal tube may be required if the child cannot tolerate an NP airway. Continuous positive airway pressure (CPAP) is often effective in upper airway obstruction. Long-term CPAP is not without problems, however (18), and may not be a satisfactory long-term solution for a child. There are some unfortunate children who do not respond to conventional therapies. For these patients, one must consider tracheotomy for relief of obstruction.

REFERENCES

1. Guilleminault C, Eldridge FL, Simmons FB, Dement WC. Sleep apnea in eight children. *Pediatrics* 1976;58:23–30.
2. Miyazaki S. Sleep-induced respiratory disturbance in children with adenotonsillar hypertrophy: the obstructive sleep dyspnea syndrome. *Oper Tech Otolaryngol Head Neck Surg* 1991;2:69–72.
3. Potsic WP. Comparison of polysomnography and sonography for assessing regularity of respiration during sleep in adenotonsillar hypertrophy. *Laryngoscope* 1987;97:1430–1437.
4. Grundfast KM, Wittich DJ. Adenotonsillar hypertrophy and upper airway obstruction in evolutionary perspective. *Laryngoscope* 1982;92:650–656.
5. Handler SD, Miller L, Richmond KH, Baranak CC. Post-tonsillectomy hemorrhage: incidence, prevention and management. *Laryngoscope* 1986;96:1243–1247.
6. Potsic WP, Pasquariello PS, Baranak CC, Marsh RR, Miller LM. Relief of upper airway obstruction by adenotonsillectomy. *Otolaryngol Head Neck Surg* 1986;94:476–480.
7. Crepeau J, Patriquin HB, Poliquin JF, Tetreault L. Radiographic evaluation of the symptom-producing adenoid. *Otolaryngol Head Neck Surg* 1982;90:548–554.
8. Laurikainen E, Erkinjuntti M, Alihanka J, Rikalainen H, Suonpää J. Radiological parameters of the

bony nasopharynx and the adenotonsillar size compared with sleep apnea episodes in children. *Int J Pediatr Otorhinolaryngol* 1987;12:303–310.

9. Brodsky L, Adler E, Stanievich JF. Naso- and oropharyngeal dimensions in children with obstructive sleep apnea. *Int J Pediatr Otorhinolaryngol* 1989;17:1–11.

10. Lind MG, Lundell BPW. Tonsillar hyperplasia in children: a cause of obstructive sleep apneas, CO_2 retention, and retarded growth. *Arch Otolaryngol* 1982;108:650–654.

11. Leiberman A, Tal A, Brama I, Sofer S. Obstructive sleep apnea in young infants. *Int J Pediatr Otorhinolaryngol* 1988;16:39–44.

12. Brouillette RT, Fernbach SK, Hunt CE. Obstructive sleep apnea in infants and children. *J Pediatr* 1982;100:31–40.

13. Mealer WR, Fisher JC. Cor pulmonale and facio-auriculo-vertebral sequence. *Cleft Palate J* 1984; 21:100–103.

14. Puckett CL, Pickens J, Reinisch JF. Sleep apnea in mandibular hypoplasia. *Plast Reconstr Surg* 1982;70:213–216.

15. Sher AE, Shprintzen RJ, Thorpy MJ. Endoscopic observations of obstructive sleep apnea in children with anomalous upper airways: predictive and therapeutic value. *Int J Pediatr Otorhinolaryngol* 1986;11:135–146.

16. Frank Y, Kravath RE, Pollak CP, Weitzman ED. Obstructive sleep apnea and its therapy: clinical and polysomnographic manifestations. *Pediatrics* 1983;71:737–742.

17. Strome M. Obstructive sleep apnea in Down syndrome children: a surgical approach. *Laryngoscope* 1986;96:1340–1342.

18. Guilleminault C, Nino-Murcia G, Heldt G, Baldwin R, Hutchinson D. Alternative treatment to tracheostomy in obstructive sleep apnea syndrome: nasal continuous positive airway pressure in young children. *Pediatrics* 1986;78:797–802.

19. Shapiro J, Strome M, Crocker AC. Airway obstruction and sleep apnea in Hurler and Hunter syndromes. *Ann Otol Rhinol Laryngol* 1985;94:458–461.

20. Sasaki CT, Ruiz R, Gaito R Jr, Kirchner JA, Seshi B. Hunter's syndrome: a study in airway obstruction. *Laryngoscope* 1987;97:280–285.

21. Kravath RE, Pollak CP, Borowiecki B, Weitzman ED. Obstructive sleep apnea and death associated with surgical correction of velopharyngeal incompetence. *J Pediatr* 1980;96:645–648.

22. Orr WC, Levine NS, Buchanan RT. Effect of cleft palate repair and pharyngeal flap surgery on upper airway obstruction during sleep. *Plast Reconstr Surg* 1987;80:226–232.

23. Simmons FB, Hill MW. Hypersomnia caused by upper airway obstructions: a new syndrome in otolaryngology. *Ann Otol Rhinol Laryngol* 1974;83:670–673.

24. Kravath RE, Pollak CP, Borowiecki B. Hypoventilation during sleep in children who have lymphoid airway obstruction treated by nasopharyngeal tube and T and A. *Pediatrics* 1977;59:865–871.

25. Williams EF III, Woo P, Miller R, Kellman RM. The effects of adenotonsillectomy on growth in young children. *Otolaryngol Head Neck Surg* 1991;104:509–516.

26. Guarisco JL, Littlewood SC, Butcher RB III. Severe upper airway obstruction in children secondary to lingual tonsil hypertrophy. *Ann Otol Rhinol Laryngol* 1990;99:621–624.

27. Mauer KW, Staats BA, Olsen KD. Upper airway obstruction and disordered nocturnal breathing in children. *Mayo Clin Proc* 1983;58:349–353.

28. Schiffmann R, Faber J, Eidelman AI. Obstructive hypertrophic adenoids and tonsils as a cause of infantile failure to thrive: reversed by tonsillectomy and adenoidectomy. *Int J Pediatr Otorhinolaryngol* 1985;9:183–187.

29. Weider DJ, Hauri PJ. Nocturnal enuresis in children with upper airway obstruction. *Int J Pediatr Otorhinolaryngol* 1985;9:173–182.

30. Bresolin D, Shapiro GG, Shapiro PA, et al. Facial characteristics of children who breathe through the mouth. *Pediatrics* 1984;73:622–625.

31. Hultcrantz E, Larson M, Hellquist R, Ahlquist-Rastad J, Svanholm H, Jakobsson OP. The influence of tonsillar obstruction and tonsillectomy on facial growth and dental arch morphology. *Int J Pediatr Otorhinolaryngol* 1991;22:125–134.

32. Klein JC. Nasal respiratory function and craniofacial growth. *Arch Otolaryngol Head Neck Surg* 1986;112;843–849.

33. Thach BT. Pediatric aspects of the sleep apnea syndrome. *Ear Nose Throat J* 1984;63:214–221.

34. Brouilette [sic] R, Hanson D, David R, et al. A diagnostic approach to suspected obstructive sleep apnea in children. *J Pediatr* 1984;105:10–14.

35. Mahboubi S, Marsh RR, Potsic WP, Pasquariello PS. The lateral neck radiograph in adenotonsillar hyperplasia. *Int J Pediatr Otorhinolaryngol* 1985;10:67–73.

36. Marsh RR, Potsic WP, Pasquariello C. Recorder for assessment of upper airway disorders. *Otolaryngol Head Neck Surg* 1983;91:584–585.
37. Marsh RR, Potsic WP, Pasquariello PS. Reliability of sleep sonography in detecting upper airway obstruction in children. *Int J Pediatr Otorhinolaryngol* 1989;18:1–8.
38. Brown OE, Manning SC, Ridenour B. Cor pulmonale secondary to tonsillar and adenoidal hypertrophy: management considerations. *Int J Pediatr Otorhinolaryngol* 1988;16:131–139.
39. McColley SA, April MM, Carroll JL, Naclerio RM, Louglin GM. Respiratory compromise after adenotonsillectomy in children with obstructive sleep apnea. *Arch Otolaryngol Head Neck Surg* 1992;118:940–943.
40. Derkay CS, Bray G, Milmoe GJ, Grundfast KM. Adenotonsillectomy in children with sickle cell disease. *South Med J* 1991;84:205–208,218.
41. Handler SD, Keon TP. Difficult laryngoscopy/intubation: the child with mandibular hypoplasia. *Ann Otol Rhinol Laryngol* 1983;92:401–404.
42. Hultcrantz E, Svanholm H, Ahlqvist-Rastad J. Sleep apnea in children without hypertrophy of the tonsils. *Clin Pediatr* 1988;27:350–352.
43. Reilly JS. Tonsillar and adenoid airway obstruction: modes of treatment in children. *Int Anesthesiol Clin* 1988;26:54–57.

Snoring and Obstructive Sleep Apnea, Second Edition,
edited by D.N.F. Fairbanks and S. Fujita.
Raven Press, Ltd., New York © 1994.

15

Oral Devices for the Management of Snoring and Obstructive Sleep Apnea

Arthur M. Strauss

*Sleep Disorders Center, Crozer-Chester Medical Center,
Upland, Pennsylvania 19013-3995*

WHAT ARE ORAL DEVICES AND HOW DO THEY WORK?

An oral device for the management of snoring and obstructive sleep apnea (OSA) is a small plastic dental appliance, similar to an orthodontic retainer or an athletic mouthguard. It is worn in the mouth during sleep to prevent the oropharyngeal tissues and base of tongue from collapsing and obstructing the airway. Most of the literature refers to these oral devices as dental appliances; therefore, throughout this chapter the terms will be used interchangeably.

Most oral devices may be held in place by gripping the teeth with wire clasps or with the flexible plastic material of which they are constructed. This is usually a methylmethacrylate, polyvinyl, or other thermoplastic material that has been FDA-approved for intraoral use. Tongue-retaining devices are held in place by the appliance's conformity to the contour and position of the dental arches. The tongue is held in the tongue-retaining bulb by suction.

Oral devices essentially function in three ways. First, by bringing the mandible and base of tongue forward or by acting as scaffolding to support a drooping soft palate and uvula. A "combination" appliance may perform two or more of these functions simultaneously. Second, by stabilizing the mandible and preventing it from opening during sleep. This assists the geniohyoid muscle in dilating the airway through protraction of the hyoid bone (1). Third, by altering mandibular position through downward rotation, thereby causing an increase in baseline genioglossus muscle activity which, it is postulated, is related to maintenance of a patent airway (2–4).

OVERVIEW AND HISTORICAL PERSPECTIVES

A detailed examination of the evolution of these dental appliances and OSA can be found in an article by Clark (5), who notes that the first reported use of a dental appliance was in 1934, when Pierre Robin described a monoblock functional appliance that was used to pull the jaw and, therefore, tongue forward. Robin's appliance was utilized for cases of micrognathia in both children and adults. One limitation of the intraoral appliance approach that Robin noted was that it was not usable in the newborn without any teeth (6).

The concept of directly pulling the tongue forward to prevent airway obstruction was first published by Shukowsky (7) in 1911. His article described micrognathia with airway obstruction in infants and related a 1903 case where he sutured the tongue to the lower lip to tie the tongue forward. In 1982 Cartwright and Samelson (8) published a paper describing a dental appliance that nonsurgically accomplished what Shukowsky had accomplished utilizing sutures 79 years earlier. This appliance, the tongue-retaining device (TRD), captured the tongue, by suction, within a small plastic bulb and held it in the forward position.

In 1984, Meier-Kwert et al. (9) reported on treatment of OSA with a mandibular protracting device. In 1985 Soll and George (10) reported effective treatment with a similar type of appliance, the nocturnal airway patency appliance (NAPA). In 1988 Schmidt-Nowara, Meade, and others (11,12) reported effective treatment of snoring and OSA with another modification of an anterior mandibular positioner, the Snore Guard. Also, in 1988 Viscomi, Toone, and others (13) reported successful treatment of five cases with yet another modification of a mandibular anterior positioner, the sleep and nocturnal apnea reducer (SNOAR). Again in 1988, Rider (14) and Clark et al. (15) separately reported successful treatments with still another appliance (an adaptation of the Herbst, a functional orthodontic appliance) that anteriorizes the mandible.

Throughout the remainder of the 1980s and into the present, additional studies of the above-noted dental appliances, and other variations of them, have been reported. These are discussed in greater depth by Alan Lowe in Meier Kryger's 1993 revised edition of *The Principles and Practice of Sleep Medicine* (16).

One can expect ongoing modification, variation, and improvement in the design of these dental appliances coming from practicing dentists. In an attempt to coordinate this with therapy, the Sleep Disorders Dental Society (SDDS) was formalized as an organization in 1991.

The objective of the SDDS is to further dental appliance therapy as an integral part of overall therapy. Its goal is to facilitate a coordinated approach to research, education, and treatment with the medical community.

There are four basic types of oral devices: the soft palate lifters, the TRDs, the mandibular repositioning devices (MRDs), and the tongue posture training devices. There are differences in the way each of these devices functions. Within these types there are variations in design that also affect the workability of each. Needed research will provide information that will enhance the effectiveness of oral devices. What we presently know and suspect about the four basic types of appliances will be conveyed by elaborating on them individually.

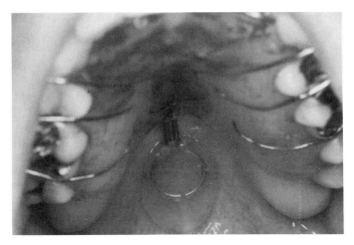

FIG. 1. Adjustable soft palate lifter. The acrylic button supporting the soft palate can be adjusted in three dimensions. (Courtesy of Herb Paskow, Longboat, Florida.)

SOFT PALATAL LIFTERS

Soft palatal lifting appliances act as scaffolding, reaching back and supporting the soft palate. This reduces the vertical drooping of the soft palate and uvula, and minimizes the fluttering effect and snoring noise. This may reduce the possibility of a long uvula getting trapped between the back of the tongue and the posterior pharyngeal wall and narrowing or occluding the oropharyngeal space. The inventor of the adjustable soft palate lifter (ASPL) (Fig. 1), Herbert Paskow, stated that he believes that the device is effective in reducing or eliminating snoring but not in treating OSA (17). To date, there are no published data on the ASPL.

TONGUE RETAINERS

The TRD (Fig. 2) and tongue-locking device (TLD) grasp the tip of the tongue and hold it forward between the front teeth. The tongue actually fits into a small flexible bulb, the size of which is related to the degree the tongue can protrude, unstrained, beyond the front teeth. When excess air is expressed from this bulb (like squeezing a bulb of a turkey baster), a suction is created. This suction holds the tongue in place. Research shows an increase in genioglossus activity directly correlated to wearing a TRD (18). It is theorized, but not yet substantiated, that TRDs are most effective when obstructions are predominantly in the oropharyngeal area. Clinicians also believe that the TRD is more suited for patients with large tongues. Studies have shown TRDs to be more effective with positional-related OSA. The TRD is a custom-made appliance, whereas the TLD is preformed (sold off the shelf). To date, there are at least six published studies on the TRD (19–24); there are no published studies on the TLD.

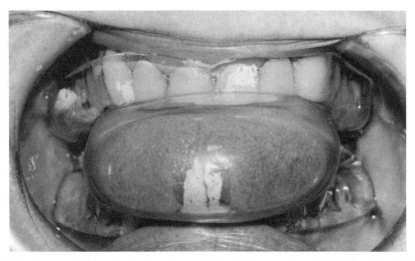

FIG. 2. Tongue-retaining device. Supplemental plastic tubes can be added to the sides to facilitate oral breathing. (Courtesy of Michael Alvarez, Freemont, California.)

MANDIBULAR REPOSITIONERS

Mandibular repositioning devices indirectly anteriorize the tongue and base of tongue by mechanically protruding the mandible. They are made of a rigid or semirigid plastic that conforms to the contour of the maxillary and mandibular arches (and teeth) and maintains them in a specific relation to one another. The devices are anchored to the teeth either by the fit and grip of wire clasps or by flexible plastic material.

The consensus on how far to anteriorize the mandible ranges from no protrusion to 1–3 mm short of the maximum unstrained protrusive range.

There are many variations in the vertical opening of the appliances. This ranges from a 5- to 7-mm interincisal distance, a minimal opening required for oral breathing, to a 13- to 17-mm interincisal distance, the opening of the SNOAR appliance (Fig. 3).

Other differences in the MRDs relate to the degree of fixation of the mandible. This ranges from total fixation of a NAPA (Fig. 4) to complete freedom of lateral and vertical movement anterior to the most protruded position of the snore guard (Fig. 5). Dr. Peter George, inventor of the NAPA, has observed return of symptoms when these appliances have become loose. He has seen these symptoms disappear again upon regaining fixation of the mandible, by tightening the grip of the NAPA clasps on the teeth. An explanation of this is described in an abstract written by George (1). In it he relates horizontal and vertical force vectors affecting the protraction of the mandible and base of tongue to vertical distance of the hyoid bone from the inferior border of the mandible. George also believes that a study by Suratt

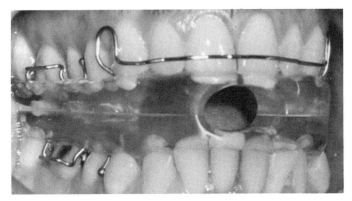

FIG. 3. Sleep and nocturnal apnea reducer. Note the larger interincisal distance of 13–17 mm. (Courtesy of Joseph Cain, Oklahoma City, Oklahoma.)

and co-workers (25) on respiratory-related recruitment of the masseter illustrates a relationship between stabilization of the mandible and the ability of an activated genioglossus muscle to dilate the upper airway.

Adjustability differs too. This ranges from nonadjustability of a mandibular repositioner monobloc-type appliance (Fig. 6) to adjustability of the Herbst appliance (Fig. 7) through incremental anteriorizing of the mandible.

There have been published studies of the above-noted mandibular anterior positioners, treating from mild to severe OSA. Combining and averaging the results shows an average reduction in mean apnea index (AI) from 45 to 16 and in mean respiratory disturbance index (RDI) from 48 to 23. Oxygen saturation and reduction of subjective symptoms seem to correlate with improvement of the AI and RDI.

TONGUE POSTURE TRAINERS

Two appliances have been designed to treat snoring and OSA by treating problems of abnormal tongue posture by strengthening the dorsal muscles of the tongue

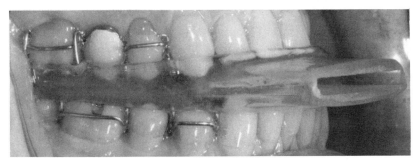

FIG. 4. Nocturnal airway patency appliance. Hollow beak facilitates oral breathing, and wire clasps grip teeth and provide total fixation of mandible. (Courtesy of Peter George, Honolulu, Hawaii.)

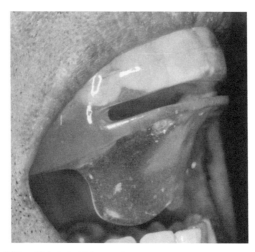

FIG. 5. Snore guard. Mandible is held forward by plastic ramp, extends behind lower front teeth, and allows some anterior, vertical, and lateral movement of mandible.

(styloglossal and palatoglossal muscles). The inventors of these appliances, the Tepper Proprioceptor Stimulator (TOPS) (Fig. 8) and the tongue positioner and exerciser (TPE), believe that they facilitate repositioning of the tongue to the soft and hard palate through proprioceptive means. The tongue then remains in a rest position so as to increase the airway space as well as the resting muscle tone. Harry Tepper, inventor of the TOPS appliance, has observed a rehabilitative effect of the appliance. To date, published data on the efficacy of these appliances are not available.

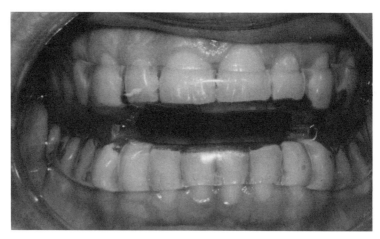

FIG. 6. A mandibular repositioner monoblock-type appliance, the "P M positioner," made of an almost-rigid thermoplastic material that anchors to teeth without clasps, not readily adjustable. (Courtesy of Jonathan Parker, St. Louis Park, Minnesota.)

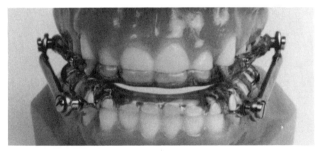

FIG. 7. Herbst appliance. Lateral metal tubes facilitate incremental anteriorization of the mandible. (Courtesy of Glen Clark, Los Angeles, California.)

DENTAL APPLIANCE THERAPY

When dentists who were utilizing more than one type of appliance in treatment began to collaborate and share their observations through the SDDS, they recognized that some dental appliances worked differently than others. They found a need to distinguish between them to determine which would be most suitable for a particular patient and condition, and why. It was also recognized that to appropriately treat patients, clinicians should be proficient in the use of the basic types of appliances.

Published studies suggest that OSA can be effectively treated by TRDs and anterior MRDs. They show a direct correlation of the degree and frequency of treatment success to the mildness of the apnea. Observations indicate that while some patients

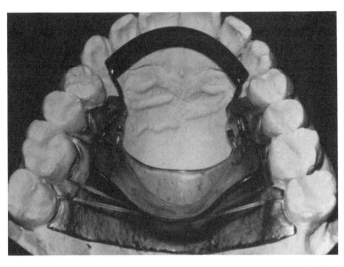

FIG. 8. Tepper proprieoceptor stimulator, which is retained by adaptation to the hard palate and gingival contours of the teeth. Tension from rubberband provides secondary ramp resistance for rehabilitative reposturing of tongue. (Courtesy of Harry Tepper, Santa Monica, California.)

can benefit from both types of appliances (TRD and MRD), others can only benefit from one or the other. Consequently, a treatment protocol for dental appliances (Fig. 9) was established to provide a therapy to select and tailor the most appropriate appliance for each patient. The appliance is customized to the patient rather than the patient having to, by chance, fit the particular appliance.

PATIENT SELECTION

The therapeutic process begins with appropriate patient selection. To facilitate the success of this, the attending physician or sleep specialist must understand what dental appliances are and how they work. They should know, statistically, when dental appliances are most effective and impart this information to the patient. For example: Dental appliances have a track record of eliminating or reducing "benign snoring" 95% of the time (12); they are most effective in treatment of mild and moderate OSA and are least effective in treatment of severe OSA (12).

The SDDS has available a brochure that explains dental appliance therapy to the lay person. The brochure is helpful to the dentist and physician/sleep disorders specialist in explaining dental appliance therapy. It is a useful supplement to other brochures on snoring and OSA available through ASDA and the American Academy of Otolaryngology—Head and Neck Surgery. It can be ordered by contacting

> Sleep Disorders Dental Society
> Wexford Professional Building, Suite 204
> 11676 Perry Highway
> Wexford, PA 15090
> Phone: (412) 935-0836
> Fax: (412) 935-0383

THE REFERRAL PROCESS

It is the position of the SDDS that snoring and sleep apnea are medical disorders that must be diagnosed by a physician or appropriate sleep specialist. The dentists' role is an adjunctive one and requires a written request from the attending physician. Accompanying information to the dentist should include the following: diagnostic history, sleep studies, prior and other anticipated treatment, and the objectives the physician has in mind for dental appliance therapy. An appropriately trained dentist is able to understand and discuss this information to collaborate in the overall treatment.

THE INITIAL VISIT

At the initial visit, patients begin a screening process, which includes their assessment of whether they are able or willing to wear any removable dental appliance while sleeping. They have an opportunity to observe and handle sample appliances.

SLEEP DISORDERS DENTAL SOCIETY

> ## Clinical Procotol for Dental Appliance Therapy
> ### for
> ## Snoring and/or Obstructive Sleep Apnea

The following therapy sequence is suggested by the SDDS for the management of dental appliances in patients who are being treated for snoring and/or OSA.

1. Medical assessment by the attending physician or sleep specialist
2. Overnight polysomnogram as required by physician or sleep specialist
3. Written referral or prescription and diagnostic report sent to dentist
4. Dental Examination
   - A. medical/dental histories
   - B. soft tissue/intra-oral assessment
   - C. peridontal evaluation
   - D. TMJ/occlusal examination
   - E. intra-oral habit assessment
   - F. examination of teeth and restorations, including prosthesis
   - G. initial dental radiographic survey
     - (1). panoramic and/or full mouth survey
     - (2). baseline cephalometric radiographic survey
   - H. diagnostic models
5. Trial appliances
   - A. design, fabrication, fitting, instructions and training
   - B. trial and evaluation (wear three to seven nights for each appliance)
   - C. final appliance design selection
     - (1). subjective symptom assessment
     - (2). cephalometric radiographic examination as required
     - (3). sleep study by attending physician as required
6. Final appliance design, fabrication, fitting and placement
7. Final appliance evaluation over 2-3 months of regular use
   - A. final adjustments to appliance
   - B. adjustment of patient to wearing appliance
   - C. subjective symptom evaluation
   - D. cephalometric radiographic examination (optional)
8. Refer patient back to attending physician for repeat overnight study
9. Possible modification, redesign or remake of appliance as required
10. Repeat adjustment and evaluation process
11. Refer back to physician for ongoing evaluation
12. Recall appointments and maintenance as requested by patient and/or physician

FIG. 9. Dental appliance therapy treatment protocol. (Courtesy of Sleep Disorders Dental Society, Wexford, Pennsylvania.)

Next, the dental condition and its relation to fitting and wearing a dental appliance must be considered. Are there enough sound teeth in strategic locations to hold or anchor the dental appliance in place? Are there dental conditions [temporomandibular joint (TMJ) dysfunction, tooth decay, periodontal disease] that may be aggravated by the use of an intraoral device?

Patients are provided with feedback regarding the relation between their current dental condition and the potential fit, including comfort and stability of various dental appliances. They also may obtain feedback on how dental treatment might affect or be affected by dental appliances. All of this assists them in their screening.

TRIAL PROCEDURES (TRIAL APPLIANCE THERAPY)

Trial procedures often begin at the initial visit and culminate in the design of a definitive appliance. Ongoing feedback is required throughout the trial process, including training and orientation sessions. This provides information for modifying the trial devices (trial TRD and trial MRD) to maximize the effectiveness. The patient can assess the relative comfort and convenience associated with wearing the trial device and interpolate this to wearing the definitive counterpart. Clinical effectiveness may be assessed through empirical feedback (observed snoring and breathing cessation, reduction of excessive daytime sleepiness, morning headaches, and other signs and symptoms), review of voice-activated tape recordings while sleeping with the trial devices and without them, and interpretation of overnight sleep studies while wearing them.

During trial procedures, patients also have the opportunity to get used to wearing a dental appliance. This includes experiencing excessive salivation or a dry mouth for a time period of a few days to a few weeks, as their body adapts to the appliance.

DEFINITIVE DENTAL APPLIANCE FABRICATION, FITTING, PLACEMENT

The process of fabrication of the definitive dental appliance is usually accomplished in a dental laboratory. Each device is custom made according to the dentist's prescription. It fits models of the teeth and gums (made of dental stone) that have been oriented in a maxillary to mandibular relationship (bite) determined through the trial procedures. When fitting the appliance, the dentist may need to modify and adjust its contour or shape for comfort and function. After wearing the appliance for several nights, the patient may return for further minor modifications. Adjustments continue until, through subjective symptom assessment, it is equal to or better than the optimized trial device. Throughout this adjustment process, clinical effectiveness can be evaluated through tests used in the trial procedures.

DEFINITIVE APPLIANCE EVALUATION

A 3-month adaptation period of nightly wearing the adjusted device should provide enough time for maximizing the effects of therapy. This occurs through habituation and through physical benefits derived from the shrinkage of previously edematous oropharyngeal tissues. The patient is then referred back to the attending physician for reevaluation including an overnight sleep study while wearing the device.

FOLLOW-UP CARE

Because these appliances are custom-fitted to the teeth and dental arches, changes in the teeth and tissues can affect their fit and necessitate adjustment. Most often the patient will be aware of symptomatic changes that can be associated with the device. An example of this may be a return of snoring or apnea symptoms associated with movement of the mandible and narrowing of the airway. This can occur with loosening of an appliance that has been locking the mandible into a static position. Further loss of muscle and tissue tone can also decrease the airway size.

Side effects, characterized by symptoms such as pain of the TMJ or masticatory muscles or a change in the bite, may necessitate temporarily or permanently discontinuing use of the device and/or modifying the design of the device.

Other side effects may be less obvious. Therefore, it is prudent for the patient to be examined by the attending dentist initially semiannually and then annually. Here, assessment of the fit of the oral device and its side effects helps determine whether modification of the device or the therapy is indicated. Some harmful side effects that may not be obvious to the patient are: changes in the bite, loosening of teeth, tissue hyperplasia, dental caries, or periodontal disease.

SUMMARY

Oral devices are similar in appearance to orthodontic retainers and athletic mouthguards. Two particular types have demonstrated effectiveness in treating OSA. They are the tongue-retaining device (TRD) and the mandibular repositioning device (MRD). Both are most effective in treating primary snoring and mild and moderate apnea.

Their designs can be modified and combined. To maximize the effectiveness of therapy, one should customize the type and design of the appliance to the patient. The treatment protocol that facilitates this involves a diagnostic process of testing the patient with trial TRDs and trial MRDs. The designs of these trial devices are modified to maximize their individual effectiveness. The trial device type and design that appears to most effectively treat the apnea becomes the basis for constructing the final/definitive appliance.

Oral devices are most often used alone. However, they also have been used in conjunction with surgery and nasal continuous positive airway pressure (CPAP).

They provide a substitute for nasal CPAP, on occasions when CPAP is inconvenient. They also may provide a means for assessing the potential success of surgery. The treatment is reversible and noninvasive. Research to date suggests that the effect of oral devices occurs only while they are being worn. No appliance has demonstrated a carry-over effect to non-use nights.

Because snoring and OSA are medical conditions, primary responsibility for diagnosis and care falls under the jurisdiction of the physician/sleep specialist. The role of the dentist is secondary and adjunctive. Therefore, the commencement of dental appliance therapy requires a written prescription by the attending physician/sleep specialist.

REFERENCES

1. George PT, Pearce JW, Kapuniai LE, Crowell DH. Stabilization of the mandible in the prevention of snoring and obstructive sleep apnea [Abstract]. *Sleep Res* 1992:21:202.
2. Lowe AA. Neural control of tongue posture. In: Taylor A. *Neurophysiology of the jaws and teeth.* London: McMillan Press, 1990;322–368.
3. Lowe AA, Fleetham J, Ryan J, Matthews B. Effects of a mandibular repositioning appliance used in the treatment of obstructive sleep apnea on tongue muscle activity. In: Suratt PM, Remmers JE, eds. *Sleep and respiration.* New York: Wiley–Liss, 1990;395–405.
4. Lowe AA. The tongue and airway. *Otolaryngol Clin North Am* 1990;23:677–698.
5. Clark GT. OSA and dental appliances. *Calif Dent Assoc J* 1988:16:26–33.
6. Robin P. Glossoptosis due to atresia and hypotrophy of the mandible. *Am J Dis Child* 1934;48:541–547.
7. Shukowski W. Zur atiologie des stridor inspiratorius congenitus. *Jahrb Kinderheilk* 1911;73:459–474.
8. Cartwright RD, Samelson CF. The effects of a nonsurgical treatment for obstructive sleep apnea—the tongue retaining device. *JAMA* 1982;248:707–709.
9. Mier-Ewert K, Schafer H, Kloss W. Treatment of sleep apnea by a mandibular protracting device. *Berichtsband 7th Eur Congr Sleep Res Munchen* 1984:217.
10. Soll BA, George PT. Treatment of obstructive sleep apnea with a nocturnal airway-patency appliance. *N Engl J Med* 1985;313:386.
11. Schmidt-Nowara WW, Meade TE, Wiggins RV. Treatment of snoring with a dental orthosis [Abstract]. *Am Rev Respir Dis* 1988;137:312.
12. Schmidt-Nowara WW, Meade TE, Hays MB. Treatment of snoring and obstructive sleep apnea with a dental orthosis. *Chest* 1991;99:1378–1385.
13. Viscomi VA, Walker JM, Farney RJ, Toone K. Efficacy of a dental appliance in patients with snoring and sleep apnea [Abstract]. *Sleep Res* 1988;17:266.
14. Rider EA. Removable Herbst appliance for treatment of obstructive sleep apnea. *J Clin Orthod* 1988;22:256–257.
15. Clark GT, Arand D, Chung E. Respiratory distress index changes with an anterior mandibular positioning device for obstructive sleep apnea. *Soc Neurosci Abstr* 1988;#1762.
16. Lowe AA. Dental appliances for the treatment of snoring and/or obstructive sleep apnea. In: Kryger M, ed. *The principles and practice of sleep medicine*, 2nd ed. 1992.
17. Paskow H, Paskow S. Dentistry's role in treating sleep apnea and snoring. *J NJ Dent Assoc* 1991; 88:815–817.
18. Ono T, Par EK, Lowe AA. Tongue retaining device effects on genioglossus muscle activity. *J Dent Res* 1993;72:261.
19. Cartwright RD. Predicting response to the tongue retaining device for sleep apnea syndrome. *Arch Otolaryngol* 1985;111:385–388.
20. Cartwright RD, Samelson CF, Lilie J, Kravitz H, Knight S, Stefoski D, Caldarelli D. Testing the tongue retaining device for control of sleep apnea [Abstract]. *Sleep Res* 1986;15:111.

21. Samelson CF. Successful use of the TRD in replacing a 27 month tracheostomy, a case report [Abstract]. *Sleep Res* 1986;15:159.
22. Cartwright RD, Stefoski D, Caldarelli D, Kravitz H, Knight S, Lloyd S, Samelson CF. Toward treatment logic for sleep apnea: the place of the tongue retaining device. *Behav Res Ther* 1988; 26:121–126.
23. Samelson CF. A survey of the effectiveness of the tongue retaining device for the control of snoring and/or obstructive sleep apnea [Abstract]. *Sleep Res* 1989;18:229.
24. Cartwright RD, Ristanovic R, Diaz F, Caldarelli D, Alder G. A comparative study of treatments for positional sleep apnea. *Sleep* 1991;14:546–552.
25. Hollowell DE, Pradmore RB, Funsten AW, Suratt PM. Respiratory-related recruitment of the masseter: response to hypercapnia and loading. *J Appl Physiol* 1991;70(6):2508–2513.

Snoring and Obstructive Sleep Apnea, Second Edition,
edited by D.N.F. Fairbanks and S. Fujita.
Raven Press, Ltd., New York © 1994.

16

Challenges and Future Trends in the Management of Obstructive Sleep Apnea

Aaron E. Sher

Division of Otolaryngology—Head and Neck Surgery, Albany Medical College, Albany, New York 12203; and Capital Region Sleep Wake Disorders Center of Albany Medical Center and St. Peter's Hospital, Albany, New York 12203

Sleep-disordered breathing is felt to be the sleep disorder that has the greatest medical and social impact. Of the approximately 75,000 patients annually seen in accredited sleep disorders centers, 75% are diagnosed with sleep apnea. Current projections of the prevalence of sleep apnea syndrome in the United States range from 7 to 18 million people. Currently, at a time when sleep apnea is just emerging as a clinically recognized entity, the cost for hospitalization is approximately $42 million. The direct cost of sleep apnea in 1990 was estimated to be 275 million dollars. This does not include the cost of reduced quality of life, lower productivity in school and the workplace, increased morbidity and mortality, and the loss of life and property due to accidents caused by excessive sleepiness (1).

Obstructive sleep apnea syndrome (OSAS) is in its infancy as a recognized disorder. Unlike many other health problems, OSAS has not had time to develop a long tradition as a health issue. Where such tradition does exist, it can exert significant influence on the public, both lay and medical. The tradition tends to relate to (a) perceived truths about the clinical significance of the disorder and (b) other perceived truths about the potential benefits and risks of available treatments, or lack of treatment. At best, these perceptions are based on scientific data. At worst, the science is obscured by the tradition itself, with the result that expectation of patients and recommendation of physicians reflect not only the science, but the tradition as well.

As a new disorder whose science (and tradition) are evolving in an era of new health policy, an era in which such tradition is being seriously challenged, OSAS can serve as a pioneer disorder developing on the frontier of a new perspective in medicine. Its estimated prevalence, its purported impact on those afflicted, and the impressive projections of its financial cost to the public all mandate that OSAS be viewed in that light. OSAS can serve as a model for the investigative approach that will hopefully dictate health policy in the future.

Major issues to be researched involve the following aspects of OSAS: its incidence and prevalence, pathophysiology, morbidity and mortality, techniques of diagnosis, techniques of treatment, and finally its cost to society in terms of human and fiscal issues.

Potential health consequences of OSAS are cardiovascular disease (including hypertension, coronary heart disease, myocardial infarction, and stroke) and neuropsychiatric problems (including depression, cognitive dysfunction, and injury due to accidents). While these associations have been inferred from a number of studies, data from prospective studies of broad segments of the population are required to define the degree to which sleep apnea is an independent risk factor for vascular and neuropsychological morbidity. Confounding influences of such co-morbidity as obesity will have to be teased out (1).

The impact of OSAS on quality of life must be investigated. Disruption of family and social relationships is a potentially significant quality of life issue for OSAS, as is interference with professional attainment and ability to earn a living.

Investigation regarding the health implications of different degrees of severity of sleep apnea is required. It remains to be determined whether there is a threshold level of sleep apnea severity above which there are adverse effects on health and quality of life. Factors that would increase susceptibility to the consequences of sleep apnea, such as age and coexisting cardiovascular, pulmonary, or psychiatric dysfunction, need to be considered. Such data would help to define an OSAS threshold, or different OSAS thresholds for patients with different patterns of co-morbidity, above which levels of morbidity and mortality would justify intervention itself, or different types and magnitude of intervention.

The search for thresholds of severity of OSAS is a complex task, since severity of OSAS is defined in terms of multiple variables. For instance, disease severity can be defined by variables associated with the respiratory disturbances during sleep: the apnea index or apnea–hypopnea index, the duration of the apneas or hypopneas, and the degree of decrease in levels of oxygen in the blood. It can also be defined by the degree of disruption of normal sleep and the degree of excessive daytime sleepiness which results from the sleep disruption. Defining clinically significant severity thresholds requires the identification of those physiological data which most closely relate to prognosis, and then incorporating these variables into an algorithm which can be applied to individual patients or to patient populations with OSAS. This would facilitate acquisition of data regarding incidence and prevalence, natural history, and effectiveness of therapy for OSAS.

The costs of OSAS and its treatment, including also the costs of associated conditions which may be exacerbated by OSAS (such as disorders of the cardiovascular system and their treatments), are potentially high and must be studied. Issues which will require study are the relative efficacy, acceptability, and cost of the various therapeutic regimens. The goal will be maximum efficacy and acceptability at minimum cost. At this point, the long-term efficacy of therapy in general, the efficacy of specific therapeutic approaches, and the natural history of OSAS, with or without therapy, are all relatively lacking in documentation.

No study to date has attempted to randomize subjects to different treatment versus control protocols, and thus there are no data to determine the influence of various treatment modalities on long-term outcomes, such as longevity, overall function, and quality of life.

While continuous positive airway pressure is effective when applied under laboratory conditions, there are significant questions relating to long-term patient compliance.

Surgical approaches have become more complex as our understanding of the nature of OSAS has increased. As the surgical armamentarium has come to include not only the soft tissue alterations of the pharynx, but also orthognathic procedures of the craniofacial skeleton, the scope of the surgical treatment team will often need to include an otolaryngologist and a maxillofacial surgeon. Indeed, a comprehensive approach to the diagnosis and treatment of OSAS will mandate a team approach, not dissimilar to the model of the craniofacial disorders team. Team members will include specialists in sleep disorders medicine, pulmonology, otolaryngology, maxillofacial surgery, bariatric medicine, bariatric surgery, pediatrics, neurology, orthodontics, and dentistry. Each team will need a director or coordinator who will be knowledgeable in all aspects of the diagnosis and treatment of OSAS, and who, with input from his panel of specialty experts, will direct the diagnostic and therapeutic course of each patient.

Along with the critical assessment and improvement of therapeutic approaches, there is a need for further evaluation of the various techniques for diagnosis of sleep apnea. Among the criteria to be studied are the accuracy, feasibility, and cost of alternative diagnostic approaches. An attempt should be made to identify those physiological parameters that correlate most closely with the diagnosis of OSAS and with the definition of its severity. The role of home monitoring as either a screening or diagnostic tool needs to be researched in terms of adequacy of identification of OSAS and its severity, degree to which coexisting pathology is missed, and relative cost when compared to traditional, in-lab polysomnography. The goal will be to maximize the adequacy of diagnosis and minimize the costs.

REFERENCE

1. National Commission on Sleep Disorders Research. Report of the National Commission on Sleep Disorders Research, Washington, DC: Superintendent of Documents, U.S. Government Printing Office, 1993.

Subject Index